Step-Up to Surgery

Step-Up to Surgery

STANLEY ZASLAU, MD, MBA, FACS
Urology Residency Program Director
Associate Professor
Division of Urology
Department of Surgery
West Virginia University
Morgantown, West Virginia

DAVID W. McFADDEN, MD, FACS
Stanley S. Fieber Professor and Chair
Department of Surgery
University of Vermont College of Medicine
Surgical Services Leader, Surgeon-in-Chief
Fletcher Allen Health Care
Burlington, Vermont

Wolters Kluwer | Lippincott Williams & Wilkins
Health
Philadelphia · Baltimore · New York · London
Buenos Aires · Hong Kong · Sydney · Tokyo

Acquisitions Editor: Charley Mitchell
Senior Managing Editor: Stacey Sebring
Marketing Manager: Jennifer Kuklinski
Production Editor: Kevin Johnson
Compositor: International Typesetting and Composition
Printer: Data Reproductions Corp.

Printed in the United States of America

Library of Congress Cataloging-in-Publication Data

Step-up to surgery / [edited by] Stanley Zaslau, David W. McFadden.
        p. ; cm. —(Step up series)
  ISBN-13: 978-0-7817-7454-3
  ISBN-10: 0-7817-7454-3
  1. Surgery—Outlines, syllabi, etc.   I. Zaslau, Stanley.   II. McFadden, David W., MD.   III. Series.
  [DNLM: 1. Surgical Procedures, Operative—Outlines.   2. Surgical Procedures, Operative—Problems and Exercises.   WO 18.2 S827 2009]
  RD37.3.S738 2009
  617—dc22
                                        2008014717

Dedication

To our students, whose interest in surgery fuels our energy and enthusiasm to further our own knowledge of this great specialty.

Preface

Step-Up to Surgery evolved from our desire to provide medical students with a concise, easy-to-read, up-to-date overview of the key concepts of general surgery, applicable to students taking the third-year clerkship rotation. We wanted our book to be different from others currently available in the following ways:

1. Provide a core overview of not only general surgery topics, but key concepts in the surgical subspecialties
2. Provide numerous "quick hits" to illustrate important points for licensure examinations
3. Provide authentic case-based questions to further illustrate concepts and allow students to apply them to typical patient presentations
4. Provide many pictures, figures, and tables to further illustrate key concepts and allow for easy recall when students are questioned on rounds, in the operating room, and on written examinations

To this end, we have recruited the authors from our department of surgery faculty and residents. These dedicated teachers are our front-line educators for our students and have provided didactic education to them.

Because of our location in rural West Virginia and three campuses throughout the state, it is our hope that *Step-Up to Surgery* will allow a standardization of general surgical clerkship education at all sites. We are hopeful that our readers will share the same enthusiasm for surgical education as we do.

With best regards,
SZ
DWM

Contributing Authors

Laura Buchanan, MD
Resident
Department of Surgery
West Virginia University
Morgantown, West Virginia

Riaz Cassim, MD
Assistant Professor
Department of Surgery
West Virginia University
Morgantown, West Virginia

Adam Cassis, MD
Resident
Department of Otolaryngology
West Virginia University
Morgantown, West Virginia

Felix Cheung, MD
Resident
Department of Orthopedic Surgery
West Virginia University
Morgantown, West Virginia

Alexandre D'Audiffret, MD
Associate Professor
Division of Vascular Surgery
Department of Surgery
West Virginia University
Morgantown, West Virginia

Kevin Day, MD
Resident
Department of Surgery
West Virginia University
Morgantown, West Virginia

Bruce Freeman, MD, PhD
Chief
Division of Plastic Surgery
Associate Professor
Department of Surgery
West Virginia University
Morgantown, West Virginia

Charles Goldman, MD
Associate Professor
Department of Surgery
West Virginia University
Morgantown, West Virginia

Cynthia Graves, MD
General Surgery Residency Program Director
Assistant Professor
Department of Surgery
West Virginia University
Morgantown, West Virginia

Syed Hashmi, MD
Assistant Professor
Division of Trauma
Department of Surgery
West Virginia University
Morgantown, West Virginia

Hannah Hazard, MD
Instructor
Division of General Surgery
Department of Surgery
West Virginia University
Morgantown, West Virginia

Marissa Howard-McNatt, MD
Assistant Professor
Division of General Surgery
Department of Surgery
West Virginia University
Morgantown, West Virginia

Antony Joseph, MD
Resident
Department of Surgery
West Virginia University
Morgantown, West Virginia

Kamran Karimi, MD
Resident
Department of Surgery
West Virginia University
Morgantown, West Virginia

Jennifer Knight, MD
Resident
Department of Surgery
West Virginia University
Morgantown, West Virginia

Tarun Kumar, MD
Instructor
Division of Pediatric Surgery
Department of Surgery
West Virginia University
Morgantown, West Virginia

James Longhi, DO
Assistant Professor
Division of General Surgery
Department of Surgery
West Virginia University
Morgantown, West Virginia

Matthew Loos, MD
Resident
Department of Surgery
West Virginia University
Morgantown, West Virginia

Christopher McCullough, MD
Chief
Division of Transplantation Services
Professor
Department of Surgery
West Virginia University
Morgantown, West Virginia

David W. McFadden, MD, FACS
Stanley S. Fieber Professor and Chair
Department of Surgery
College of Medicine
University of Vermont
Morgantown, West Virginia
Surgical Services Leader, Surgeon-in-Chief
Fletcher Allen Health Care
Burlington, Vermont

Stephen McNatt, MD
Associate Professor
Division of General Surgery
Department of Surgery
West Virginia University
Morgantown, West Virginia

Bradford Mitchell, MD
Assistant Professor
Division of General Surgery
Department of Surgery
West Virginia University
Morgantown, West Virginia

Muhammad Nazim, MD
Resident
Department of Surgery
West Virginia University
Morgantown, West Virginia

Matthew Oliverio, MD
Resident
Department of Otolaryngology
West Virginia University
Morgantown, West Virginia

Jessica Partin, MD
Resident
Department of Surgery
West Virginia University
Morgantown, West Virginia

Kumar Pillai, MD
Chief
Division of Vascular Surgery
Associate Professor
Department of Surgery
West Virginia University
Morgantown, West Virginia

Ganga Prabhakar, MD
Assistant Professor
Division of Cardiovascular Surgery
Department of Surgery
West Virginia University
Morgantown, West Virginia

Irfan Rizvi, MD
Resident
Department of Surgery
West Virginia University
Morgantown, West Virginia

Larry Roberts, MD
Associate Professor
Division of Trauma
Department of Surgery
West Virginia University
Morgantown, West Virginia

Daniel Rossi, DO
Resident
Department of Surgery
West Virginia University
Morgantown, West Virginia

Walter Samora, MD
Resident
Department of Orthopedic Surgery
West Virginia University
Morgantown, West Virginia

Susan E. Saunders, MD
Resident
Division of Urology
Department of Surgery
West Virginia University
Morgantown, West Virginia

Farooq Shahzad, MD
Resident
Department of Surgery
West Virginia University
Morgantown, West Virginia

Santosh Shenoy, MD
Resident
Department of Surgery
West Virginia University
Morgantown, West Virginia

Magesh Sundaram, MD
Chief
Division of Surgical Oncology
Associate Professor
Department of Surgery
West Virginia University
Morgantown, West Virginia

Richard Vaughan, MD
Chairman
Department of Surgery
Professor
West Virginia University
Morgantown, West Virginia

Giridhar Vedula, MD
Resident
Department of Surgery
West Virginia University
Morgantown, West Virginia

Alison Wilson, MD
Director
Jon Michael Moore Trauma Center
Assistant Professor
Department of Surgery
West Virginia University
Morgantown, West Virginia

Stanley Zaslau, MD, MBA, FACS
Urology Residency Program Director
Associate Professor
Division of Urology
Department of Surgery
West Virginia University
Morgantown, West Virginia

Pamela Zimmerman, MD
Instructor
Department of Surgery
West Virginia University
Morgantown, West Virginia

Jamshed Zuberi, MD
Assistant Professor
Division of Trauma
Department of Surgery
West Virginia University
Morgantown, West Virginia

Acknowledgments

To Stacy Sebring and Donna Balado for their support and guidance throughout this process. To our wives and families who allowed us to spend more time on our laptops writing chapters instead of being with them.

Contents

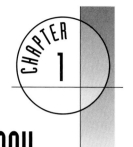

Surgical Physiology

Larry Roberts, MD
Jamshed Zuberi, MD
Farooq Shahzad, MD

FLUIDS AND ELECTROLYTES

All surgical patients need intravenous access and most receive intravenous fluids. The general surgeon must be well versed in the kinds and quantities of fluids to be used, the differences in crystalloids, colloids, and blood products, and the electrolyte disturbances common in surgical diseases.

I. Body Water and Distribution

A. The human body is 45% to 60% water by weight. For a 70-kg adult, there are 31.5 to 42 liters of water throughout the body. Body mass and habitus play roles in percentage of water, as does gender (females have a slightly lower water percentage than males).

B. The total body water (TBW) is distributed in the following ways:
  1. Extracellular compartment (40% TBW).
     a. Intravascular/plasma space (25% extracellular water).
     b. Extravascular/interstitial space (75% extracellular water).
  2. Intracellular compartment (60% TBW).

C. The extracellular water electrolyte composition is primarily that of sodium, chloride, and bicarbonate. The intracellular water electrolyte composition is primarily that of potassium, organic phosphate, and sulfate.

D. The intravascular water also has many proteins (mostly albumin), which account for plasma colloid oncotic pressure.

E. The kidneys maintain volume and composition of body fluid by two mechanisms: regulation of water excretion via antidiuretic hormone (ADH), and reabsorption of sodium.
  1. By regulating sodium and water metabolism, the kidneys maintain volume and body fluid composition body in a very narrow range.
  2. Osmolality throughout all compartments remains similar even if the solutes are different. Regulation is primarily by the kidneys: if water intake decreases, the kidneys can concentrate the urine to a solute concentration four times that of the plasma, thus maintaining body osmolality.

II. Volume Disorders

A. Starling fluid flux equation
  1. The movement of fluids and proteins between the intravascular and interstitial spaces is governed by the Starling fluid flux equation:

$$Q = K_f (P_{mv} - P_t) - \sigma(p_{mv} - p_t)$$

where σ is the osmotic reflection coefficient, p_{mv} is the capillary colloid osmotic pressure, p_t is the tissue interstitial colloid osmotic pressure, K_f is the filtration coefficient, P_{mv} is the capillary hydrostatic pressure, and P_t is the tissue interstitial hydrostatic pressure.

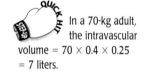

In a 70-kg adult, the intravascular volume = $70 \times 0.4 \times 0.25$ = 7 liters.

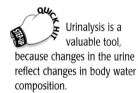

Urinalysis is a valuable tool, because changes in the urine reflect changes in body water composition.

2. The net fluid flux in normal patients favors movement of fluid from the intravascular to the interstitial space.
3. *Example*: During hemorrhage, the initial P_{mv} drops, favoring the influx of fluid from the interstitial to the intravascular space. In cardiac failure, P_{mv} increases, and fluid flux into the interstitial space can result in pulmonary edema.

B. Volume overload
1. Syndrome of inappropriate antidiuretic hormone secretion (SIADH). This syndrome can occur after head injury, some cancers, and burns. The patient is hyponatremic, and hypervolemic (the extracellular fluid volume is increased). The patient also has concentrated urine and high urine sodium concentrations. Lethargy and coma can ensue. Treatment includes free-water intake restriction, replacing lost sodium with intravenous saline infusion, and a loop diuretic such as furosemide (Lasix).
2. Iatrogenic conditions. In the majority of hospitalized surgical patients, volume overload is iatrogenic (caused by management of the health care team). Attention to the volume of administered fluids is required, and can be anticipated by the increase in patient weight.

C. Volume depletion
1. Diabetes insipidus (DI) occurs in head trauma patients due to damage in the hypothalamic nuclei or hypophyseal stalk. Large urine outputs that may reach 2 liters/hour are characteristic. Urine sodium is low, and the patient is hypernatremic and hyperosmolar.
   a. Treatment is supportive, with replacement of free water as guided by the following estimate:

   (Body weight) × (% water) = normal TBW
   (140/current serum sodium) × TBW = current body water
   TBW − current body water = water deficit

   b. *Example:* In a 70-kg man with a serum sodium of 156 meq/L,

   (70) × (0.6) = 42 L normal TBW
   (140/156) × (42 L) = 37.7 L current TBW
   42 L − 37.7 L = 4.3 L water deficit

2. Gastrointestinal (GI) fluid losses
   a. Table 1-1 lists the typical electrolyte compositions and volumes of different gastrointestinal fluids. Often, this can aid in fluid and electrolyte replacement strategy.
   b. *Example:* In a patient on a proton-pump inhibitor, or H_2 blocker therapy (that is, low acid stomach fluid), who has emesis, the typical replacement fluid would be 0.45% normal saline with 20 mEq KCl ($Na^+ = 72$, $Cl^- = 92$, $K^+ = 20$), and to maintain isotonicity, the commercially available fluid adds 5% dextrose. Therefore, D5$^1/_2$ NS with 20 mEq KCl is the typical crystalloid fluid replacement for protracted emesis.
   c. Choosing fluids and amounts. In response to a fall in blood pressure and intravascular volume, angiotensin I is released, converted to angiotensin II by angiotensin converting enzyme. This causes vasoconstriction. Angiotensin II also stimulates the release of aldosterone from the adrenal gland. Aldosterone affects the kidney by reabsorbing more sodium and thereby "holding onto" more water. A byproduct is renal potassium wasting, or excretion of potassium in the urine.
      (1) In most surgical patients, a balanced isotonic salt crystalloid solution is used for intravenous fluid replacement and management. The body loses water in the urine, stool, and via insensible (evaporative) losses. Open wounds dramatically increase the latter. It is estimated that during open abdominal surgery, up to 1 L insensible losses occur per hour.

TABLE 1-1 Electrolyte Composition and Volumes of Gastrointestinal Fluids					
	Na$^+$ (mEq/L)	K$^+$ (mEq/L)	Cl$^-$ (mEq/L)	HCO$_3^-$ (mEq/L)	Volume (mL/24 hr)
Stomach, high acid	20	10	120	0	1,000–9,000
Stomach, low acid	80	15	90	15	1,000–2,500
Pancreas	140	5	75	80	500–1,000
Bile	148	5	100	35	300–1,000
Proximal small bowel	110	5	105	30	1,000–3,000
Distal small bowel	80	8	45	30	1,000–3,000
Colon/diarrhea	120	25	90	45	500–17,000

(2) In resuscitation, blood loss volume is estimated, and three times that volume is replaced with a crystalloid. (Crystalloids readily leave the intravascular space within 20 minutes after a one-liter infusion of crystalloid, and only 200 mL remain intravascularly!) However, the clinical scenario must guide the volume of fluid resuscitation. In blunt trauma patients, the volume tends to be greater initially than that given to penetrating trauma victims.

(3) In the adult, fluid maintenance requirements approximate 30 mL/kg body weight/24 hours. Maintenance fluid after resuscitation is also estimated using the 4-2-1 formula:

4 L/kg for the first 10 kg body weight.
2 mL/kg for the second 10 kg body weight.
1 mL/kg for all additional weight.

(4) The postoperative, or physiologically stressed, patient is glucose intolerant as a result of high circulating glucagon levels and relative insulin resistance. Diabetics tend to be particularly hyperglycemic at these times, and the high serum glucose can function as an osmotic agent to promote inappropriate diuresis. During the first 48 to 72 hours postsurgery and after trauma, it is unlikely that exogenous glucose will provide an energy substrate. Therefore, crystalloid solutions with dextrose should be avoided during this time. See the nutrition section later in the chapter for guidance. Commonly, lactated Ringers or normal saline solutions are appropriate choices for surgical patients until specific restrictions are necessary.

QUICK HIT Based on an estimated need of 30 mL/kg/hr, a 70-kg man requires 2,100 mL crystalloid per day replacement and maintenance fluid, or approximately 88 mL fluid per hour. The patient's temperature, degree of GI fluid losses (urine output), and overall cardiovascular state may favor a higher replacement rate.

III. Electrolyte Abnormalities

A. Hypernatremia. Commonly, hypernatremia is seen in free water deficit. This condition may occur as a result of DI or a significant renal condition. Please refer to the section on volume deficit.

B. Hyponatremia. This condition, which may occur as a result of isotonic fluid loss, can be seen in SIADH (discussed above), in adrenal insufficiency, or in hyperglycemia, where the osmotic effects of glucose lead to inappropriate fluid loss from the kidney. In usual circumstances, a balanced salt solution can be used to replace sodium deficits.

C. Hyperkalemia
1. This serious condition mandates prompt attention. It can result from any catabolic state, such as crush injuries in trauma, burns, prolonged illness, hemolysis, renal failure, and from adrenal insufficiency (addisonian crisis). Depolarizing paralytics such as succinylcholine (commonly used

for rapid-sequence induction anesthesia) can cause massive muscle potassium release and acute hyperkalemia. In acute scenarios, most clinical manifestations are absent. However, an abnormal electrocardiogram (EKG) demonstrating progressive peaked T-waves and widening of the QRS complex can ultimately lead to cardiac arrest. Hyperkalemia also occurs in acidosis (see later in the chapter).

   2. Treatment is based on rapidity of rise of serum potassium and the underlying cause.

      a. Serum potassium is actively transported intracellularly with insulin. Therefore, initial treatment is administration of intravenous glucose (1 ampule of $D_{50\%}$) and intravenous regular insulin (20 U).

      b. Correcting a metabolic acidosis with sodium bicarbonate can lower serum potassium levels.

      c. Calcium gluconate is another option—calcium antagonizes the tissue effects of hyperkalemia and thereby minimizes cardiac effects. The infusion of calcium does not by itself lower serum potassium levels.

      d. If hyperkalemia is due to adrenal insufficiency, hydrocortisone can be administered. Hyperkalemia due to renal failure may require hemodialysis or peritoneal dialysis.

      e. A slower treatment is Kayexalate (sodium polystyrene sulfonate, a cation exchange resin), which can be given orally or by enema, and binds potassium in the GI tract in exchange for sodium.

  D. Hypokalemia

    1. Obligatory potassium losses occur in both the urine (30–60 mEq/day) and stool (30–90 mEq/day). Increased potassium loss can result from emesis, diarrhea, diuretic use, DI, and metabolic alkalosis.

    2. Increased urinary excretion of potassium occurs when the serum potassium level rises above 4 mEq/L. Aldosterone release is increased as a result of hyperkalemia, promoting excretion of potassium in the distal tubule of the kidney. In patients with emesis, the loss of hydrogen ion in the emesis results in potassium retention in the kidney (to maintain electrical neutrality) at the expense of hydrogen ion excretion. The emesis causes a hypochloremic, hypokalemic metabolic alkalosis, worsened paradoxically over time by the kidney, leading to a paradoxical aciduria.

    3. Another cause of hypokalemia is potassium loss, primarily from the kidney. This is called renal wasting of potassium. Greater than 30 mEq/L of urinary potassium when the serum potassium is <3.5 mEq/L defines renal potassium wasting. The three causes of renal potassium wasting are diuretic therapy, effects of aldosterone, or alkalosis.

    4. When assessing for hypokalemia, the acid-base status of the patient must be ascertained first. If the patient is alkalemic, the hypokalemia may simply be an ion exchange issue; the more alkalemic the intravascular space is, the more hydrogen ion is shifted intravascularly and potassium shifts extravascularly. Figure 1-1 suggests a replacement strategy for potassium when alkalosis exists. Often correcting the underlying alkalosis resolves the hypokalemia and should be considered first. This is depicted in Table 1-2.

    5. Treatment most often consists of potassium replacement once the acid–base status of the patient has been ascertained. Intravenous potassium (usually potassium chloride) generally is given at rates of 20 mEq/hour, and causes local discomfort if given peripherally. A preferable route is through a central venous line. If the patient can tolerate it, oral administration is preferred. If the cause of hypokalemia is diuretic therapy, consider alternatives to that therapy.

  E. Hypercalcemia. This condition occurs with hyperparathyroidism, cancer, hyperthyroidism, adrenal insufficiency, and prolonged immobilization. Serum calcium levels of 12 g/dL and greater are a medical emergency and should be managed with intravenous saline. Loop diuretics, steroids, and calcitonin are additional treatments.

FIGURE
1-1 **Relationship of serum potassium to total body potassium stores at different blood pH levels.**

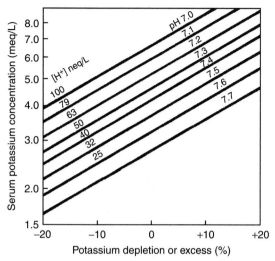

(Reprinted, with permission, from Scribner B, ed. *University of Washington Teaching Syllabus for the Course on Fluid and Electrolyte Balance.*)

F. Hypocalcemia. This is a more common calcium abnormality in surgical patients and may result from hypoparathyroidism, pancreatitis, severe trauma and crush injuries, necrotizing fasciitis, and severe renal failure. Clinically, patients develop hyperactive deep tendon reflexes and a Chvostek sign (an abnormal reaction to stimulation of the facial nerve), abdominal cramps, and carpopedal spasm. Treatment initially involves treating a metabolic alkalosis if it exists, then replacing calcium with calcium chloride or gluconate.

G. Hypermagnesemia. Hypermagnesemia is rare in surgical patients, but can occur with renal disease. Iatrogenic hypermagnesemia can occur in these patients with excessive magnesium intake through antacid and laxative therapy. Patients with hypermagnesemia are lethargic and weak. EKG abnormalities are similar to those in hyperkalemia. Progressive hypermagnesemia result in the loss of deep tendon reflexes, somnolence, coma, and death. Treatment consists of intravenous normal saline, calcium infusions (similar to hyperkalemia, calcium antagonizes the neuromuscular effects of hypermagnesemia), and possibly dialysis if the patient has severe renal failure.

TABLE 1-2	Prediction of Serum Potassium Concentrations in Acid–Base Abnormalities Assuming No Potassium Wasting
If Serum pH is:	**The Predicted Serum K⁺ (mEq/L)**
7.10	5.9
7.20	5.1
7.30	4.7
7.40 (normal)	4.1
7.50	3.8
7.60	3.1
7.70	2.6

H. Hypomagnesemia
   1. This abnormality occurs as a result of poor dietary intake, malabsorption in the GI tract, excessive GI loss (for example, diarrhea), enteric fistulas, chronic alcohol use and abuse, acute pancreatitis, severe burns, prolonged use of total parenteral nutrition (TPN) with insufficient magnesium, hyperaldosteronism, and hypercalcemia. Symptoms are similar to those of hypocalcemia (hyperactive deep tendon reflexes, Chvostek sign, tremors, delirium, and seizures).
   2. Treatment consists of replacing magnesium. Oral replacement is best. Intravenous magnesium in the form of magnesium sulfate is often used, especially in more severe deficiencies. While replacing magnesium, the EKG should be monitored, and in renal failure, any magnesium must be given with great caution.
I. Hypophosphatemia. This condition occurs in hyperparathyroidism and malnourished patients (for example, alcoholics). Neuromuscular effects (fatigue, weakness, convulsions, and even death) predominate when serum phosphorus levels fall below 1 mg/dL. Replacement is accomplished either orally or parenterally (potassium phosphate).
J. Hyperphosphatemia. This disorder occurs in severe trauma, muscle breakdown, and in severe renal failure. Elevated serum phosphorus decreases intravascular calcium. Phosphate-binding antacids (such as aluminum hydroxide) can be used, as well as diuretics to promote urinary excretion of phosphorus. In severe renal failure, hemodialysis may be necessary.

IV. Acid–Base Disorders
A. General principles
   1. Hydrogen ions are generated in the body at a rate of about 70 mEq/kg/day. Carbon dioxide is formed from aerobic metabolism. The Henderson–Hasselbalch equation depicts the relationship of bicarbonate to carbonic acid and pH:

$$pH = pK + \log \left(\frac{[HCO_3^-]}{(0.03 \; p \times CO_2)} \right)$$

   A simpler form of this same equation is:

$$[H^+] = \frac{(24 \times pCO_2)}{[HCO_3^-]}$$

   and it must be remembered that:

$$H_2O + CO_2^- = H_2CO_3 = HCO_3^- + H^+$$

   2. The serum pH is a reflection of the amount of carbon dioxide that is produced, the efficiency of elimination in the lung (ventilation), and the buffering capability (in the serum, and either elimination or retention of bicarbonate by the kidney) according to the equations above. Hydrogen ion can also be excreted by the kidney in the form of ammonium ion.
B. Respiratory disorders
   1. Acidosis. Patients who inadequately eliminate CO_2 develop respiratory acidosis. As a result, hydrogen ion accumulates as the equation above is forced to the "right." Treatment acutely is to improve ventilation and elimination of CO_2. Patients with a metabolic alkalosis (high HCO_3^-) drive the equation to the right, resulting in a compensatory respiratory acidosis.
   2. Alkalosis. Patients may hyperventilate for many reasons, including anxiety, hypoxia, sepsis, and a mechanically induced small tidal volume. Elimination of excessive CO_2 results in the equation being driven to the "left," causing an alkalosis. Patients who have a metabolic acidosis (high H^+) also drive the equation to the left, prompting hyperventilation and a compensatory respiratory alkalosis.
C. Metabolic disorders
   1. Acidosis. Excessive production of hydrogen ion or increased excretion of bicarbonate results in a metabolic acidosis. The decrease in bicarbonate is

exchanged for an increase in serum chloride, maintaining a normal anion pap. The anion gap (AG) is simply measured by:

$$[HCO_3 + Cl^-] - Na < 15 \text{ mEq/L}$$

If the AG is greater than 15, an unmeasured anion (such as lactate or ketoacid) is present.

  a. Distinguishing AGA (anion gap acidosis) from NAGA (non-anion gap acidosis) is critical in evaluating a patient with a metabolic acidosis. Treating the underlying cause of the acidosis is most relevant. In NAGA, bicarbonate depletion is primarily the cause.

  b. *Example:* In AGA, the presence of lactate may signify inadequate perfusion and anaerobic metabolism, generating lactate. In this case, treatment is directed at restoring perfusion.

2. Alkalosis. The kidneys play a significant role in acid–base homeostasis. Active hydrogen ion secretion occurs in response to acidosis, and bicarbonate combines with hydrogen ion to form carbonic acid and CO_2, thereby facilitating reabsorption of bicarbonate.

D. Mixed disorders. In the acute phase of injury or surgery, many acid–base disorders are purely respiratory or metabolic. However, patients with premorbidities and medical conditions, as well as those who are beyond the acute phase of their disease, often manifest mixed acid–base disorders.

1. *Example:* A patient who suffers an injury and is in shock develops lactic (metabolic) acidosis (AGA). The patient hyperventilates to remove CO_2 and develops a compensatory respiratory alkalosis. However, it is uncommon for the compensation to ever exceed the primary process. Therefore, despite the patient's best efforts, he or she remains acidotic with a primary metabolic acidosis and compensatory respiratory acidosis until the shock and poor perfusion are corrected with resuscitation.

2. *Example:* A patient suffers acute respiratory distress syndrome, and this results in the inability of the lungs to ventilate adequately. Therefore, the $PaCO_2$ rises, resulting in a respiratory acidosis. Over time (more than 24 hours), the kidneys respond and excrete hydrogen ion and chloride in order to retain bicarbonate. This results in a compensatory metabolic alkalosis. However, until the lung condition improves, the compensation is partial, and the patient remains slightly acidotic.

3. *Example:* A patient who has diarrhea and chronic obstructive pulmonary disease may have a high respiratory rate and therefore a respiratory alkalosis. However, the diarrhea causes loss of fluid and bicarbonate, and results in a metabolic acidosis.

4. *Example:* A patient with vomiting may present with a metabolic alkalosis. The patient may also be breathing rapidly due to abdominal pain, and may also have a respiratory alkalosis.

E. Arterial blood gas and interpretation

1. Co-oximeter analyzer separately can measure oxyhemoglobin, methemoglobin, and carboxyhemoglobin. A normal ABG is: $PaO_2 = 100$ mm Hg, $PaCO_2 = 40$ mm Hg, pH = 7.40, bicarbonate = 24 mEq/L, base excess/deficit = 0, and $HbO_2 = 100\%$.

2. In a pure metabolic condition, the $PaCO_2$ remains normal at 40, but the pH is low (in a metabolic acidosis) or high (in a metabolic alkalosis). The calculated base deficit or excess, respectively, reflects the degree of metabolic derangement. It is important to remember that base deficit and excess are a reflection of the metabolic acidosis or alkalosis, respectively, and not a reflection of respiratory acid–base conditions.

3. In mixed acid–base disorders, the base deficit/excess as seen on an ABG helps sort out the primary disorder. With metabolic acidosis, the AG further helps sort out the abnormality and direct treatment.

QUICK HIT

In pure respiratory disorders, a rise in $PaCO_2$ by 10 lowers the pH by 0.08. Therefore, in respiratory acidosis, a $PaCO_2 = 50$ results in a pH = 7.32. In respiratory alkalosis, a $PaCO_2 = 30$ results in a pH = 7.48. In both cases, the calculated bicarbonate is still 24 and the base excess/deficit is still 0.

TABLE 1-3 Solute Concentrations of Standard Crystalloid Solution							
Crystalloid	Na$^+$ (mEq/L)	Cl$^+$ (mEq/L)	K$^+$ (mEq/L)	HCO$_3^-$ (mEq/L)	Ca$^+$ (mEq/L)	Glucose	Lactate
Normal saline (0.9%)	154	154					
Lactated Ringers	130	109	4	28	2.7		
D5$_{1/2}$NS	77	77				50	
D5$_{1/2}$NS + 20KCl	77	97	20			50	

V. Fluid Therapy

A. Crystalloids. The solute concentrations of four typical crystalloids are presented in Table 1-3.

1. Normal saline is ubiquitously used for dehydration and hypovolemia. It is compatible with blood product transfusion and most medications. It is the most commonly used fluid in trauma resuscitation.

2. Lactated Ringers provides less sodium than normal saline and offers a small amount of other solutes as well. Some studies suggest that lactated Ringers stimulates the immune system. In severely underperfused patients, the increase in circulating lactate may exacerbate an acidosis. Lactated Ringers is not compatible with blood product transfusions and with some medications. Despite these considerations, lactated Ringers is widely used and has equal efficacy in most circumstances to normal saline. The L-lactate is converted to bicarbonate in the perfusing liver, thereby helping to resolve acidosis.

3. D5$^1/_2$ NS.

   a. This mildly hypotonic fluid provides a small amount of dextrose along with hypotonic salt. Adding 20 mEq/L of KCl results in an almost isotonic solution whose solute concentrations approach that of stomach fluid. The small amount of dextrose helps decrease the hypotonicity and may help with minimizing ketoacidosis. However, the dextrose is not a nutritional substrate in this setting.

   b. *Example:* Initially in the resuscitative management of the patient with emesis, normal saline should be used. Once stabilized, maintenance with D5$^1/_2$ NS with 20 KCl is often used as the replacement fluid.

4. Other crystalloids. Another crystalloid solution is 3% NaCl, which can be used as a resuscitation fluid (for example, with burns), as well as occasionally in traumatic brain injury and intracranial hypertension. Hypertonic saline solutions of various concentrations have been studied.

B. Colloids

1. Plasmanate is a dilute colloid consisting of 5% albumin in saline. It is occasionally used in anesthesia but is not common in other settings.

2. A solution of 25% albumin (formerly called salt-poor albumin) is a concentrated form of albumin derived from human serum. Albumin has limited indications. When colloid osmotic pressure is low, albumin can be used in some circumstances. Associated irradiation and infectious complications are very rare.

C. Synthetic colloids

1. The hetastarch (Hespan) synthetic colloids have the greatest application in surgery and trauma. They are excellent volume expanders; the volume infused remains intravascularly longer than crystalloids. In addition, there are few side effects. However, large quantities of hetastarch can interfere with coagulation, and therefore its use must be limited in the trauma patient.

2. Dextran 40 and 70. These two synthetic colloids were once popular as both volume expanders and as hemorheologic modifiers (making the blood less viscous and promoting perfusion). They are still used in some vascular situations.

3. Gelatin synthetic colloids are available in Europe and Asia, but not in the United States.

D. Blood products. U.S. blood banks provide an array of blood products, and transfusion is based on clinical need. Although viral and other infections are well-known transmissible complications of blood product transfusions, they occur rarely (1 in 200,000 units for hepatitis B, and 1 in 1.6 million units for hepatitis C or human immunodeficiency virus (HIV)). Transfusion reactions are significantly more common (1 in 200 units), can be morbid, and on rare occasion, anaphylaxis can be life threatening. Judicious transfusion with a clear clinical indication is always warranted.

1. Whole blood is not approved in the United States by the American Red Cross. In the United States, blood component therapy is the standard. Interestingly, the U.S. military has used whole blood transfusions overseas in combat, with excellent results.

2. Each unit of packed red blood cells (PRBCs) is a volume of approximately 550 mL and weighs 400 g. Generally speaking, one unit of transfused blood equates to a patient hemoglobin rise of 1 g/dL, but depends on the donor's initial hemoglobin.

3. Platelets are pooled from multiple donors and generally are provided in a six-pack. Because the platelets are pooled from multiple donors, their transfusion must be for clinically appropriate reasons only.

4. Fresh frozen plasma (FFP) is rich in fibrinogen, coagulation factors, and protein. When there is a need for a colloid, as well as to reverse a coagulopathy, FFP is transfused. Often, the amount is determined by the clinical appearance of bleeding and the prothrombin time (PT).

5. Cryoprecipitate is pooled from multiple donors, and similarly to platelets, its administration must be guided by a true need. Cryoprecipitate is especially rich in fibrinogen.

6. Recombinant factor VIIa (rFVIIa) is a U.S. Food and Drug Administration (FDA)-approved agent for hemophilia. However, its use has recently gained popularity in bleeding patients. Some data exist regarding its utility in cardiac surgery. There are no conclusive studies in trauma and in surgery, but rFVIIa appears promising as an adjunct in the bleeding patient, especially one who is already acidotic from hypoperfusion. It is sometimes administered at a dose of 90 µg/kg body weight. rFVIIa currently is quite expensive.

E. Blood substitutes have been investigated for 40 years. At the moment, there is no FDA-approved blood substitute.

HEMOSTASIS/COAGULATION

I. **General Principles.** Hemostasis is a complex interaction of multiple components in the body. Usually, it occurs in an ordered way as the body's response to injury, but can also occur in a dysfunctional manner, leading to significant morbidity.

A. Vasoconstriction is the initial response to injury. It occurs as a reflex to most stimuli.

B. Platelet aggregation results from the release of platelet factors and fibrin. This leads to formation of a platelet plug that acts as a physical barrier to further bleeding.

C. Coagulation is an interaction of factors that leads to the formation of a fibrin and platelet plug. It is a series of enzymatic reactions that can be slowed with hypothermia or a deficiency of factors.

D. Fibrinolysis is the final step in the coagulation cascade. Its main effect is to prevent the thrombosis from going unchecked. It also helps break down the clot once bleeding has been controlled and leads to improved blood flow in the vessel.

II. **Testing the Surgical Patient for Hemostatic Risk Factors**

A. For minor surgical procedures, all that is needed is a thorough history and physical. It is especially important to ask about excessive bruising after minor injuries or significant bleeding after small cuts or abrasions. Medications are also an important factor.

B. If the history and physical are unrevealing, but the patient is to undergo a major surgical procedure (one that involves a large part of the body), or the operation is to involve a part of the body where even a small amount of excessive bleeding would have disastrous complications (that is, involving the eye or brain), then additional tests need to be ordered. In most circumstances, checking a prothrombin time (PT), prothromboplastin time (PTT), and platelets suffices. However, if these are normal, but the history or physical suggest some bleeding abnormalities, then tests such as bleeding time can be ordered.

C. Other tests that are useful include a hematocrit and a platelet count (although this gives no information on the function of the platelets).

III. Tests of Hemostasis and Coagulation

A. PT measures mostly the extrinsic factors that lead to clotting. Extrinsic refers to the interaction between platelets, and specifically, factors outside the blood vessel, leading to initiation of the clotting cascade. It is also used as a surrogate to reflect the function of the liver.

B. PTT refers to the function of the intrinsic pathway.

C. Bleeding time is not useful as an initial screening test because it is labor intensive, and the results can be subjective. It is useful though when the bleeding disorder is caused by factors that are not measured by the PT or PTT.

IV. Congenital Defects

A. Hemophilia A, or classic hemophilia, is caused by an abnormality in factor VIII. It occurs as a sex-linked recessive trait that occurs almost exclusively in males. Although history may lead to the diagnosis, levels of factor VIII confirm it. Patients also have an elevated PTT, with a normal PT. Treatment is with factor VIII or cryoprecipitate.

B. Hemophilia B, or Christmas disease, is caused by a factor IX abnormality. It is also sex-linked and recessive, and so occurs exclusively in males. The disease has a similar presentation to classic hemophilia. Treatment is with factor IX concentrate.

C. Von Willebrand disease is secondary to abnormalities with von Willebrand factor (vWF). Normally vWF helps in platelet adhesion to collagen and cross-linking platelets in clot aggregation. It is commonly inherited in an autosomal dominant pattern with variable penetrance. Affected people usually have episodes of mucocutaneous bleeding. Bleeding time is commonly prolonged, although the PTT can also be prolonged. Treatment is with cryoprecipitate.

V. Acquired Defects

A. Platelet defects can occur secondary to drugs, uremia, or thrombocytopenia (which may be related to massive blood transfusion or platelet destruction).

B. Fibrinogen deficiency usually occurs with disseminated intravascular coagulation (DIC). DIC can be brought on by multiple causes, including retained placenta, sepsis, or amniotic fluid embolism. Treatment is to remove the underlying cause, if possible.

VI. Hepatic and Renal Disease

A. Liver disease, especially if severe, can lead to depletion in coagulation factors by a decrease in production. All factors, except for factor VIII and von Willebrand factor, which are produced by the endothelium, are produced by the liver. This can lead to a severe coagulopathy that is difficult to correct. Vitamin K should be administered first. If that fails, then FFP may be necessary. Platelet transfusion may be warranted if concomitant thrombocytopenia is present. A prolonged PT is usually present.

B. Renal failure leads to a uremic state. This occurs typically when the patient has not undergone dialysis and the blood urea nitrogen has increased significantly. The uremia interferes with the aggregation of platelets and leads to a diffuse bleeding diathesis. The best way to correct this is through dialysis. If that is not immediately available, then intravenous 1-deamino-8-D-arginine vasopressin or conjugated estrogens have been shown to work.

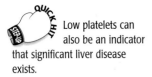 Low platelets can also be an indicator that significant liver disease exists.

VII. Anticoagulation

A. Heparin is a naturally occurring heterogeneous mixture of glycosaminoglycans with differing molecular weights. It accelerates the effect of antithrombin III, leading to a systemically anticoagulated state. It is given intravenously or subcutaneously. The heparin antithrombin III complex inactivates several factors in the anticoagulant cascade, especially thrombin and factor X. The level of anticoagulation achieved can be measured by checking the PTT.

B. Low-molecular-weight heparin (LMWH), which is made by fractionating heparin into its lower-weight molecules, acts primarily by inhibiting factor X. It is always administered subcutaneously. The lower-weight molecule is incapable of inactivating thrombin or antithrombin. Because of this, LMWH does not prolong PTT.

C. Warfarin leads a deficiency of vitamin K, resulting in a decrease in production by the liver of factors II, VII, IX, X, protein C, and S. The drug is given orally, with a half-life of about 1.5 days, and so it takes a few days to take effect and to reverse. The level of anticoagulation can be measured by checking the PT (the international normalized ratio [INR] is an indirect measure of the PT).

D. Heparin-induced thrombocytopenia (HIT) occurs in two forms:

1. HIT type I, which occurs frequently. It usually occurs with a drop in platelet count of more than 100,000. It occurs by a nonimmune-mediated phenomenon. There is no risk of thrombosis, and discontinuation of heparin is not necessary.

2. HIT type II, which occurs far less frequently (in 2–10% of all exposed patients). It should be suspected when the platelet count drops by more than 50% from baseline, or to a total less than 100,000. The diagnosis can be confirmed by checking for antibodies to HIT antibody. The cause is an immune-mediated reaction against heparin-platelet factor antibodies. This results in aggregation of platelets, leading to thrombocytopenia and possibly arterial and venous thrombosis. Because up to 30% of patients with HIT type II develop thrombosis even after discontinuation of heparin, anticoagulation with a nonheparinoid product is essential.

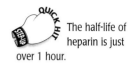 The half-life of heparin is just over 1 hour.

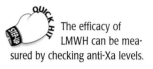 The efficacy of LMWH can be measured by checking anti-Xa levels.

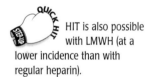 Because proteins C and S lead to systemic anticoagulation, their deficiency can lead to a prothrombotic state if the patient is given warfarin compounds. For this reason, heparinization should always be performed prior to administering warfarin.

HIT is also possible with LMWH (at a lower incidence than with regular heparin).

VIII. Management of Bleeding.
Local control of bleeding is especially important during, and sometimes after, surgical procedures. The most frequent cause of surgical bleeding is inadequate hemostasis in the wound. Less likely causes include coagulopathies.

A. Direct pressure is a very effective way to control and slow most bleeding. Ligature of vessels also controls most surgical bleeding. Tourniquets can be used for small periods of time under dire circumstances.

B. Electrocautery leads to hemostasis by the denaturation of proteins, resulting in coagulation over a large surface area, secondary to the diffusion of the electrical current.

C. Chemical agents can act as procoagulants and vasoconstrictors (epinephrine). New agents are being tested; they lead to a mild thermal burn, resulting in coagulation.

IX. Replacement Therapy

A. Typing and cross-matching is performed to establish serologic compatibility—to establish A, B, O, and the Rh status of the patient. This may take upward of an hour or so to do. If no knowledge about the patient's blood type is available, but PRBCs are urgently needed, then type O Rh-negative blood can be given to women, and type O Rh-positive can be given to men. If time permits, a type-and-screen be done, and type-specific blood can be infused.

B. Component therapy has mostly replaced fresh whole blood because of cost and efficiency; the American Red Cross does not approve of its usage.

C. Platelet concentrates are given for either a significant deficiency in platelet function or quantity. Each unit raises the count by about 10,000/μL.

D. Volume expanders are isotonic or hypertonic crystalloid products, such as lactated Ringers, 0.9% normal saline, or 3% normal saline. Artificial colloids such as hetastarch, or natural ones such as albumin, are also useful for volume expansion.

E. Concentrates of factors such as FFP, or concentrates of specific factors such as factor VIII, are useful for replacement of deficiencies or dysfunction.

X. Indications for Replacements of Blood and Its Substitutes

A. Volume replacement is best performed based on amount of blood loss. Initially, isotonic crystalloid solutions are best. As significant amounts of blood are lost, replacement should be completed using a combination of PRBCs and crystalloid solutions. If massive bleeding is occurring, and large amounts of transfusions are needed, then FFP is also needed, secondary to the dilutional effect of crystalloid solutions and the PRBCs.

B. Oxygen-carrying capacity can be impaired if severe anemia exists. This is especially significant if an area of ischemia exists in the body. However, in most other circumstances, hemoglobin as low as 5 g/dL may be tolerated well. For the elderly or those with ischemic disease, minimum hemoglobin levels such as 7 to 8 g/dL are desirable.

C. Massive transfusion refers to the transfusion of more than 10 units of PRBCs, or the entire blood volume over a 24-hour period. This can lead to problems such as hypothermia, coagulopathies, and acid–base disturbances.

XI. Complications of Transfusions

A. Febrile and allergic reactions.
1. Acute hemolytic transfusion reactions occur because the wrong blood type is given, usually because of clerical error. Typical symptoms include anxiety, chest pain, chills, flank pain, and headaches. The treatment is to stop the transfusion, alert the blood bank, and ensure adequate hydration and diuresis.
2. Nonhemolytic transfusion reactions are secondary to antibodies against donor white blood cells. Patients might become anxious, pruritic, and dyspneic, and they may also develop fevers, flushing, and mild hypotension. Treatment includes ruling out a hemolytic transfusion and stopping the transfusion, followed by supportive therapy.

B. Transmission of bacteria and viruses. Screening for viruses is performed on all donated units, which has led to a significant decrease in infection risk.
1. The estimated risk of infection with hepatitis B is 1 case in 60,000 units transfused, whereas the estimated risk of infection with hepatitis C is 1 case per 100,000 units transfused.
2. The estimated risk of HIV is about 1 case in 450,000 units transfused.
3. Bacterial infections are not common secondary to blood being stored at 4°C. Transfusion-acquired sepsis carries a high mortality rate, usually secondary to the size of the inoculum and impaired immunocompetence of the host.

C. Morbidity and mortality. Emerging data show increased morbidity and even mortality with each unit of blood transfused. Each unit of foreign blood transfused leads to an immunologic suppressed state, which in turn, leads to a higher risk of infection. Cell-mediated immunity can be impaired. Also, blood products tend to be given by the blood bank with a "last in, first out" strategy in mind, so some of their functionality may be lost due to time in storage.

SURGICAL NUTRITION

I. Nutritional Assessment

A. History: weight loss, chronic illnesses, dietary habits, social habits (predisposing to malnutrition), and medications (that influence food intake).

B. Physical examination: loss of muscle or adipose tissue, organ dysfunction, and changes in skin, hair, or neuromuscular function.

C. Anthropometric data: weight change, triceps skin fold thickness, and midarm circumference.

D. Biochemical data: albumin, prealbumin, transferrin, total lymphocyte count, and creatinine excretion.

II. Estimation of Nutritional Requirements

A. Energy requirements
   1. Energy is needed for metabolic processes, core temperature maintenance, and tissue repair.
   2. Energy requirements can be estimated by indirect calorimetry and urinary nitrogen excretion.
   3. Basal energy expenditure may be estimated by the Harris–Benedict equation.
   4. Most postsurgical patients have an energy requirement of 30 kcal/kg per day. If the degree of surgical stress increases secondary to trauma or sepsis, this requirement goes up to 1.2 to 2.0 times the resting energy expenditure (Table 1-4).

B. Protein requirements
   1. Proteins are required for wound healing.
   2. A nonprotein calorie:nitrogen ratio of 150:1 is needed to prevent the utilization of protein as a source of energy.
   3. In stress, more protein is required, so that a ratio of 90:1 to 120:1 is beneficial.

III. Nutritional Requirements in Specific Conditions

A. Renal failure
   1. Renal failure results in an impaired ability to clear the byproducts of protein metabolism.
   2. These patients are given nutrients in a restricted volume with great care not to overfeed proteins.
   3. Administration of essential amino acids and high biologic value protein, such as egg albumin, results in less frequent need for dialysis.

B. Hepatic failure
   1. Liver damage and portosystemic shunting results in a derangement in the level of amino acids in the blood, resulting in an increase in the aromatic to branched-chain amino acids.
   2. The aromatic amino acids are precursors of false neurotransmitters that contribute to hepatic encephalopathy.
   3. Patients with hepatic failure are therefore given diets enriched in branched-chain amino acids and deficient in aromatic amino acids.

C. Respiratory failure
   1. Carbohydrate metabolism produces more CO_2 (respiratory quotient [RQ] = 1) as compared to fat (RQ = 0.7) or protein (RQ = 0.8).
   2. Production of higher amounts of CO_2 results in more need for ventilatory support.
   3. It is therefore important to prevent overfeeding patients. The amount of carbohydrate intake can be reduced, and that of fat may be increased. However, this must be done cautiously, because high-fat diets may exacerbate lung injury.

D. Cardiac failure
   1. Fluid overload may exacerbate cardiac failure.
   2. Concentrated solutions are therefore given to these patients to limit the amount of fluid administered.

TABLE 1-4 Caloric and Protein Requirements in Hypermetabolic Conditions

Condition	Kcal/kg per day	Adjustment over Basal Energy Expenditure	Grams of Protein/ kg per Day	Nonprotein Calories: Nitrogen
Normal/ moderate malnutrition	25–30	1.1	1.0	150:1
Mild stress	25–30	1.2	1.2	150:1
Moderate stress	30	1.4	1.5	120:1
Severe stress	30–35	1.6	2.0	90–120:1
Burns	35–40	2.0	2.5	90–100:1

SURGICAL PHYSIOLOGY

IV. Enteral Nutrition

A. General principles

1. Nutrition via the enteral route is preferred over the parenteral route.
2. Feeding the GI tract functions to preserve the "gut mucosal barrier." This barrier prevents the translocation of bacteria and bacterial toxins across the gut into the host portal venous circulation.
3. Maintenance of the gut mucosal barrier requires (a) normal perfusion, (b) an intact epithelium, and (c) normal mucosal immune mechanisms.
4. Luminal contact of food prevents intestinal mucosal atrophy and stimulates intestinal production of immunoglobulin A (IgA).
5. Surgical patients who are adequately nourished and have not suffered a major complication, can tolerate 10 days of partial starvation before any significant protein catabolism occurs. Therefore, most patients can be maintained on a 5% dextrose solution before return of feeding after surgery, with no detrimental outcome.
6. Initiation of enteral feeding should occur immediately after adequate resuscitation.

B. Enteral formulas

1. Wide arrays of formulas are commercially available. The choice of an enteral formula is influenced by the degree of organ dysfunction and nutrient needs.
2. Patients who have not been fed for a prolonged period of time are less likely to tolerate complex solutions.
3. Patients with malnutrition benefit from provision of dipeptides, tripeptides, and medium-chain triglycerides, because these substances are more easily absorbed.
4. Major categories of enteral formulas are:
   a. Low-residue isotonic formulas
      (1) These first-line formulas for stable patients with an intact GI tract contain no fiber bulk and so leave minimal residue.
      (2) They provide a caloric density of 1 kcal/mL, and a nonprotein calorie:nitrogen ratio of 150:1.
   b. Isotonic formulas with fiber
      (1) The formulas contain fiber, which delays intestinal transit time and reduces the incidence of diarrhea.
      (2) The fiber stimulates pancreatic lipase activity and is degraded by gut bacteria into short-chain fatty acids.
   c. Immune-enhancing formulas
      (1) The formulas contain special nutrients such as glutamine, arginine, branched-chain amino acids, omega-3 fatty acids, nucleotides, and beta carotene.
      (2) The addition of amino acids generally doubles the amount of protein.
   d. Calorie-dense formulas
      (1) The formulas provide 1.5 to 2 kcal/mL, and are therefore used in fluid-restricted patients.
      (2) They have a higher osmolarity than standard formulas, and are therefore used for intragastric feedings.
   e. High-protein formulas
      (1) The formulas are used in critically ill patients with high protein requirements.
      (2) They provide nonprotein calorie:nitrogen ratios of 80:1 to 120:1.
   f. Elemental formulas
      (1) The formulas contain predigested nutrients, and are thus easy to absorb.
      (2) They are deficient in fat, vitamins, and trace elements that limit their long-term use. Instead, they are used in patients with malnutrition, gut impairment, and pancreatitis.
   g. Renal failure formulas
      (1) These formulas contain protein exclusively in the form of essential amino acids and have a high nonprotein:calorie ratio.
      (2) They require lower fluid volumes and contain lower concentrations of potassium, magnesium, and phosphorus.

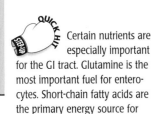

Certain nutrients are especially important for the GI tract. Glutamine is the most important fuel for enterocytes. Short-chain fatty acids are the primary energy source for colonocytes.

h. Pulmonary failure formulas
  (1) These formulas have a reduced content of carbohydrate and a corresponding increased content of fat up to 50% of the total calories.
  (2) This aims to reduce the amount of CO_2 produced, to decrease the burden of ventilation.
i. Hepatic failure formulas. These formulas have an increased quantity of branched-chain amino acids and reduced aromatic amino acids.
C. Access for enteral nutrition
  1. Nasoenteric tubes (nasogastric and nasoduodenal tubes)
    a. Intragastric feeding permits bolus feeding, due to the reservoir capacity of the stomach.
    b. Feeding the stomach results in stimulation of the biliary-pancreatic axis, which is trophic for the small bowel.
    c. Gastric secretions also have a dilutional effect on the osmolarity of the feedings decreasing the incidence of diarrhea.
    d. Nasogastric feeding should be administered to patients with intact mental status and protective laryngeal reflexes to minimize the risk of aspiration.
    e. Nasoduodenal feedings decrease the risk of aspiration pneumonia by 25%.
    f. Placement of tubes past the pylorus is technically difficult. However, fluoroscopic-guided placement has a high success rate.
  2. Percutaneous endoscopic gastrostomy (PEG)
    a. This technique is used for long-term enteral nutrition access.
    b. Catheters are placed in the stomach percutaneously using endoscopic guidance.
    c. Relative contraindications to PEG include ascites, coagulopathy, gastric varices, gastric neoplasm, and lack of suitable abdominal site.
  3. Percutaneous endoscopic gastrostomy-jejunostomy (PEG-J) and direct percutaneous endoscopic jejunostomy (DPEJ)
    a. These techniques are used for patients who cannot tolerate gastric feedings or are at risk of aspiration.
    b. PEG-J is performed by passing a tube past the pylorus into the jejunum using an existing PEG tube. This is done endoscopically or fluoroscopically. PEG-J has a more than 50% malfunction rate due to retrograde tube migration, clogging, and kinking.
    c. DPEJ is performed using the same techniques as PEG, but requires the enteroscope to reach the jejunum.
  4. Surgical gastrostomy and jejunostomy
D. Complications of enteral nutrition
  1. Abdominal distension and cramps. This is managed by temporarily discontinuing feeds and resuming at a lower infusion rate.
  2. Pneumatosis intestinalis and small bowel necrosis
    a. This occurs as a result of bowel distension, and consequent reduction in bowel wall perfusion.
    b. Factors implicated include hyperosmolarity of tube feeds, bacterial overgrowth, fermentation, and metabolic breakdown products.
    c. Initiation of enteric tube feedings in critically ill patients should be delayed till they have been adequately resuscitated, so that an already hypoperfused bowel is not stressed further.
    d. Tube feeds can also be diluted, or solutions with low osmolarity can be used so that less digestion is needed by the GI tract.

V. Parenteral Nutrition

A. General principles. Parenteral nutrition consists of infusion of a hyperosmolar solution containing carbohydrates, proteins, fats, and other important nutrients.
B. Indications:
  1. Prolonged ileus (less then 7–10 days) after a major operation
  2. Hypermetabolic patients in whom enteral nutrition is not possible or adequate (e.g., critically ill patients, cancer patients)

DPEJ has a lower rate of malfunction than PEG-J, but is technically much more challenging.

3. Short bowel syndrome
4. High-output enterocutaneous fistulas (output >500 mL/day)
5. Malabsorption (for example, pancreatic insufficiency, celiac disease, inflammatory bowel disease)
6. Functional gastrointestinal disorders (for example, esophageal dyskinesia, anorexia nervosa)

C. Routes of parenteral nutrition
   1. Total parenteral nutrition (TPN; also called central parenteral nutrition)
      a. These solutions are hyperosmolar, and must therefore be delivered into a high-flow system (that is, a central vein) to prevent venous sclerosis.
      b. A standard TPN solution contains 15% to 25% dextrose, 10% amino acid, lipids and electrolytes, minerals, and vitamins.
      c. Lipids are primarily in the form of long-chain triglycerides, which provide essential fatty acids (linoleic acid). However, the high content of these polyunsaturated fatty acids has harmful effects on pulmonary and immune function.
   2. Peripheral parenteral nutrition (PPN)
      a. These solutions can be administered via peripheral veins, because they have low osmolarity; secondary to reduced levels of dextrose (5–10%) and protein (3%).
      b. Some nutrients cannot be administered due to inability to concentrate them into small volumes.
      c. Typically, PPN is used for nutritional support for short periods (less than 2 weeks), when central venous access is not available or feasible.

D. Complications of TPN
   1. TPN is associated with more complications, compared with enteral feeding, due to intestinal bacterial overgrowth and increased gut permeability leading to bacterial translocation. However, parenteral feeding still has fewer infectious complications compared with no feeding at all.
   2. Complications of TPN can be divided into mechanical, metabolic, and infectious.
      a. Mechanical
         (1) Pneumothorax
         (2) Subclavian artery injury
         (3) Air embolism
         (4) Catheter embolization
         (5) Venous thrombosis
         (6) Catheter malposition
      b. Metabolic
         (1) Hyperglycemia: treated by adding insulin to the formulation, or decreasing the amount of glucose
         (2) Hypoglycemia: due to sudden cessation of TPN. Treated by administering dextrose
         (3) Carbon dioxide retention: due to excess glucose administration. Treated by decreasing glucose calories and replacing with fat.
         (4) Azotemia: due to excess amino acid administration. Treated by decreasing amino acids and increasing glucose calories.
         (5) Hypertriglyceridemia: due to rapid fat infusion. Treated by decreasing rate of fat infusion.
         (6) Liver enzyme elevation: mild elevation of transaminases, alkaline phosphatase, and bilirubin may occur. However, this is transient, and if liver enzymes do not plateau or return to normal over 7 to 14 days, another cause of the enzyme elevation should be investigated. Excess glucose is stored in the form of fat, and results in hepatic steatosis. Long-term TPN administration results in cholestasis and formation of gallstones.
         (7) Mineral, vitamin, and essential fatty acid deficiencies
      c. Infectious. Sepsis can occur due to line infection or contamination of the solution.

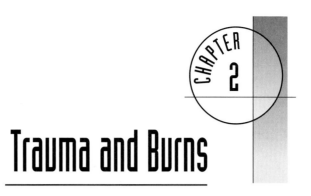

Trauma and Burns

Alison Wilson, MD
Daniel Rossi, DO

I. General Principles

A. Primary examination of the injured patient

   A = Airway maintenance with cervical spine immobilization

   B = Breathing and ventilation

   C = Circulation with hemorrhage control

   D = Disability: neurologic status

   E = Exposure/environment control: undress patient; then prevent hypothermia

   1. Airway

     a. Airway protection is needed in patients with the following conditions:

       (1) Decreased level of consciousness

       (2) Severe maxillofacial fractures

       (3) Risk of aspiration such as bleeding or vomiting

       (4) Risk of obstruction such as stridor, neck hematoma, laryngeal or tracheal injury

     b. Airway maintenance techniques include chin lift, jaw thrust, oropharyngeal airway, and nasopharyngeal airway

     c. Definitive airway. **Be sure to provide in-line cervical spine immobilization**

       (1) Endotracheal intubation

       (2) Nasotracheal intubation

       (3) Surgical airway: cricothyrotomy, tracheostomy.

   2. **Ventilation: adequate CO_2 exchange.** Assisted ventilation may be required with apnea due to neuromuscular paralysis, decreased level of consciousness, or inadequate respiratory efforts.

B. **Secondary examination**

   1. Head-to-toe evaluation with reassessment of all vital signs

   2. Complete neurologic examination, including the Glasgow Coma Scale (GCS) Pertinent x-rays: lateral cervical spine, chest x-ray, and pelvis

   3. History includes AMPLE: Allergies, Medications, Past Illness, Last Meal, Events

C. **Shock**

   1. Hemorrhagic shock (Table 2-1)

     a. A type of hypovolemic shock

     b. The most common cause of shock in the trauma patient

   2. Nonhemorrhagic shock

     a. Cardiogenic shock: myocardial dysfunction from blunt cardiac injury, myocardial infarction

     b. Obstructive shock: obstruction to normal flow, causing inadequate perfusion

       (1) Cardiac tamponade

       (2) Tension pneumothorax

       (3) Pulmonary embolism

     c. Neurogenic shock: loss of sympathetic tone causing hypotension without tachycardia

     d. Septic shock: very uncommon in acute trauma

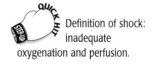

QUICK HIT
Airway and breathing are the most important priorities in the trauma patient. Facial fractures and injuries can severely compromise and complicate the airway.

QUICK HIT
Signs and symptoms of airway compromise include stridor, hoarseness, subcutaneous emphysema, obvious fractures, noisy breathing, and displacement of the trachea.

QUICK HIT
Definition of shock: inadequate oxygenation and perfusion.

TABLE 2-1 Categories of Hypovolemic Shock

	Class I	Class II	Class III	Class IV
Blood loss (mL)	Up to 750	750–1,500	1,500–2,000	>2,000
Blood loss (% blood volume)	Up to 15%	15–30%	30–40%	>40%
Pulse rate	<100 bpm	>100 bpm	>120 bpm	>140 bpm
Blood pressure	Normal	Normal	Decreased	Decreased
Urine output (mL/hr)	>30	20–30	5–15	None
Mental status	Normal	Anxious	Confused	Lethargic
Fluid replacement	Crystalloid	Crystalloid	Crystalloid and blood	Crystalloid and blood

> **QUICK HIT**
> The primary focus in caring for patients with severe brain injury is to prevent secondary injury. Secondary injury is caused by hypoxia and hypotension.

> **QUICK HIT**
> Monro–Kellie doctrine: The total volume of the intracranial contents must remain constant. This means that a small increase in any of the intracranial contents can cause a large increase in intracranial pressure.

II. Head and Neck

A. Traumatic brain injury

1. Anatomy

 a. The scalp is made of five layers and is very vascular. Can be a source of significant blood loss.

 b. The skull is a bone composing cranial vault and base.

 c. The meninges are three layers that cover the brain (dura mater, arachnoid, and pia mater).

 d. The brain consists of cerebrum, cerebellum, and brain stem.

 e. The cerebrospinal fluid is produced by choroids plexus in the ventricles. It exits ventricles into subarachnoid space, and then is reabsorbed into venous circulation.

 f. The third cranial nerve, which runs along the edge of the tentorium and is compressed with temporal herniation. Compression causes pupil dilatation due to unopposed sympathetic activity.

2. Assessment

 a. The severity of injury is based on the **Glasgow Coma Scale** (GCS; Fig. 2-1).

 b. Types of head injury:

FIGURE 2-1 Glasgow Coma Scale.

Eye Opening

Spontaneous	4
To speech	3
To pain	2
None	1

Verbal Response

Oriented	5
Confused	4
Inappropriate words	3
Moans	2
None	1

Motor Response

Follows commands	6
Localizes pain	5
Withdrawals	4
Decorticate (Flexion)	3
Decerebrate (Extension)	2
None	1

Note: Glasgow Coma Scale score = E + V + M; minimum score is 3, maximum is 15.

(1) Skull fracture requires significant force and increases the risk of an underlying brain injury.

(2) Physical signs associated with basal skull fractures are periorbital ecchymosis (raccoon eyes), retroauricular ecchymosis (Battle sign), and rhinorrhea (cerebrospinal fluid leakage from the nose).

(3) Intracranial lesions can be focal or diffuse, although both commonly occur together.

   (a) Diffuse injuries include hypoxia or ischemia

      i. Computed tomography (CT) scan of the brain may appear normal or diffusely swollen.

      ii. **Diffuse axonal injury** includes punctuate hemorrhages throughout both hemispheres primarily at the gray-white matter junction.

   (b) Focal injuries

      i. **Epidural hematomas** are usually located in temporal regions, outside the dura and are biconvex in shape. Usually, a result of a tear in the middle meningeal artery.

      ii. **Subdural hematomas** are a result of a tearing of the small surface vessels of the cortex, and can cover the entire surface of the hemisphere.

(4) Contusions and intracerebral hematomas can evolve with time, and therefore are best detected by follow-up CT scan at 12 to 24 hours.

3. Management of brain injuries

   a. Mild (GCS 14 to15). CT of the brain for patients who have loss of consciousness for greater than 5 minutes, amnesia, severe headaches, GCS less than 15, or focal neurologic deficit.

   b. Moderate (GCS 9 to 13)

   (1) Perform detailed neurologic examination and prevent secondary injury.

   (2) CT scan should be performed, and neurosurgeon consulted.

   (3) Follow-up CT scan should be performed if the initial is abnormal or if the patient's neurologic status deteriorates.

   (4) Hourly neurologic checks should be performed.

   c. Severe (GCS less than 8)

   (1) Perform detailed neurologic examination and prevent secondary injury.

   (2) Early endotracheal intubation should be performed to protect the airway, and ensure adequate oxygenation and ventilation.

   (3) Hypotension is not a result of brain injury, and a source of bleeding must be sought. Hypotension with severe brain injury doubles the mortality.

   (4) GCS and pupil examination must be performed prior to sedating or paralyzing the patient.

   (5) **A mass effect causing a midline shift of 5 mm or greater seen on the CT often indicates the need for emergency craniotomy and decompression.**

   (6) For patients with a GCS less than 8, intracranial pressure monitoring is essential.

4. Intracranial pressure monitoring. **An intracranial pressure of greater than 20 mm Hg requires intervention.** Therapies may include mannitol, diuretics, sedation, barbiturates, or cerebrospinal fluid (CSF) drainage via ventriculostomy.

B. Facial fractures

   1. Neurologic, airway, and ocular examinations are important.

   2. Mandible and midface fractures can compromise the airway.

   3. Orbital wall and sinus fractures may cause muscle entrapment or nerve injury.

   4. Parotid duct injuries can occur with lateral facial lacerations.

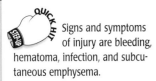

TRAUMA AND BURNS

Signs and symptoms of injury are bleeding, hematoma, infection, and subcutaneous emphysema.

All patients with a radiographic abnormality, neurologic deficit, or decreased level of consciousness should be considered to have an unstable spine and should be completely immobilized.

C. Neck
1. **Zones of the neck**
   a. Zone I: thoracic outlet, cricoid cartilage down to the clavicle
   b. Zone II: cricoid cartilage up to the angle of the mandible
   c. Zone III: angle of the mandible to the base of the skull
2. Diagnosis and evaluation
   a. **Ensure adequate airway and breathing while maintaining cervical immobilization.** Document a complete neurologic assessment that includes GCS, sensory, motor, pupil, and cranial nerve examination.
   b. Key tests for hemodynamically stable patients with zone I or III trauma are arteriography, endoscopy of the airway and esophagus, and a barium swallow. Injuries found on these tests are then repaired.
   c. Penetrating injuries to zone II that violate the platysma often were evaluated by operative exploration, although these injuries are now being selectively evaluated as above.
   d. **Do not probe a penetrating wound, because this can dislodge a clot.** All unstable patients with expanding hematomas, shock, or uncontrolled bleeding should be taken directly to the operating room.
D. Spine and spinal cord injuries
1. Anatomy
   a. Spinal column consists of 7 cervical, 12 thoracic, and 5 lumbar vertebrae.
   b. Cervical spine is most prone to injury.
   c. Ten percent of patients with a cervical spine fracture have a noncontiguous vertebral column fracture.
2. Examination. The examination consists of a sensory examination, including pain, temperature, proprioception, vibration, and light touch, as well as the motor examination throughout all dermatomes and myotomes (Table 2-2).
3. Classification of spinal cord injury
   a. Level: defined at the most caudal segment of the spinal cord with normal sensory and motor function on both sides of the body.
   b. Severity
      (1) Injuries are defined as incomplete paraplegia, complete paraplegia, incomplete quadriplegia, and complete quadriplegia.
      (2) Signs of incomplete injury include the following:
         (a) Sacral sparing: perianal sensation or voluntary anal sphincter contraction.
         (b) Voluntary movement or sensation distal to the injury.

TABLE 2-2 **Nerve Root Association with Myotomes and Dermatomes**

Dermatomes	Myotomes
C5: area over deltoid muscle	C5: deltoid
C6: thumb	C6: wrist extensors
C7: third digit	C7: elbow extensors (triceps)
C8: fifth digit	C8: flexor digitorum profundus
T4: nipple	T1: abductor digiti minimi
T10: umbilicus	L2: hip flexors
T12: symphysis pubis	L3,4: knee extensors
L5: web space between first and second toes	L4,5,S1: knee flexion
S1: lateral border of the foot	L5: ankle dorsiflexor
S4,5: perianal region	S1: gastrocnemius

4. Spinal cord syndromes
   a. **Central cord syndrome** shows greater motor loss in upper versus lower extremities with various sensory losses, and is often seen with hyperextension injury in a patient with preexisting cervical canal stenosis.
   b. **Anterior cord syndrome** includes paraplegia with loss of pain and temperature, but preserved position, vibration, and deep pressure. Usually due to infarction of anterior spinal artery.
   c. **Brown–Séquard syndrome** is caused by hemisection of the cord, resulting in ipsilateral motor loss and proprioception with contralateral loss of pain and temperature.
5. Anatomic injury. Injuries can be described as stable or unstable, fractures, fracture dislocations, or spinal cord injury without radiographic abnormality (**SCIWORA**).
   a. **Atlanto-occipital dislocation** is usually fatal due to brain-stem injury. Survivors tend to be quadriplegic and ventilator dependent.
   b. C1 fracture/**Jefferson fracture** is a burst fracture of the ring often not associated with spinal cord injury.
   c. C2 fracture is a hangman's fracture involving posterior elements of C2.
   d. **Chance fractures** are transverse fractures through the lumbar vertebral body.
      (1) Often associated with lap belt.
      (2) High association with retroperitoneal and bowel injuries.
6. Evaluation and treatment
   a. **Methylprednisolone is given in nonpenetrating spinal cord injury within the first 8 hours of injury.**
   b. Dose is 30 mg/kg in the first 15 minutes, then 5.4 mg/kg/hr for 24 hours.

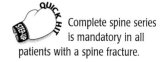

Complete spine series is mandatory in all patients with a spine fracture.

III. Thoracic Trauma

A. Sternal and scapular fractures (usually direct blow with large force), underlying cardiac or pulmonary contusions
B. Rib fractures can impair oxygenation and ventilation, and are very painful.
   1. Ribs 1 to 3 imply significant force transmitted, with the underlying lung and great vessels at increased risk of injury.
   2. Ribs 4 to 9 are the most common location in blunt injury, and can cause underlying pulmonary contusion.
C. Flail chest occurs when more than two ribs are fractured in two or more places.
   1. Paradoxical movement of the chest when breathing
   2. May require mechanical ventilation
   3. High risk of pneumonia and pulmonary contusion
D. Pulmonary contusion
   1. Can be immediate, or occur over 24 to 48 hours
   2. Can cause severe hypoxia and respiratory failure
   3. Try to minimize intravenous fluids
E. Hemothorax
   1. Can be from blunt or penetrating trauma.
      a. Blunt trauma intercostal artery injury is a common source of massive bleeding.
      b. Penetrating anterior wound medial to nipple line and posterior wounds medial to scapula, are at risk for severe injury to great vessels, hilum, or heart.
   2. Treatment
      a. 36 Fr chest tube in fifth intercostal space
      b. **Chest tube output is an indication for emergency operative intervention.**
         (1) Greater than 1,500 mL immediately when chest tube placed
         (2) Evidence of ongoing bleeding
         (3) Greater than 200 mL/hr over 4 hours

F. Pneumothorax: air between the parietal and visceral pleura causing lung collapse
  1. Simple pneumothorax: air only between pleura
     a. Diagnosed on chest x-ray (CXR); if possible upright, expiratory film most sensitive
     b. Can convert to tension pneumothorax if patient is on mechanical ventilation
     c. Treatment: chest tube placed in fifth intercostal space, anteriorly
  2. **Tension pneumothorax:** one-way valve air leak into thoracic cavity
     a. Life-threatening!!!!
     b. Collapse of affected lung
     c. Mediastinum shifts to opposite side
     d. Decreases venous return and compresses opposite lung
     e. Clinical diagnosis: **do not wait for CXR before treating**
        (1) The signs are respiratory distress, tachypnea, tachycardia, hypotension, tracheal deviation, unilateral absence of breath sounds, neck vein distention.
        (2) Treatment
           (a) Immediate decompression
           (b) 18-gauge needle placed in second intercostal space at midclavicular line
           (c) Follow up with placement of chest tube in fifth intercostal space
  3. Open pneumothorax is a sucking chest wound
     a. Large defect in chest wall causing equilibration between intrathoracic and atmospheric pressure
     b. Cover defect, and tape on three sides
     c. Complete occlusion will cause a tension pneumothorax
     d. Place chest tube as remote from the wound as possible
G. Tracheobronchial tree injuries are injuries to trachea or bronchus.
  1. Blunt trauma injury usually occurs within 1 inch of the carina.
  2. Signs and symptoms: hemoptysis, tension pneumothorax, pneumothorax with massive air leak, CXR with completely collapsed, nonventilated lung.
  3. Diagnosis is made with bronchoscopy.
  4. Treatment is to intubate main-stem bronchus of opposite lung.
     a. Place chest tube on affected side.
     b. Immediate surgical intervention.
H. Cardiac injuries
  1. **Cardiac tamponade**
     a. Pericardium fills with blood preventing cardiac filling and constricting the heart causing hemodynamic collapse.
     b. Penetrating trauma is a more common cause.
  2. Signs
     a. **Beck triad**
        (1) Elevated central venous pressure, decreased blood pressure, and muffled heart tones
        (2) May not be apparent in hypovolemic patient
     b. **Kussmaul sign**, which is a rise in venous pressure with inspiration when breathing spontaneously
  3. Diagnosis is made with transthoracic ultrasound
  4. Treatment
     a. Fluid bolus to help venous return and cardiac output
     b. Temporizing maneuver is with pericardiocentesis
     c. Operative repair is with thoracotomy or median sternotomy, depending on injury
I. Blunt cardiac injury
  1. Etiology: can result from myocardial muscle contusion, valve disruption, and chamber rupture
  2. Signs and symptoms
     a. Chest pain

   b. Arrhythmias which may become progressively worse
   c. Pump failure, leading to low cardiac output, respiratory distress
3. Diagnosis
   a. 12-lead electrocardiogram: if any new abnormalities, patient should be monitored for 24 hours.
   b. Common dysrhythmias include premature ventricular contractions, right bundle branch block, may progress to ventricular tachycardia.
   c. Patient may show ischemic changes.
   d. An echocardiogram may show wall dysfunction. Order in cases of symptoms of failure.
4. Treatment is supportive. Inotropes, diuretics, antiarrhythmics, and a balloon pump may be needed.
J. **Traumatic aortic injury**
   1. This is a common cause of sudden death after deceleration blunt injury. There is a transection of the aorta at the ligamentum arteriosum (distal to the left subclavian artery).
   2. Signs and symptoms
      a. High index of suspicion in deceleration injuries.
      b. Fractures of first, second ribs, scapula.
   3. Diagnosis
      a. CXR: wide mediastinum (Fig. 2-2)
      b. **Arteriography, which is a traditional gold standard**
      c. Helical contrast-enhanced CT, which is a screening tool, and an emerging technique
K. Esophageal injuries
   1. Signs and symptoms
      a. An early sign or symptom is a left pneumothorax without a rib fracture, particulate matter in chest tube, or mediastinal air.
      b. A late sign or symptom is shock, or sepsis out of proportion to injury after epigastric blow.

QUICK HIT

Signs of possible traumatic aortic injury on CXR: wide mediastinum, obliteration of aortic knob, deviation of trachea to the right, obliteration of aortopulmonary window, depression of left mainstem bronchus, deviation of esophagus to right, wide paratracheal stripe, pleural cap.

FIGURE 2-2 Plain CXR demonstrating signs of traumatic aortic injury. Note the wide mediastinum, esophageal deviation, and blurring of the aortic knob.

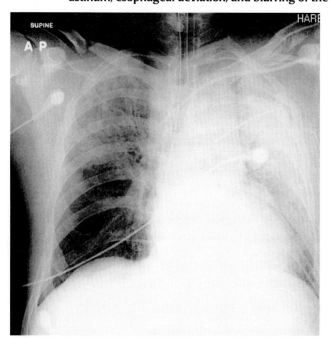

(Reprinted, with permission, from *Greenfield's Surgery*, 4th ed. Philadelphia: Lippincott Williams & Wilkins; 2006:415.)

2. Diagnosis (**both of these are required to complete the workup**):
   a. Esophagoscopy
   b. Gastrografin swallow
3. Treatment
   a. Early treatment includes primary repair and drainage.
   b. Late treatment includes wide pleural drainage and proximal diversion.

IV. Abdomen/Pelvis

A. Evaluation
1. Blunt force injury
   a. Hemodynamically stable indicates CT abdomen/pelvis, serial abdominal exams, focused abdominal sonography in trauma (FAST).
   b. Hemodynamically unstable indicates laparotomy, FAST, diagnostic peritoneal lavage (DPL).
2. Penetrating injury
   a. Hemodynamically stable
      (1) Stab wound includes local wound exploration, serial abdominal examinations, laparotomy.
      (2) Gunshot wound includes laparotomy.
   b. Hemodynamically unstable indicates laparotomy.

B. Liver injuries
1. Signs and symptoms
   a. Abdominal pain, hypotension
   b. Most commonly injured organ in blunt trauma
2. Diagnosis
   a. CT abdomen/pelvis
      (1) May show subcapsular hematoma, laceration, and arterial blush
      (2) Grades I to VI, mild to severe based on findings on CT
3. Treatment:
   a. Grades I to III: often heals spontaneously over 6 weeks, manage conservatively.
   b. Grades III to V: more severe injuries, and a higher risk of bleeding.
      (1) ICU management, bed rest, serial hematocrits, possible arteriogram and embolization
      (2) A laparotomy is indicated if continued bleeding or hemodynamic instability.
         (a) The most common technique is packing the abdomen to stop bleeding.
   c. Grade VI: complete avulsion of liver, which is lethal

C. Spleen injuries
1. Anatomy
   a. Located under ninth to eleventh ribs on left
   b. Blood supply
      (1) Arterial, which includes splenic artery, short gastric arteries. **Dual arterial supply permits embolization of main splenic artery with preservation of immune function.**
      (2) Venous, which includes splenic vein, short gastric veins.
2. Signs and symptoms
   a. Left upper quadrant (LUQ) pain, hypotension.
   b. Kehr sign-referred pain to left shoulder from diaphragm.
   c. Balance sign-enlarged tender LUQ mass from splenic hematoma.
3. Diagnosis
   a. Unstable patients need a history, physical, FAST, DPL, laparotomy.
   b. Stable patients need a history, physical, CT, abdomen/pelvis.
4. Treatment
   a. Unstable patients
      (1) Laparotomy: splenorrhaphy versus splenectomy.
      (2) More often associated with grade IV to V injuries.

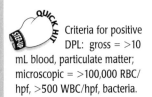

Criteria for positive DPL: gross = >10 mL blood, particulate matter; microscopic = >100,000 RBC/hpf, >500 WBC/hpf, bacteria.

b. Stable patients
   (1) Bed rest, serial examinations, and hematocrit.
   (2) Grade I to III injuries usually heal spontaneously.
   5. Complications
      a. Postsplenectomy sepsis, which is rare (2% occurrence).
      b. Injury to tail of the pancreas.
      c. Delayed rupture, which can occur 10 to 14 days after injury.
D. Diaphragm injuries
   1. Blunt injuries include large radial tears, usually on left.
   2. Penetrating injuries include small holes that may enlarge and herniate over time.
   3. The signs and symptoms are chest or abdomen pain, respiratory distress, severe nausea, gastric dilatation, hemodynamic compromise.
   4. Diagnosis
      a. CXR, which may show elevated hemidiaphragm, air–fluid level above the diaphragm, nasogastric (NG) tube in chest, displacement of mediastinum to right (Fig. 2-3).
   5. Treatment
      a. Acute
         (1) Approach through laparotomy as there are a high incidence of associated injuries.
         (2) Blunt injuries. With a large defect, try primary repair with horizontal mattress sutures. Mesh may be needed.
      b. Chronic
         (1) Approach through chest
E. Pancreas injuries
   1. Often associated with direct blow to epigastrium.
   2. Signs and symptoms include severe abdominal pain, peritonitis, nausea, vomiting, elevated pancreatic isoenzymes.
   3. Diagnosis
      a. A CT abdomen/pelvis, which often may show midbody transection after blunt trauma.
F. Bowel injuries
   1. Duodenum

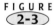

For both liver and spleen trauma, the presence of an arterial blush on CT is associated with higher risk of failure of nonoperative management but may also respond to selective embolization.

FIGURE 2-3 **CXR demonstrating evidence of a traumatic diaphragmatic hernia. Note the cardiac deviation to the right and the elevated air-fluid level in the chest.**

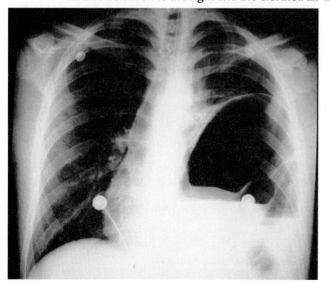

(Reprinted, with permission, from *Greenfield's Surgery*, 4th ed. Philadelphia: Lippincott Williams & Wilkins; 2006:473.)

a. The risk factors are penetrating trauma, crush to epigastrium, and pancreatic injury.
b. Diagnosis
   (1) Hemodynamically unstable
      (a) Laparotomy, right upper quadrant (RUQ) retroperitoneal hematoma, bile staining.
      (b) DPL may be negative because duodenum is retroperitoneal.
   (2) Hemodynamically stable
      (a) CT of abdomen/pelvis or UGI series with water-soluble contrast.
c. Treatment
   (1) Intramural hematoma indicates NG tube, total parenteral nutrition (TPN).
   (2) Perforation
      (a) Transverse primary two-layer repair.
      (b) In all cases, use wide drainage and consider feeding access.

2. Small bowel (jejunum and ileum)
   a. Penetrating trauma is the most common cause
   b. Blunt trauma, which occurs at ligament of Treitz, distal ileum, or areas of adhesions.
   c. Diagnosis
      (1) Positive DPL
   d. Treatment
      (1) Primary repair in transverse fashion if less than 50% of wall is involved.
      (2) Resection and anastomosis
         (a) Loss of more than 50% circumference
         (b) Multiple perforations in single segment
         (c) Devascularized segment

3. Colon
   a. The diagnosis is the same as small bowel
   b. Treatment
      (1) Right colon
         (a) Repair if less than 50% wall is involved.
         (b) Resect and primary anastomosis for larger or devascularized injuries.
      (2) Left colon
         (a) If hemodynamically stable, minimal contamination, and normal temperature, then repair, or resect and anastomosis is needed.
         (b) If hemodynamically unstable, significant other injuries, hypothermic, then a diverting colostomy is needed.
      (3) Rectum
         (a) For intraperitoneal, a repair and diverting colostomy is indicated.
         (b) For extraperitoneal, a diverting colostomy is indicated.

G. Retroperitoneum
   1. **Zones**
      a. Zone 1: central and medial aspects; contains great vessels.
      b. Zone 2: flanks.
      c. Zone 3: pelvis.
   2. Treatment
      a. Zone 1. Must be explored and injury repaired in both penetrating and blunt trauma.
      b. Zone 2. If the hematoma is stable, do not explore.
      c. Zone 3
         (1) With blunt trauma, do not explore the hematoma.
         (2) With penetrating trauma, explore and repair.

H. Kidney
   1. Signs and symptoms: **hematuria indicates possible injury.**

A bucket handle injury results from blunt trauma causing a shearing and tearing of the mesentery and vessels, usually occurring at the ileocolic junction, and resulting in ischemia.

Retroperitoneum is very important because it contains the great vessels in the abdomen.

    a. In adults, gross hematuria.
    b. In children, gross or microscopic hematuria.
  2. Diagnosis is made with a CT in hemodynamically stable patients.
I. Ureteral injuries
  1. These injuries are rare in blunt trauma, and are more likely to occur with stab or gunshot wounds.
  2. Diagnosis is with intravenous pyelogram.
  3. Treatment
    a. If possible, primary repair over stent.
J. Urethral injuries
  1. Most commonly due to blunt trauma with associated pelvic fracture.
  2. Signs and symptoms.
    a. Blood at the meatus.
    b. Inability to void.
    c. High-riding prostate on digital rectal examination.
  3. Diagnosis is with a retrograde urethrogram.
  4. Treatment is with early realignment over catheter.
K. Bladder injuries
  1. Types of injuries include intraperitoneal, extraperitoneal, and combined. They are often associated with pelvic fractures.
  2. The signs and symptoms are abdominal pain, gross hematuria, anuria, or low urine output.
  3. Diagnosis is with cystography or CT cystogram.
    a. In an intraperitoneal rupture, the contrast outlines bowel loops.
    b. In an extraperitoneal rupture, the contrast is contained in the pelvis, and may track along the muscles.
  4. Treatment
    a. In an intraperitoneal rupture, the treatment is operative, with a two-layer repair.
    b. In an extraperitoneal rupture, the treatment is conservative; Foley 10 to 14 days with follow-up cystography.
L. Pelvis fractures
  1. Anterior fractures.
    a. May cause injury to urethra, bladder, prostate, vagina.
    b. If isolated, usually hemodynamically stable.
  2. Posterior fractures
    a. May cause severe injury to pelvis arteries, veins, and nerves.
    b. May be source of massive pelvic hematoma, bleeding, and death.
  3. Treatment
    a. Stabilize the patient with a sheet, pelvic binder, external fixator.
    b. Angiography with embolization. Selective if identified or hypogastric artery.

V. Extremity Injuries
A. Assessment
  1. History and physical, with special attention to neurologic and vascular examination.
  2. X-rays of extremity, which include the joint above and below the injury.
  3. Mangled extremity severity score
    a. Tool to assess viability for limb salvage.
    b. The score is based on bone/soft tissue loss, shock, ischemia, age.
  4. Vascular compromise
    a. **Hard signs of vascular compromise.**
      (1) No pulse in extremity.
      (2) No or poor capillary refill.
      (3) Expanding hematoma.
      (4) Pale, blue extremity. Proceed to operative repair of vessel.

b. Decreased pulses or signs of mild ischemia.
  (1) Realign and splint extremity.
  (2) Ankle brachial index.
    (a) Compare systolic blood pressure (SBP) of dorsalis pedis/posterior tibialis pressures to SBP of brachial artery.
    (b) Normal = 1, and each side within 10%.
  (3) The arteriogram is the gold standard, but is invasive.

B. Open fractures/joints
  1. Any laceration that communicates with a fracture.
  2. Treatment must occur within 6 hours to minimize risk of infection.
    a. Grades I and II: first-generation cephalosporin.
    b. Grade III: first-generation cephalosporin and aminoglycoside.

C. **Compartment syndrome**
  1. Risk factors
    a. Tibial and forearm fracture.
    b. Fractures in tight dressings, casts.
    c. Severe crush injury to muscle.
    d. Localized, prolonged external pressure to an extremity.
    e. Reperfusion after ischemia.
    f. Burns.
  2. Signs and symptoms
    a. Pain on passive motion.
    b. Paresthesias and lack of pulse are late signs, and damage is irreversible.
  3. Diagnosis
    a. Clinical examination.
    b. Compartment pressures can be measured, and should be less than 30 mm Hg.
  4. Treatment is with fasciotomy.

VI. Burns

A. Anatomy
  1. Skin layers
    a. Epidermis
      (1) Acts as a barrier to environment, protecting from infection, toxins, ultraviolet light, and fluid evaporation.
      (2) Epidermal layers superficial to deep: stratum corneum → stratum lucidum → stratum granulosum → stratum spinosum → stratum basale (germinativum).
    b. Dermis
      (1) Consists of the papillary dermis and reticular dermis.
      (2) Majority of the dermis consists of the reticular dermis.

B. Burn types
  1. **Thermal**
    a. Zones of injury
      (1) Zone of coagulation is the central, most severely injured area. The tissue is necrotic and constitutes a full-thickness burn.
      (2) Zone of stasis consists of vasoconstriction and ischemia, and is immediately adjacent to the zone of coagulation. It constitutes a partial-thickness burn.
      (3) Zone of hyperemia is the most superficial area and heals quickly without scarring. It constitutes a superficial partial-thickness burn.
  2. **Chemical**
    a. Alkali burns occur from cement, lime, potassium/sodium hydroxide, and bleach.
    b. Acid
      (1) Seen often with formic and hydrofluoric acid.
      (2) Do not penetrate as deeply as alkaline.

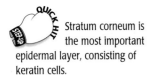
Stratum corneum is the most important epidermal layer, consisting of keratin cells.

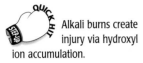
Alkali burns create injury via hydroxyl ion accumulation.

(3) Hydrofluoric acid results in calcium chelation, which leads to insoluble salt formation, which leads to hypocalcemia, dysrhythmia. The treatment with calcium gluconate is used to treat the dysrhythmia, not the burn.

   c. Hydrocarbon in organic solvents create injury by causing cell membrane dissolution and skin necrosis.

   d. Treatment involves copious irrigation with water for 30 minutes (15–20 L).

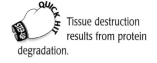

Tissue destruction results from protein degradation.

3. **Electrical**

   a. High-voltage burns due to greater than 1,000 watts (W) require a full trauma evaluation.

      (1) Check for rhabdomyolysis. and complete an ophthalmologic examination to exclude cataract formation.

      (2) Monitor median nerve function (lies within carpal tunnel).

      (3) Treatment may require escharotomy or fasciotomy.

      (4) Extent of injury is actually greater than the visible areas of tissue necrosis.

   b. Low-voltage burns due to less than 1,000 W

      (1) Systemic sequelae are rare and are not transmitted to deeper tissues.

      (2) Typically, the result of a child chewing on an electric cord, and causing burns to the corner of the mouth.

   c. Lightning is another source of electrical burn injury.

4. **Inhalation**

   a. Upper airway thermal injury

      (1) Due to heat or chemical toxins, upper airway injury occurs more often than lower airway injury because heat is absorbed by the oropharynx.

      (2) Diagnosis is confirmed by direct laryngoscopy.

      (3) Symptoms manifest within first 6 hours of injury. The most sensitive sign is lip edema.

      (4) Therapy includes the use of humidified oxygen, pulmonary toileting, and bronchodilators. Endotracheal intubation is indicated if posterior pharyngeal swelling, mucosal sloughing, or carbonaceous sputum are present.

   b. Lower airway burn injury

      (1) Results from the combustion products in smoke.

      (2) Mucosal damage and loss of ciliary clearance leads to parenchymal inflammation, pulmonary edema, pneumonia, and acute respiratory distress syndrome (ARDS).

      (3) Diagnosis is via bronchoscopy or xenon ventilation–perfusion scan.

C. Burn classification

  1. Superficial (first-degree) burn

    a. Burn injury is confined to the epidermis.

    b. Burns are painful, erythematous, and blanch to the touch. However, the epidermal barrier is intact.

    c. Examples of first-degree injuries include minor scalds or sunburn.

    d. Treatment involves the use of salves or nonsteroidal anti-inflammatory drugs.

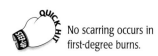

No scarring occurs in first-degree burns.

  2. Partial-thickness (second-degree) burns

    a. Involve the dermis to varying degrees.

    b. Superficial partial-thickness burns

      (1) Burns present as erythematous, painful, blanching, or blisters, and no scarring occurs.

      (2) Scalding and flash flame injuries are examples of superficial partial-thickness burns.

      (3) Reepithelialization occurs spontaneously in 7 to 14 days.

    c. Deep partial-thickness burns

      (1) Burn injury extending into the reticular dermis.

      (2) Appearance of burn is described as pale, mottled, nonblanching, or painful.

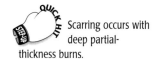

Scarring occurs with deep partial-thickness burns.

(3) Healing occurs in 2 to 4 weeks by reepithelialization from hair follicles and sweat glands.

(4) Healing begins at the central epidermal appendages and extends peripherally.

3. Full-thickness (third-degree) burns

a. Injury extends into the subcutaneous fat.

b. Burns appear as a painless, hard leathery eschar, and color varies from black, white, or cherry.

c. No epidermal or dermal appendages remain, and thus healing occurs by reepithelialization from wound edge peripherally, extending centrally.

d. Treatment for third-degree burns consists of burn or eschar excision and skin grafting.

4. Fourth-degree burns: involves other organs beneath the skin such as muscle, brain, and bone.

D. Burn size

1. **Rule of nines (Color Fig. 2-4). First-degree burns are not included in burn calculations.**

a. Adults

(1) Each arm equals 9% of the total body surface area (TBSA).

(2) Each leg equals 18% TBSA.

(3) Anterior and posterior trunk each equal 18% TBSA.

(4) Head equals 9% TBSA.

(5) Perineum equals 1% TBSA.

(6) An alternative method for calculating burn quantity utilizes the palm, including the digits, to represent 1% TBSA.

b. Children

(1) Each arm equals 9% TBSA.

(2) Each leg equals 14% TBSA.

**FIGURE
2-4** Rule of nines diagram for estimating burn size for both pediatric and adult use.

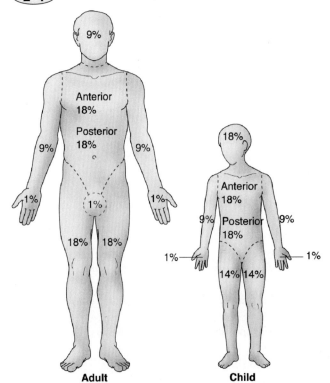

Adult   Child

(Reprinted, with permission, from *Greenfield's Surgery*, 4th ed. Philadelphia: Lippincott Williams & Wilkins; 2006:245.)

TABLE 2-3 Resuscitation Formulas

Formula	Crystalloid Volume	Colloid Volume	Free Water
Parkland	4 mL/kg per % total body surface area (TBSA) burn	None	None
Galveston (pediatric)	5,000 mL/m^2 TBSA burned + 1500 mL/m^2 TBSA	None	None
Brooke	1.5 mL/kg per % TBSA burned	0.5 mL/kg per % TBSA burned	2.0 L

    (3) The anterior and posterior trunk each equal 18% TBSA.

    (4) Head equals 18% TBSA.

E. Resuscitation

  1. **Resuscitation formulas (Table 2-3)**

    a. Parkland formula: reportedly underestimates needs.

      (1) Half of the total volume is given in the first 8 hours.

      (2) The remaining half is given over the next 16 hours.

      (3) Lactated Ringers is used to avoid hyperchloremic metabolic acidosis, associated with large infusions of 0.9% normal saline.

    b. Brooke formula: uses colloid, question if increased ARDS.

    c. In children, the Galveston formula is used because children require more resuscitation fluid per kilogram.

      (1) Dextrose is not used in adults for initial burn resuscitation. However, it should be used in the children weighing less than 20 kg due to inadequate hepatic glycogen reserves.

      (2) Maintenance fluid for children should consist of D5 0.45% half normal saline at a rate of 3 to 4 mL/kg/hr.

    d. Colloid can be used after the initial 24 hours, because less capillary leak/ permeability occurs.

  2. Transfer criteria to burn center (Table 2-4)

QUICK HIT Urine output must be maintained at 0.5 mL/kg/hr in adults and 1 to 2 mL/kg/hr in children; fluid resuscitation should be adjusted accordingly to maintain these goals.

TABLE 2-4 American Burn Association Criteria for Patient Transfer to a Burn Center

1	Partial-thickness burns greater than 10% total body surface area.
2	Burns that involve the face, hands, feet, genitalia, perineum, or major joints.
3	Third-degree burns in any age group.
4	Electrical burns, including lightning burns.
5	Chemical burns.
6	Inhalation injury.
7	Burn injury in patients with preexisting medical conditions that could increase mortality or morbidity.
8	Concomitant burn and trauma in which the burn poses the greatest risk. If the trauma poses the greatest threat, patient may be stabilized initially at a trauma center prior to burn center transport.
9	Burned children at hospitals not equipped to deal with pediatric population.
10	Patients who will require special social, emotional, or long-term rehabilitative services.

F. Systemic complications
   1. Constrictive eschar
      a. These tight, circumferential bands of skin around the extremities, thoracic and abdominal cavities result in neurovascular, respiratory and end-organ (renal) compromise.
      b. Treatment
         (1) Extremity escharotomy
            (a) Escharotomy is performed by extending incisions through the skin only, without involving the fascia.
            (b) In anatomic position, medial and lateral incisions are made extending across the wrist.
            (c) Eschar of the dorsal hand must be released to restore flow through the palmar arch.
         (2) Thoracic escharotomy (Color Fig. 2-5). The skin incision extends along each anterior axillary line, connecting cephalad at the infraclavicular midline and caudally at the subcostal midline.
   3. Extremity compartment syndrome
      a. If compartment pressure is greater than 30 mm Hg, perform a fasciotomy.
      b. Suspect extremity compartment syndrome if pain is out of proportion, pain is present with passive movement, or an ischemia time greater than 6 hours.
   4. **Rhabdomyolysis**
      a. Rhabdomyolysis may be caused by myoglobinuria, resulting in acute tubular necrosis.
      b. Laboratory values indicative of rhabdomyolysis, include positive urine myoglobin, elevated muscle enzymes, and normal serum haptoglobin.
      c. Rhabdomyolysis is treated by maintaining a urine output of 100 mL/hr; urine alkalinization with intravenous NaHCO$_3$ (0.12–0.5 mEq/kg/hr osmotic diuresis with mannitol as a last resort).
G. Burn healing and management
   1. Stages of wound healing
      a. Inflammatory phase

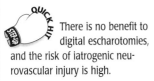

There is no benefit to digital escharotomies, and the risk of iatrogenic neurovascular injury is high.

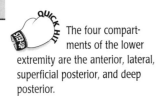

The four compartments of the lower extremity are the anterior, lateral, superficial posterior, and deep posterior.

FIGURE 2-5 Torso escharotomy can be useful to improve compliance and ventilation. Appropriate lines for torso escharotomy are depicted.

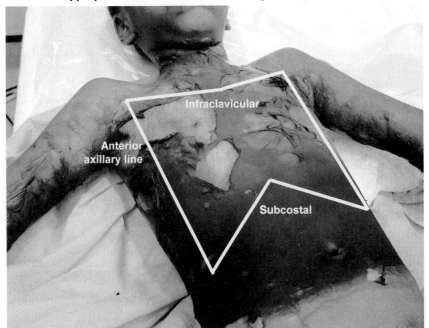

(Reprinted, with permission, from *Greenfield's Surgery*. 4th ed. Philadelphia: Lippincott Williams & Wilkins; 2006:251.)

(1) Begins immediately and lasts up to 7 to 10 days.
(2) Infiltration by neutrophils occurs up to 24 hours, followed by macrophage infiltration over the next 2 to 3 days, and completed by lymphocyte recruitment.
b. Proliferative phase
(1) Occurs from day 5 through 3 weeks postinjury.
(2) Begins with formation of a provisional matrix consisting of fibrin and fibronectin.
(3) Fibroblasts present by day 3, initiating collagen synthesis.
(4) Macrophages release growth factors inducing angiogenesis.
(5) Vitamin C is necessary for collagen cross-linking and stabilization via hydroxylation of proline and lysine.
c. Remodeling phase
(1) Collagen equilibrium is attained, beginning at approximately three weeks and lasting up to one year.
(2) Type I collagen predominates type III by a ratio of 4:1.
(3) Collagen remodeling occurs, and wound color changes from purple/pink to pale.
(4) Scarring occurs, in which collagen fibrils align longitudinally along lines of stress with less degree of order than normal skin.
(5) 70% of the strength of unwounded skin is achieved by 84 days.
2. Burn wound management
a. **Topical antimicrobials (Table 2-5)**

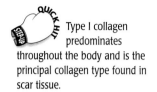

Type I collagen predominates throughout the body and is the principal collagen type found in scar tissue.

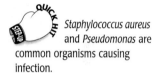

Staphylococcus aureus and *Pseudomonas* are common organisms causing infection.

TABLE 2-5 Topical Antimicrobial Agents for Burns			
Antimicrobial Agent	**Coverage**	**Advantages**	**Disadvantages**
Silver sulfadiazine (Silvadene)	Broad spectrum, especially *Pseudomonas*	Painless	Neutropenia. Does not penetrate eschar. Discolors skin from silver. Inhibits epithelialization.
Mafenide acetate (Sulfamylon)	Broad spectrum, including *Clostridium*	Excellent eschar penetration	Painful. Carbonic anhydrase inhibitor with secondary metabolic acidosis.
Silver nitrate	Broad spectrum	Excellent prophylaxis	Poor eschar penetration. Hyponatremia, hypochloremia. Methemoglobinemia. Stains skin.
Bacitracin	Gram-positive bacteria	Good for shallow facial burns	Expensive.
Mupirocin (Bactroban)	Gram-positive bacteria, especially *Staphylococcus*	Good coverage, methicillin-resistant *Staphylococcus aureus*	Expensive.
Neomycin	Broad spectrum	Painless	Nephrotoxic.
Polymyxin B	Gram-negative bacteria, including *Pseudomonas*	Painless	Nephrotoxic.
Nystatin	Fungus	Fungal coverage	Cannot be used with mafenide acetate.
Acticoat silver-impregnated dressing	Broad coverage	Good for shallow burns.	Nonadhesive, can slip.

b. Systemic antibiotics should be used for diagnosed infection only, which occurs in approximately 80% of patients with large burns.

c. Tetanus prophylaxis. Tetanus toxoid is given for all patients with burns greater than 10% TBSA. If no prior immunization has been given, or last booster was given more than 10 years prior, immunoglobulin should be administered.

3. Wound closure

a. All eschar or nonviable tissue should be excised as soon as possible, ideally within the first week and closed with an autograft.

b. Full-thickness grafts are not typically used in burn patients with large TBSA burns.

c. **Autograft**

(1) The skin graft harvested from the patient's own tissue.

(2) The patient's own tissue is the preferred coverage material if feasible, because of less risk of rejection and poor wound healing.

d. **Human allograft (cadaveric)**

(1) Grafts can be meshed, and applied to an excised wound bed.

(2) Graft vascularizes and engrafts, providing coverage for 2 to 4 weeks before rejection.

e. **Xenograft (porcine)**. This graft will not vascularize or engraft.

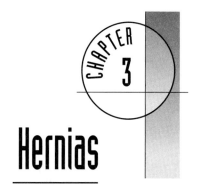

Hernias

Cynthia F. Graves, MD
Jessica Partin, MD

I. Abdominal Wall Hernias

A. Anterior abdominal wall
   1. Skeletal support includes the lowest ribs, pelvic brim, lumbar spine.
   2. Compresses and contains abdominal viscera, and contributes to support and movement of spine and pelvis.
   3. Lamination of the muscles and aponeurosis precludes evisceration; hernias most commonly form between laminations (where only peritoneum and fascia exist).
   4. Fascial layers
      a. Superficial layers include Camper; continuous inferiorly with the outer peritoneal and genital fascia, and which contains dartos fascia (scrotum). It can contain a significant amount of fat (panniculus adiposis).
         (1) Blood vessels include superficial epigastric and superficial circumflex iliac (both arise from femoral vessels).
         (2) Lymphatic drainage to inguinal lymph nodes inferior to inguinal ligament.
         (3) Superficial fascia fuses with fascia innominata, which invests the external abdominal oblique, binds to inguinal ligament, and continues onto the fascia lata. It includes Hesselbach triangle superiorly, and is the weakest part of the groin.
      b. Deep: Scarpa fascia is compressed fibrous components of superficial fascia, where it forms the fundiform ligament of the penis, continues onto the penis and scrotum, and fuses with the superficial perineal fascia.
   5. Skin is innervated in a dermatome pattern. Nerves divide into anterior and lateral cutaneous branches of T7 to T12, and L1 to L2 ventral rami.
      a. Fields overlap, so disruption is not normally noticed.
      b. Nerves course between the flat lateral muscles and pierce the rectus sheath.
B. Lateral abdominal wall
   1. Three muscles with large aponeurosis (tendon of insertion and forms rectus sheath)
   2. The linea alba is the midline decussation of the three aponeuroses.
   3. Aponeurosis is the fiber-containing portion of the muscle, present at insertion points.
   4. Muscles (Color Fig. 3-1)
      a. The external abdominal oblique (EAO) is the most superficial.
         (1) From the posterior lower eight ribs, it inserts on the anterior iliac crest, and interdigitates with the serratus and latissimus.
         (2) Mostly horizontal fibers above, oblique below. The lower oblique fibers fold onto themselves and form the inguinal ligament. The remainder inserts onto the linea alba and anterior rectus sheath.
         (3) Medial fibers divide into medial and lateral crus, and form the external or superficial inguinal ring (spermatic cord, and ilioinguinal and genitofemoral nerves, pass through).

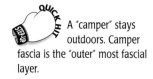

A "camper" stays outdoors. Camper fascia is the "outer" most fascial layer.

F I G U R E
3-1   **Muscles of the lateral anterior abdominal wall.**

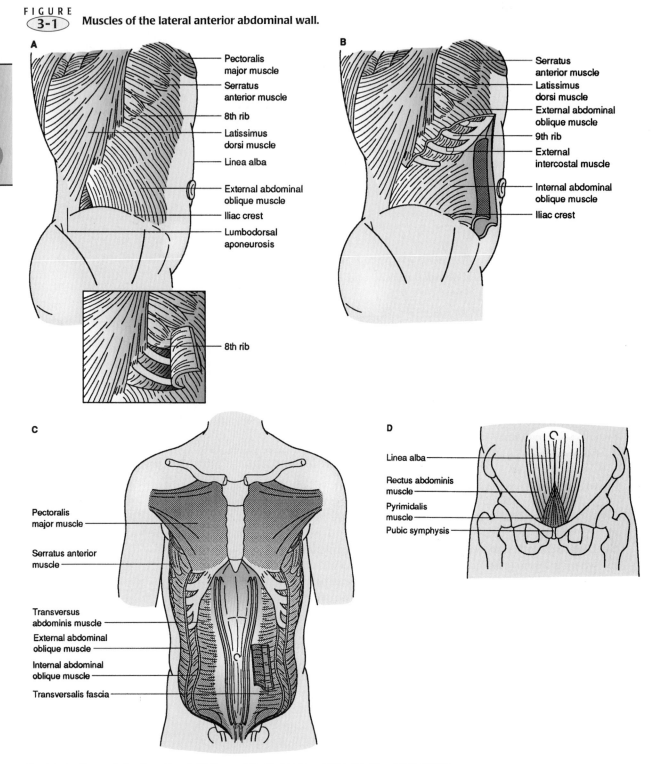

(Reprinted, with permission, from *Greenfield's Surgery: Scientific Principles and Practice,* 4th ed. Philadelphia: Lippincott Williams & Wilkins; 2006:1175.)

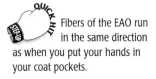 Fibers of the EAO run in the same direction as when you put your hands in your coat pockets.

(4) The inguinal ligament is from obliquely oriented anteroinferior aponeurotic fibers of EOA. Lateral attachment is the anterior superior iliac crest, medial attachment is the pubic tubercle.

b. The internal abdominal oblique (IAO) is the middle layer of the lateral abdominal muscles.

(1) It arises from iliac fascia along the crest, and fuses with the iliac ligament.

(2) Fibers run obliquely toward the lower "floating" ribs and fan out along iliac crest. Lower fibers in the male join transversus abdominis and form the cremaster muscle.

(3) The internal oblique aponeurosis is superior to the umbilicus, splits to envelop the rectus muscle, reforms in the midline and joins the linea alba. Inferior to the umbilicus, the fibers run anterior to (do not split) and join the rectus sheath before they contribute to the linea alba.

c. Transversus abdominis muscle

(1) It arises from the iliac crest and inguinal ligament and six costal ribs. Interdigitates with lateral diaphragmatic fibers, runs horizontally, and inserts on the crest and pecten of pubis.

(2) The aponeurosis is above the umbilicus, joins the posterior lamina of IAO, and forms a portion of posterior rectus sheath.

    (a) Below the umbilicus, the aponeurosis is a component of anterior rectus sheath.

    (b) Medial aponeurotic fibers insert on pecten pubis and form falx inguinalis.

    (c) True conjoined tendon forms only infrequently when joined by a portion of the IAO aponeurosis.

(3) Aponeurotic arch is the termination of aponeurosis of transversus abdominis. If the area beneath the arch is large, may predispose to direct inguinal hernia.

d. Rectus abdominis

(1) Central and anchoring muscle mass.

(2) Arises from the fifth to seventh costal cartilages, and inserts on pubic symphysis and tendinous intersections at xiphoid, umbilicus, and a point midway between.

(3) The principal blood supply are the superior and inferior epigastric arteries. Also, the anterior branches of intercostal are coming in laterally.

(4) Innervation: the seventh to twelfth intercostals nerves pierce the sheath laterally.

(5) The semilunar line is a slight depression in aponeurosis at lateral edge of muscle.

e. The pyramidalis is a small muscle which arises from the pubic symphysis, lies within the rectus sheath, and tapers to attach at the linea alba.

f. Rectus sheath

(1) The semilunar line is a lateral depression, and site of insertion of aponeurotic tendons of lateral abdominal muscles.

(2) Tendinous inscriptions divide each rectus muscle into three parts; the linea alba is midline confluence.

(3) The anterior sheath is superior to the umbilicus, EAO aponeurosis, and anterior lamina of IAO. No transversalis; inferior to the umbilicus is a composite of all layers.

(4) The posterior sheath is superior to the umbilicus, the posterior lamina of IAO aponeurosis and transversus aponeurosis. No EAO; inferior to umbilicus; fibers attenuate gradually and sheath is primarily transversalis fascia.

(5) Arcuate line (of Douglas) is a transfer of connective tissue away from the the posterior sheath.

g. Innervation of anterior abdominal wall

(1) Lower intercostal and upper lumbar (T7 to T12, L1, L2) nerves; pass between IAO and transversus abdominis and pierce the lateral sheath.

(2) EAO receives intercostal branches.

(3) Anterior ends of nerves form cutaneous branches.

(4) First lumbar nerve divides into ilioinguinal and iliohypogastric.

    (a) Ilioinguinal passes through external ring to run with the spermatic cord.

    (b) Iliohypogastric pierces EAO to innervate skin above the pubis.

(5) Genitofemoral nerve (L1, L2) innervates cremasteric muscles.

    h. Blood supply
      (1) Lateral muscles: primarily from lower three or four intercostals, deep circumflex iliac, lumbar arteries.
      (2) Rectus: superior epigastric (continuation of inferior mesenteric artery), inferior epigastric (off external iliacs); these anastomose near umbilicus; lower intercostals also contribute.

C. Posterolateral (lumbar) abdominal wall
    1. Borders of the lumbar abdominal wall include the twelfth rib (superior), iliac crest (inferior), erector spinae muscles (medial), and eight muscles in three layers.
    2. Most superficial layer is the EAO, and latissimus dorsi.
      a. The latissimus arises from the posterior iliac crest, sacral and lumbar spinous processes, and lumbodorsal fascia.
      b. The inferior (Petit) triangle is a space formed between the EAO and latissimus dorsi, and iliac crest.
    3. The middle layer consists of the erector spinae (significant portion), IAO, and serratus posterior inferior (thin, insignificant).
      a. The superior lumbar triangle (Grynfelt) is a more common hernia site than the inferior triangle.
      b. Borders are margin of the twelfth rib (superior), serratus posterior inferior and superior lumbocostal ligaments, upper border of IAB (inferiorly), and erector spinae (medially).
    4. The deep layer consists of the quadratus lumborum (posterior iliac crest to the twelfth rib) and psoas major (vertebrae T12-L5) to lesser trochanter, and transverse abdominis.

D. Clinical features of hernias
    1. All ages (neonate to elderly), with a 10% incidence in premature infants, and varies by gender.
      a. Inguinal hernias have 7:1 male-to-female ratio.
      b. Femoral hernias have 1.8:1 female predominance.
    2. Types of hernias
      a. Inguinal hernias: 80%
      b. Femoral hernias: 5%
      c. Incisional, umbilical, and epigastric hernias: 15%
    3. Duration of symptoms vary (chronic versus acute).
    4. Present with history of lump or swelling that occurs on straining.
    5. Complications include incarceration, obstruction, or strangulation. Annual risk ranges from 0.002 to 0.0037.
    6. In incarceration, the hernia is "trapped."
      a. Clinically, an irreducible hernia. The hernia sac contents may vary (omentum, ovary, nonobstructed bowel), and are irreducible due to adhesions.
      b. Must differentiate between a hydrocele and a hernia.
        (1) One can get one's examining fingers above a hydrocele, but not a hernia.
        (2) A hydrocele transilluminates, whereas a hernia does not.
      c. Treatment of incarcerated hernia is surgical.
    7. Strangulation
      a. Serious and life-threatening condition.
        (1) The contents of the hernia sac are ischemic and nonviable.
        (2) Pressure on the bowel trapped in the hernia sac produces venous congestion, which leads to edema of the bowel, and subsequent pressures so high that arterial inflow is obstructed and the bowel becomes gangrenous.
      b. Strangulated hernias present with tender irreducible masses as well as toxicity, dehydration, and fever.
        (1) The hernia is tense and very tender, and may have overlying skin changes (reddish or bluish tinge).
        (2) Bowel sounds are absent in the hernia.
        (3) Leukocytosis is common, and metabolic acidosis may be present.

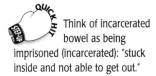

Think of incarcerated bowel as being imprisoned (incarcerated): "stuck inside and not able to get out."

c. Strangulated hernias should not be reduced.
 (1) Patients should receive nasogastric tube suction, fluid and electrolyte replacement, and antibiotics.
 (2) Surgery follows, with exposure of the hernia, opening of the sac, and resecting any gangrenous viscera, followed by hernia repair.
8. Intestinal obstruction
 a. Once the most common cause of obstruction, hernia is now the third most common cause (first is adhesions, second is cancer).
 b. Adequate exposure for physical examination is imperative, with evaluation of entire abdomen (nipples to knees) with proper lighting. An obstructed hernia is tense and irreducible; the abdomen is distended, and high-pitched bowel sounds are heard with frequent rushes.
 c. Plain x-ray shows classic dilated loops of bowel with air–fluid levels, and paucity of gas distal to obstruction. Bowel shadows may be apparent in region of the hernia. Computed tomography may be helpful if clinical diagnosis is uncertain.
 d. Patient is sedated in bed and placed in Trendelenburg position. The taxis maneuver (grasping hernia neck with one hand and applying intermittent pressure with other hand on distal neck of hernia) elongates the neck to allow contents to pass back into abdomen. Abort the attempt at reduction if unsuccessful after two or three tries, because reduction of gangrenous bowel or reduction en masse is possible.
 e. Reduction of hernia is followed by resuscitation, and urgent surgery via a direct approach over the hernia site.
 (1) Entire gastrointestinal (GI) tract is assessed for other causes of obstruction.
 (2) Viable bowel is reduced back into the abdomen. Nonviable bowel is resected with anastomosis prior to hernia repair.
9. Massive hernia
 a. Large portion of abdominal contents situated in hernia sac; usually chronic, hernia contents have lost their right of domain. Replacement of abdominal contents with fascial closure puts the patient at risk of abdominal compartment syndrome, skin edema, and cellulitis after closure.
 b. Pneumoperitoneum may help when returning contents to the abdominal cavity over 3 weeks prior to repair. A prosthesis is usually required because of the size of the defect.
10. Groin hernias (see Section II)
11. Periumbilical hernias
 a. Improper healing of umbilical scar, leaving a fascial defect covered by skin.
 b. Defect is commonly 1 to 2 cm in infants.
 (1) Majority heal spontaneously, and 80% close by 2 years of age.
 (2) Requires surgery if persistent.
 c. Onset is usually sudden with small defect in older patients. The underlying cause of increased intra-abdominal pressure must be found.
 d. Differential diagnosis is caput medusae, metastatic deposits of intra-abdominal tumor (via lymphatics in falciform ligament), umbilical granulomas, omphalomesenteric duct remnant cysts, and urachal cysts.
 e. Conservative management until age 2. Then repair depends on defect size (simple repair for most small defects via subumbilical semilunar incision; larger defects may require prosthesis in the preperitoneal space).
12. Epigastric hernias are a "painful nodule" in the upper midline.
 a. Occur through defect in linea alba.
 (1) Majority of patients lack normal triple decussation and have only a single decussation.
 (2) 20% are multiple.
 (3) Most contain only preperitoneal fat and are less than 1 cm.
 b. Incidence ranges from 1% to 5%, and are two to three times more common in men.

c. Repair by reducing preperitoneal fat and simple defect closure. This can become large enough to accommodate peritoneal sac if left untreated, and is prone to recur (10%).

d. In diastasis recti, the rectus muscles are widely separated, stretching the linea alba like a fin. This is easily reducible and rarely causes problems, but patients prefer repair for cosmetic reasons. Repair by removing strip of linea and reapproximating.

13. Incisional hernias
    a. Complications of prior surgeries can follow any type of surgery, regardless of incision.
    b. Midline and transverse incisions have highest incidence.
    c. Important causes include poor surgical technique, rough handling of tissue, rapidly degradable suture use, closure under tension, and infection.
    d. Patient factors associated with hernias include morbid obesity, cigarette smoking, pulmonary disease, and hypoalbuminemia.
    e. Repair depends on size.
       (1) Solitary and less than or equal to 3 cm. Primary closure with nonabsorbable suture.
       (2) Larger or multiple hernias need tension-free mesh repair. Use of a peritoneal flap or omentum reduces opportunity for erosion with fistula formation or adhesive bowel obstruction.
          (a) Infection is a major problem with prosthesis, with an incidence of about 5%.
          (b) Factors predisposing to infection.
             • Preexisting infection or ulceration of skin over hernia.
             • Obesity.
             • Incarcerated or obstructed bowel within hernia.
             • Bowel perforation at time of repair.
             • Seroma can become secondarily infected.
             • Prolonged use of suction drains.
    f. Factors leading to poor results in hernia repair.
       (1) Preexisting comorbidities.
       (2) Debilitation from cancer.
       (3) Morbid obesity.
       (4) Steroid use.
       (5) Chemotherapy.
       (6) Tension on repair.

14. Parastomal hernias
    a. Most common complication of stoma formation; more than 50% of patients followed for longer than 5 years may develop parastomal hernia.
    b. Lower rate for small bowel stomas than colon.
    c. Etiology is poor site selection or technical errors (e.g., placing stoma lateral to rectus sheath).
    d. Other contributing factors are obesity, malnutrition, advanced age, collagen abnormalities, postoperative sepsis, abdominal distention, constipation, obstructive uropathy, steroid use, and chronic lung disease.
    e. Life-threatening complications are few, and less than 20% of parastomal hernias require repair.
    f. Three general types of repair:
       (1) Fascial repair, which includes local exploration, primary closure of defect.
       (2) Stomal relocation, receiving better results than above. Indicated for skin excoriation and suboptimal construction. Mesh not recommended.
       (3) Prosthetic repair, where complications involve use of foreign body (initiating infection).
          (a) Exit of stoma must be isolated from surgical field.
          (b) May be repaired primarily via dissection to the fascia, and closure of defect with overlying buttress sutures.

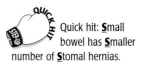
Quick hit: **S**mall bowel has **S**maller number of **S**tomal hernias.

(c) Prosthesis may be used to bridge defect (tension-free).

(d) Disadvantages of extraperitoneal approach include technical challenge of defining entire extent of hernia and seroma formation from undermining subcutaneous tissue.

(e) Intra-abdominal repair places prosthesis on peritoneal side of abdominal wall and intra-abdominal pressure helps fuse prosthesis to wall. Better adapted to laparoscopy.

15. Unusual hernias

a. Spigelian hernia, named for the Flemish anatomist Adriaan van der Spieghel, who described the semilunar line.

(1) Protrudes through weak area lateral to rectus sheath just below semilunar line.

(2) Usually intraperitoneal, rarely penetrating external oblique fascia (thus easily diagnosed at laparoscopy).

(a) May contain omentum, small or large bowel.

(b) Common complications are incarceration and strangulation.

(3) Usually presents as lower abdominal swelling lateral to rectus muscle. Pain and tenderness may be only signs.

(4) Often seen in elderly female patients, and are usually small (1 to 2 cm). Fewer than 800 cases are described in the literature.

(5) Operative treatment via transverse incision over mass, splitting external oblique. Triangular aponeurotic defect has its base near the lateral border of the rectus, and is closed by approximating the transversus and internal oblique muscles.

b. Lumbar hernia

(1) Lumbar area boundaries are twelfth rib superiorly and iliac crest inferiorly. There are three types:

(a) Superior lumbar hernia of Grynfelt: through space between latissimus dorsi, serratus posterior inferior, and internal oblique posterior border.

(b) Inferior lumbar hernia of Petit: through space between latissimus dorsi, iliac crest, and external oblique posterior border.

(c) Secondary lumbar hernia: results from trauma, surgery (renal), or infection. Seen historically in patients with paraspinal abscesses from spinal tuberculosis.

(2) Large hernias are repaired, and mesh is used. Fascia lata rotational flap may be used for inferior lumbar hernia.

c. Obturator hernia. Through obturator canal with obturator vessels and nerves.

(1) Associated with laxity of pelvic floor, and seen mostly in women.

(2) Intermittent pain is the main complaint. A mass can occasionally be palpated in upper medial thigh with hip flexed, abducted, and externally rotated, and sometimes on vaginal examination.

(3) Repair of defect is transperitoneal. Mesh is placed over defect after hernia is reduced.

d. Sciatic hernia is a very rare herniation of peritoneal sac through major or minor sciatic foramen.

(1) Presents as swelling on buttock, and may involve sciatic nerve or obstruction of ureter.

(2) Treatment is surgical, via transperitoneal or transgluteal approach, and usually requires mesh.

e. Littre hernia is a groin hernia containing a Meckel diverticulum.

(1) Sometimes also contains the appendix.

(2) If symptomatic or strangulated, the diverticulum must be resected at the time of hernia repair.

f. Perineal hernia is due to lax pelvic floor, and more common in older female patients.

(1) Anterior or posterior in location based on relation to transversus perinea muscle.
    (a) Anterior hernias present as labial or lateral vaginal wall swelling.
    (b) Posterior hernias occur between rectum and ischial tuberosity.
(2) Repaired via transperitoneal approach. Mesh required if opening is large.
g. Perivascular hernia occurs through defects between inguinal ligament and iliopubic bone.
    (1) Laugier hernia: through defect in lacunar ligament.
    (2) Cloquet hernia: through pectineal fascia.
    (3) Velpeau hernia: anterior to femoral vessels and behind the inguinal ligament.
    (4) Serafini hernia: posterior to femoral vessels.
    (5) Hesselbach hernia: lateral to femoral artery and anterior.
    (6) Partridge hernia: lateral to femoral artery and posterior.
h. Sliding hernia is a hernia in which a portion of the hernia sac is made up of an intra-abdominal organ (Fig. 3-2); most commonly sigmoid, bladder, cecum, or ovary.
i. Richter hernia is a hernia at any location in which the antimesenteric wall of the bowel is partially incarcerated (Fig. 3-3).

II. Groin Hernias

A. Anatomy of the inguinal region
  1. Anatomic connections in the groin
    a. External oblique becomes the inguinal ligament (Poupart ligament).
    b. Internal oblique becomes the cremasteric muscle.
    c. Processes vaginalis evagination of peritoneum that accompanies the testicle and gubernaculums. This forms the hernia sac in an indirect hernia.
    d. Gubernaculum attaches the testicle to the scrotum and is the anatomic equivalent of the round ligament in women.
  2. Spermatic cord contains testicular and cremasteric arteries, pampiniform venous plexus, vas deferens, and processus vaginalis (or hernia sac).

Richter hernias rarely obstruct because only partial segment of the bowel is compromised.

The ilioinguinal nerve runs along spermatic cord and must be identified and preserved during an open inguinal hernia repair.

F I G U R E
3-2 **Sliding hernia.**

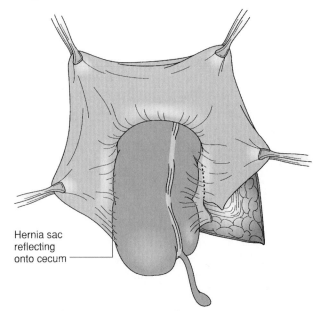

Hernia sac reflecting onto cecum

(Reprinted, with permission, from *Greenfield's Surgery: Scientific Principles and Practice,* 4th ed. Philadelphia: Lippincott Williams & Wilkins; 2006:1190.)

FIGURE
3-3   **Richter hernia.**

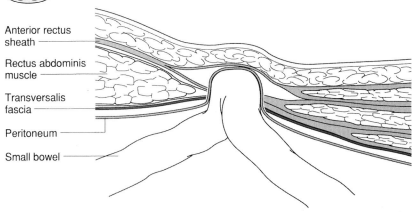

Anterior rectus
sheath

Rectus abdominis
muscle

Transversalis
fascia

Peritoneum

Small bowel

(Reprinted, with permission, from *Greenfield's Surgery: Scientific Principles and Practice,* 4th ed. Philadelphia: Lippincott Williams & Wilkins; 2006:1187.)

  3. Inguinal canal
     a. The communication between the internal and external inguinal rings.
     b. Contains spermatic cord in men and round ligament in women.
     c. Anatomic borders.
        (1) External oblique aponeurosis is the anterior wall.
        (2) Inguinal ligament is the inferior wall.
        (3) Conjoint tendon (internal oblique and transversus muscles) is the roof.
        (4) Transversalis fascia and aponeurosis are the floor.
  4. Hesselbach triangle (Color Fig. 3-4) is an area bounded by (a) inferior epigastric vessels, (b) inguinal ligament, and (c) lateral border of the rectus sheath.
  5. The femoral canal contains the femoral nerve, femoral artery, femoral vein, and lymphatics.

> **QUICK HIT** Contents of the femoral canal can be remembered from lateral to medial with the mnemonic NAVEL (**N**erve, **A**rtery, **V**ein, **E**mpty space [location of a femoral hernia], and **L**ymphatics).

FIGURE
3-4   **Hesselbach's triangle.**

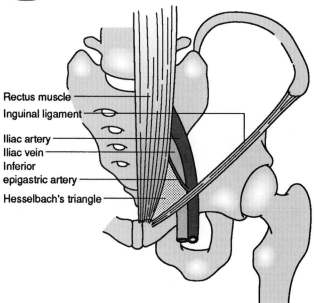

Rectus muscle
Inguinal ligament
Iliac artery
Iliac vein
Inferior
epigastric artery
Hesselbach's triangle

(Reprinted, with permission, from *Greenfield's Surgery: Scientific Principles and Practice,* 4th ed. Philadelphia: Lippincott Williams & Wilkins; 2006:1181.)

FIGURE
3-5   **Indirect inguinal hernia.**

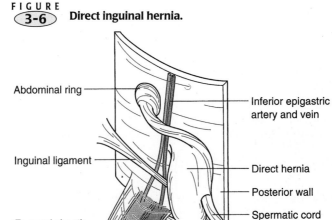

Abdominal ring

Inferior epigastric artery and vein

Indirect sac

Posterior wall

Inguinal ligament

Spermatic cord

Cooper's ligament

Femoral sheath

(Reprinted, with permission, from *The Essentials of Surgery*, 4th ed. Philadelphia: Lippincott Williams & Wilkins;2006:231.)

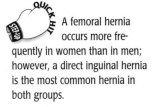 A femoral hernia occurs more frequently in women than in men; however, a direct inguinal hernia is the most common hernia in both groups.

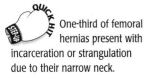 One-third of femoral hernias present with incarceration or strangulation due to their narrow neck.

B. Types of hernias
  1. Indirect inguinal hernia (Fig. 3-5)
     a. Hernia lateral to Hesselbach triangle, traveling through the inguinal canal.
     b. Etiology: caused by a patent processus vaginalis, occurring in 5% of men.
  2. Direct inguinal hernia (Fig. 3-6)
     a. Hernia within Hesselbach triangle, directly through abdominal wall without traveling through the inguinal ring.
     b. Etiology
        (1) Acquired defect occurring in 1% of men, increasing with age.
        (2) Most common hernia in men and women.
  3. Femoral hernia
     a. Hernia under inguinal ligament, medial to the femoral vessels.
     b. Frequently has a narrow neck, and is prone to incarceration or strangulation.
     c. More common in women than men.

FIGURE
3-6   **Direct inguinal hernia.**

Abdominal ring

Inferior epigastric artery and vein

Inguinal ligament

Direct hernia

Posterior wall

Spermatic cord

Cooper's ligament

Femoral sheath

(Reprinted, with permission, from *The Essentials of Surgery*, 4th ed. Philadelphia: Lippincott Williams & Wilkins;2006:230.)

4. Obturator hernia
   a. Hernia through the obturator canal along with the obturator vessels and nerves.
   b. More common in women, associated with a laxity of the pelvic floor.
   c. Mass may be felt in the upper medial thigh.
   d. Presents with pain referred to the thigh.
5. Cooper hernia is a hernia through the femoral canal, tracking into the scrotum or labia majus.
6. Pantaloon hernia is the presence of both direct and indirect inguinal hernias straddling the inferior epigastric vessels.
7. Littre hernia is a groin hernia containing a Meckel diverticulum.

C. Clinical presentation
1. Epidemiology
   a. Inguinal hernias are the most common abdominal hernia (80% of total)
   b. Femoral hernias account for 5%
2. Presentation
   a. Groin pain and swelling
   b. Often with sudden onset while lifting or straining
3. Physical examination
   a. Swelling with a cough impulse
   b. Indirect hernias can be controlled by applying pressure over the midinguinal point (midway between the anterior superior iliac spine and the pubic tubercle); this maneuver will not control a direct inguinal hernia.
   c. During examination, the index finger is used to invaginate the scrotum, thereby placing the finger through the external inguinal ring into the inguinal canal. An indirect hernia pushes against the fingertip, whereas a direct hernia pushes against the side of the finger.
   d. Femoral hernias present with a swelling below the inguinal ligament lateral to the pubic tubercle.
   e. Obturator hernia may have a swelling on the medial thigh.
4. Differential diagnosis: hydrocele, varicocele, testicular torsion, undescended or ectopic testis, femoral artery aneurysm, lipoma of the spermatic cord, inguinal lymphadenopathy, and psoas abscess.

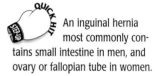

An inguinal hernia most commonly contains small intestine in men, and ovary or fallopian tube in women.

D. Repair of inguinal hernias
1. Goals of repair are to return contents into peritoneal cavity, ligation of hernia sac, and repair of defect to prevent recurrence.
2. Tissue repair includes the Bassini, Shouldice, and McVay procedures.
   a. These repairs use the patient's own tissue to reinforce the weakness in the posterior wall of the inguinal canal.
   b. These procedures may require a relaxing incision in the rectus sheath to allow approximation of conjoined tendon to inguinal ligament without tension.
   c. Tissue repair has higher incidence of recurrence than repair with prosthesis.
3. Mesh repair
   a. Reinforcement of the abdominal wall defect with prosthetic mesh.
   b. May be done with an open, preperitoneal, or laparoscopic approach.
   c. Recurrent and bilateral hernias are well suited to laparoscopic repair.
4. Truss
   a. External device that applies pressure over the hernia defect keeping the space obliterated.
   b. This may be used when surgery cannot be safely performed or when the patient refuses surgery. But this is not routinely recommended.

E. Special considerations
1. Incarceration. This is a hernia that cannot be reduced. Irreducibility is associated with adhesions to the hernia sac.
2. Intestinal obstruction. Hernia is the third most common cause of obstruction after adhesions and cancer, and presents with a tense, irreducible hernia.

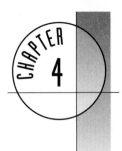

CHAPTER 4

Esophagus and Stomach

**Stephen McNatt, MD, James Longhi, DO
Irfan Rizvi, MD, Antony Joseph, MD**

ESOPHAGUS

I. Embryology
A. The esophagus develops from the foregut caudal to the pharynx.
B. The final relative length is established by the seventh gestational week.
C. Separation from the trachea is accomplished by the tracheoesophageal septum. Incomplete fusion of the tracheoesophageal folds to form the tracheoesophageal septum, or deviation of the septum, results in the formation of a tracheoesophageal fistula and esophageal atresia.
D. Initially, the epithelium proliferates and can completely obliterate the lumen of the esophagus. Recanalization then occurs, and restores the lumen of the esophagus by the end of eighth week of development.
E. The upper one-third of the esophagus contains striated muscle from the caudal pharyngeal arches.
F. The lower one-third of the esophagus contains smooth muscle derived from splanchnic mesenchyme.

II. Anatomy
A. Segments of the esophagus
  1. Cervical esophagus is approximately 5 cm in length.
    a. It begins below the cricopharyngeus muscle at the level of the sixth cervical vertebrae.
    b. It ends at approximately the first thoracic vertebrae.
  2. Thoracic esophagus is where the esophagus descends from the thoracic inlet to the level of the diaphragm in the posterior mediastinum, lying anterior to the vertebral column.
    a. In the upper chest, it passes behind the trachea and left main-stem bronchus.
    b. At the level of the aortic arch, the esophagus is posterior and to the right of the aorta.
    c. In the lower chest, at the level of the T8 to T10 vertebral bodies, the esophagus is anterior to the aorta.
  3. Abdominal esophagus is approximately 1 to 2 cm in length.
    a. It begins as the esophagus traverses the esophageal hiatus.
    b. It ends at the junction of the esophagus to the gastric cardia.
B. Neurovascular supply
  1. Arteries
    a. The inferior thyroid artery supplies the cervical esophagus.
    b. The bronchial arterial branches and small unnamed aortoesophageal arteries supply the thoracic esophagus.
    c. The left gastric and phrenic arteries supply the abdominal and lower thoracic esophagus.

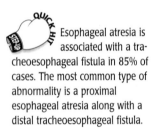

Esophageal atresia is associated with a tracheoesophageal fistula in 85% of cases. The most common type of abnormality is a proximal esophageal atresia along with a distal tracheoesophageal fistula.

2. Venous drainage parallels the segmental arterial supply, with the cervical esophagus draining to the internal jugular system, the thoracic esophagus draining to the azygous system, and the abdominal esophagus draining to the portal system.

3. Lymphatic drainage of the esophagus, in general, parallels the segmental arterial supply. The esophagus has an extensive network of submucosal lymphatics that interconnect.

   a. Cervical esophageal lymphatics drain to the internal jugular and tracheal nodes.

   b. Thoracic esophageal lymphatics drain to the tracheal nodes for the upper thoracic esophagus, and to the subcarinal and paraesophageal nodes for the lower thoracic esophagus.

   c. Abdominal esophageal lymphatics drain to the celiac and gastric cardiac nodes.

4. Innervation

   a. Recurrent laryngeal nerves innervate the cervical esophagus and the cricopharyngeal sphincter.

   b. Vagus nerves supply the thoracic esophagus and synapse with the post-ganglionic nerves in the myenteric plexus.

   c. Sympathetic innervation of the esophagus arises from the cervical, thoracic, and celiac ganglia.

C. Histology

1. Mucosa. The epithelium of the mucosal layer is composed of nonkeratinized stratified squamous cells. The junction of the stratified squamous epithelium of the esophagus and the columnar epithelium of the stomach is known as the Z-line.

2. Submucosa consists of blood vessels, nerves, lymphatics, and the ganglia of the Meissner plexus.

3. Muscularis consists of inner circular and outer longitudinal muscle layers with the myenteric plexus between.

   a. Skeletal muscle extends from the pharynx, and composes the cervical and portions of the upper thoracic esophagus.

   b. Smooth muscle predominates in the thoracic and abdominal esophagus.

4. Adventitia. No consistent serosa surrounds the esophagus.

III. **Physiology.** The esophageal body and two sphincters at either end of the esophagus regulate the passage of a food bolus from the hypopharynx to the stomach.

A. The upper esophageal sphincter (UES) is a 2- to 4.5-cm region of high pressure located between the cervical esophagus and the hypopharynx.

1. The UES, a striated muscle "sphincter," is closed at rest, and relaxes during deglutition to allow the passage of a food bolus into the upper esophagus.

2. Relaxation of the UES also occurs with belching, vomiting, and regurgitation.

3. Resting UES pressure varies from 60 to 200 mm Hg.

B. The lower esophageal sphincter (LES) is a 2- to 4-cm region of high pressure at the gastroesophageal junction that separates the lumen of the stomach from the lumen of the esophagus.

1. The LES, a smooth muscle "sphincter," is tonically contracted at rest with a pressure of 10 to 45 mm Hg.

2. The LES relaxes to a pressure equal to gastric pressure on deglutition, allowing passage of a food bolus into the stomach.

3. LES relaxation also occurs with belching, retching, vomiting, and with esophageal distention.

C. Esophageal body function is when the body of the esophagus acts to propel a food bolus from the hypopharynx to the stomach through peristaltic contractions.

1. Primary peristaltic contractions are occlusive waves of contraction that follow voluntary swallowing (deglutition).

QUICK HIT The left gastric or coronary vein drains the lower esophagus and is a source of esophageal varices in patients with portal hypertension.

QUICK HIT Because of the extensive submucosal lymphatic plexus of the esophagus, cancers of this organ can spread to lymph nodes located significant distances away from the primary tumor along the long axis of the esophagus.

QUICK HIT Afferent sensory pain fibers from the esophagus travel in the same pathways as pain fibers from the heart, which explains why heart pain and esophageal pain are at times indistinguishable.

ESOPHAGUS AND STOMACH

2. Secondary peristaltic contractions are waves of contraction that occur with esophageal distention from food or refluxed gastric contents.
3. Tertiary contractions are contractions that are not peristaltic, and their significance is a topic of debate.

IV. **Disorders of Esophageal Motility**
A. Achalasia (Greek for failure to relax). Achalasia is characterized by the failure of the smooth muscle segment of the esophagus. Aperistalsis is noted in the esophageal body along with incomplete relaxation of the LES.
1. Etiology
a. Idiopathic where the causes are unknown.
b. Chagasic, which is caused by Chagas disease, a parasitic infection of the esophageal musculature by *Trypanosoma cruzi*.
c. Pseudoachalasia, which is caused by extrinsic compression of the lower esophagus by masses (for example, tumors, hematoma, and enlarged lymph nodes).
2. Pathophysiology (idiopathic achalasia). Findings are consistent with the failure or loss of neurons of the myenteric plexus.
a. Loss of myenteric ganglia.
b. Neural fibrosis.
c. Mononuclear inflammatory cell infiltrate surrounding the myenteric plexus.
d. Variable degrees of hypertrophy of the musculature at or surrounding the LES.
3. Clinical presentation
a. Dysphagia occurs in 98% of patients with achalasia, and is defined as difficulty in the passage of solids or liquids from the mouth to the stomach. Patients often report that food sticks in their chest.
(1) They have equal difficulty in eating solids and drinking liquids.
(2) They tend to try and augment the passage of food by drinking liquids to wash down food. They may also attempt maneuvers such as extending the neck or back, or walking around during a meal to help food pass into the stomach.
b. Regurgitation occurs in 75% of patients, and is defined as the passive return of food to the mouth after eating.
(1) Often occurs with changes in position (for example, bending over or lying down).
(2) May lead to aspiration.
c. Chest pain occurs in 43% of those with achalasia.
(1) More common in patients with vigorous achalasia.
(2) Heartburn may occur as retained food and liquids in the distal esophagus ferment.
d. Weight loss occurs in up to 58% of patients.
e. Pulmonary complications include cough and chronic aspiration. They occur in 10% to 30% of those with achalasia.
4. Diagnostic criteria
a. Aperistalsis of the smooth muscle segment of the esophagus.
b. Incomplete relaxation of the LES with a residual pressure greater than 8 mm Hg.
5. Diagnostic tests
a. Barium swallow (Fig. 4-1). Classic features include esophageal dilatation, loss of peristalsis, delayed emptying with a column of barium retained within the esophagus, and symmetric narrowing of the distal esophagus (bird beaking appearance).
b. Esophagoscopy. Endoscopy is useful in evaluating the mucosa of the esophagus, and in excluding neoplasia as a cause of dysphagia. Typical findings on endoscopy include retained food and liquid within the esophagus, a dilated esophagus, and a closed or tight LES on passage of the endoscope into the stomach.

FIGURE
4-1   **Esophagogram demonstrating achalasia. The patient has a smooth, abrupt tapering of the distal esophagus and an air–fluid level proximally.**

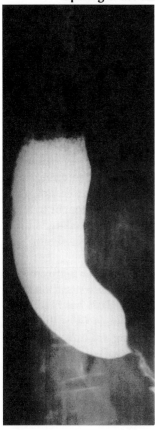

(Reprinted, with permission, from Castell, Richeter. *Esophagus,* 4th ed. Lippincott Williams & Wilkins; 362.)

    c. Esophageal manometry. **Manometry of the esophagus is the "gold standard" for diagnosing achalasia.** Classic findings include:
       (1) Aperistalsis of the smooth muscle segment of the esophagus, where the contractions are simultaneous and the contractile pressures are usually low.
       (2) Abnormal relaxation of the LES, where 70% to 80% have absent or incomplete LES relaxation. Residual LES pressures greater than 8 mm Hg with relaxation strongly suggests achalasia.
       (3) 60% of patients have hypertensive resting LES pressures.
  6. Treatment
    a. Medical therapy indicates smooth muscle relaxants.
       (1) Nitrates given sublingually can decrease LES pressure and offer short-term relief of dysphagic symptoms. However, they do not affect LES function, and efficacy decreases over time.
       (2) Calcium-channel blockers can decrease LES pressure and relieve dysphagic symptoms. However, as with nitrates, the function of the LES does not improve, side effects are common, and efficacy is short-lived.
    b. Botulinum toxin A
       (1) Botulinum toxin blocks release of acetylcholine at nerve receptors, and when injected into the LES, leads to relaxation of the LES by inhibiting the function of the unopposed neurons that cause LES contraction.
       (2) Three-fourths of patients respond to an initial injection.

(3) Response rates vary over time, with approximately half sustaining symptom recurrence after 6 months.

(4) Efficacy decreases over time with multiple treatments.

c. Pneumatic dilatation

(1) Pneumatic dilatation forcefully disrupts the hypertrophied muscle fibers of the LES leading to decreased LES pressure.

(2) Response rates typically decline over time.

(3) Complications include a 1% to 6% risk of esophageal perforation.

(4) Compared to botulinum toxin and medications, pneumatic dilatation is the most effective nonsurgical therapy.

d. Esophagogastric myotomy (Heller myotomy)

(1) The operation consists of splitting the longitudinal muscle fibers, and dividing the circular muscle fibers of the distal esophagus at the area of the LES. The myotomy is carried down onto the gastric cardia for 2 to 3 cm, and the operation can be performed through the chest or abdomen, and is most commonly done via laparoscopy.

(2) Myotomy lowers LES pressure more reliably than medication, botulinum toxin, or pneumatic dilatation.

(3) A fundoplication is usually performed along with the myotomy, because 30% to 40% of patients develop symptomatic gastroesophageal reflux disease (GERD).

e. Esophageal resection is used if there is significant esophageal dilatation and elongation, "sigmoid esophagus," or a previous failed myotomy.

B. Diffuse esophageal spasm (DES). DES is a problem of uncoordinated esophageal contractions of unknown etiology.

1. Clinical presentation indicates that the clinical features may be intermittent.

a. Chest pain commonly mimics angina, and it is not always associated with swallowing.

b. Dysphagia can occur after the swallowing of either solids or liquids, but it is not consistent with all swallows.

2. Diagnostic tests. Diagnosis is made by evaluation with esophageal manometry.

a. Required findings show 10% or more simultaneous contractions, with pressures greater than 30 mm Hg, which are accompanied by intermittent normal peristalsis.

b. Other findings include spontaneous contractions, contractions of long duration, elevated LES pressure, repetitive contractions, and multiple peaked contractions.

c. Barium swallow studies often show a "corkscrew" appearance of the esophagus (Fig. 4-2).

3. Treatment. Therapeutic strategies are geared toward relief of symptoms. However, current evidence does not support one predominant treatment.

a. Medications that relax smooth muscle: nitrates (nitroglycerin and isosorbide dinitrate), calcium-channel blockers (nifedipine and diltiazem), and antimuscarinics (dicyclomine).

b. Medications that affect the perception of visceral pain: trazodone and imipramine.

c. Botulinum toxin injection into the LES.

d. Long esophagogastric (Heller) myotomy with partial fundoplication.

V. Gastroesophageal Reflux Disease and Hiatal Hernia

A. Gastroesophageal reflux disease, or GERD, is the most common disease affecting the esophagus.

1. Pathophysiology and etiology of GERD are the result of the failure of the LES to be an effective barrier between the esophagus and the duodenogastric contents of the stomach. **Exposure of the esophagus to bile as well as gastric acid is injurious to the lining of the esophagus.** LES dysfunction,

FIGURE
4-2 **Esophagogram showing diffuse esophageal spasm.**

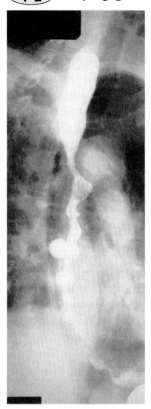

(Reprinted, with permission, from Castell, Richeter. *Esophagus*, 4th ed. Lippincott Williams & Wilkins; 372.)

impaired clearance of reflux from the esophagus, abnormal gastric emptying, and external factors contribute to the development of GERD.

  a. Normal LES function is paramount to prevent reflux. A hypocontractile LES and increased transient LES relaxations are the most common causes of GERD. Normal anatomic positioning of the LES is also important, as hiatal hernias potentiate GERD by disrupting the influence of the diaphragm on the function of the LES.

  b. Impaired esophageal motility leads to poor clearance of duodenogastric refluxate from the distal esophagus. Poor saliva production can also lead to GERD, because it normally neutralizes refluxed gastric acid.

  c. Delayed gastric emptying leads to an increase gastric pressure and a large volume of material available for reflux.

  d. External factors that can lead to GERD by decreasing LES pressure include dietary factors such as alcohol, fats, caffeine, smoking, medications, nitrates, and calcium-channel blockers. Also, hormones like progesterone. Obesity also worsens GERD by increasing abdominal pressure.

2. Clinical presentation

  a. Classic "esophageal" symptoms are heartburn (the most common symptom), regurgitation, and dysphagia. Dysphagia may result from a GERD-induced stricture of the distal esophagus, or from impaired esophageal motility.

  b. Atypical extraesophageal symptoms are coughing, hoarseness, noncardiac chest pain, and asthma. GERD is a cause of asthma in 45% to 65% of adult onset asthmatics.

3. Diagnostic tests. Various studies are used to evaluate esophageal anatomy and function, as well as to **provide objective evidence for the presence of GERD.**

  a. Barium esophagram is useful in delineating esophageal anatomy. Reflux of gastric content, strictures, ulcerations, and hiatal hernias may all be demonstrated with a barium swallow.

b. Esophagogastroduodenoscopy (EGD) is an essential study in the evaluation of those with GERD. EGD can provide objective evidence of GERD by identifying esophagitis, peptic strictures, esophageal ulcerations, or Barrett metaplasia within the esophagus. A majority of patients have normal findings on endoscopy (nonerosive esophageal reflux disease). EGD is also useful in evaluating the stomach and duodenum for other non-GERD (gastritis, peptic ulcer) causes of symptoms.

c. **Esophageal pH analysis is the "gold standard" for the diagnosis of GERD.** Findings of distal esophageal acid exposure to a pH less than 4 for more than 4.2% of a 24-hour period, or exposure of the proximal esophagus (20 cm above the LES) to a pH less than 4 for 1.3% of a 24-hour period are diagnostic for GERD.

d. Esophageal manometry is used to evaluate LES function and the peristaltic function of the esophageal body. It is also useful in eliminating achalasia as a cause of GERD symptoms.

4. Treatment. Therapy consists of controlling the exposure of the esophagus to duodenogastric reflux.

a. Medications are the mainstay of treatment. H_2-receptor antagonists are appropriate for patients with only occasional (once per week) GERD symptoms. Proton pump inhibitors (PPIs) are recommended for those with more frequent or daily symptoms. Both drugs dramatically reduce gastric acid production by the stomach. However, neither class of drug is efficacious against the reflux of bile.

b. Endoscopic therapy for GERD is in its infancy, with many techniques under investigation.

c. Surgery for GERD consists of constructing an esophagogastric fundoplication to augment the function of the LES, and to provide a barrier to duodenogastric reflux into the esophagus.

(1) Efficacy of surgical fundoplication is approximately 90%.

(2) Fundoplications can be total (Nissen 360-degree wrap of the fundus around the distal esophagus), or partial (Toupet 270-degree posterior wrap; Dor 180-degree anterior wrap). However, the Nissen total fundoplication is thought to be the best barrier to reflux.

(3) Most fundoplications are performed as laparoscopic procedures, but they may also be performed through laparotomy or thoracotomy.

(4) The presence of a hiatal hernia often requires surgery for control of GERD symptoms, because it signifies a distinct anatomic cause for GERD, which medications do not address.

5. Complications

a. Conditions that may develop include esophageal dysmotility, peptic stricture of the esophagus, erosive esophagitis, asthma, aspiration, recurrent pneumonia, and laryngitis.

b. Barrett esophagus (BE), which develops from a metaplastic process, is the end-stage manifestation of GERD. BE is defined as the replacement of the normal squamous epithelium of the esophagus with intestinal epithelium and stratified columnar epithelium, with the presence of goblet cells.

(1) **BE is a premalignant lesion that occurs in up to 7% to 10% of patients with GERD.**

(2) BE increases the risk of adenocarcinoma of the esophagus by 30 to 125.

(3) Those with BE should be followed with surveillance endoscopy.

(4) **The presence of high-grade dysplasia in BE is an indication for esophagectomy.**

B. Hiatal hernias are common, whereas paraesophageal hernias (PEHs) are relatively rare

1. Etiology. Hiatal hernias and PEHs are thought to arise as an acquired disorder of the diaphragm and the gastroesophageal junction due to chronic elevations in abdominal pressure, weakening of the musculature of the esophageal crura, and possibly shortening of the esophagus from chronic GERD.

> **QUICK HIT**
>
> Objective evidence for the diagnosis of GERD includes a positive 24-hour pH study, or the presence of erosive esophagitis, peptic stricture, or Barrett esophagus on endoscopy.

TABLE 4-1	**Types of Hiatal and Paraesophageal Hernias**			
Type	**Position of Gastroesophageal Junction**	**Hernia Contents**	**Volvulus**	**Spontaneous Reduction**
I—Sliding	Variable	Cardia, fundus	None	Common
II—True paraesophageal hernia	Intra-abdominal	Fundus, body	None or organoaxial	Uncommon
III—Mixed	Intrathoracic	Fundus, body	Organoaxial or mesoaxial	None
IV—Mixed + other organ	Intrathoracic	Fundus, body, other abdominal organ	Organoaxial or mesoaxial	None

2. Pathophysiology. There are four types of PEHs (Table 4-1).
3. Clinical presentation
   a. The majority of type I hiatal hernias are asymptomatic. However, they may predispose one to GERD and its symptomatology.
   b. Types II, III, and IV hiatal hernias and PEHs account for approximately 5% to 15% of all hiatal hernias. Common symptoms include substernal fullness, regurgitation, dysphagia, chest pain, and respiratory symptoms. GERD occurs infrequently with these types of PEHs.
   c. Uncommon complications of PEHs include anemia, secondary to ulcers in the herniated stomach, incarceration and strangulation of the herniated stomach, and perforation.
4. Diagnostic tests. Diagnostic studies are similar to those for the workup of GERD.
   a. Barium esophagram is useful to diagnose hiatal hernia and PEH. The volume of stomach herniated, position of the LES, and presence of mesoaxial (axis of rotation along the mesenteric attachment) or organoaxial (axis of rotation along the long axis of the stomach) volvulus can be determined.
   b. EGD is useful in the diagnosis of hiatal hernia and PEH, because the presence of ulceration, ischemia, and rotation of the stomach can be determined.
5. Treatment. Therapy of type I hiatal hernias is straightforward, whereas that of types II, III, and IV PEH is controversial.
   a. **Most type I hiatal hernias are asymptomatic and do not require therapy.** When symptomatic, therapy parallels that of GERD, with surgery consisting of an esophagogastric fundoplication with hiatal repair.
   b. The morbidity of surgery for patients with types II to IV PEH, who are advanced in age and have significant comorbidities, makes surgical therapy for asymptomatic patients controversial.
   c. Surgical therapy for types II to IV PEH entails reduction of the herniated stomach, resection of the hernia sac, repair of the diaphragmatic crura with mesh, and esophagogastric fundoplication.

VI. Esophageal Diverticula are rare. Classified by the region of the esophagus in which they occur.
   A. Hypopharyngeal, or Zenker diverticulum. This is a pulsion (false) diverticulum arising at the junction of the pharynx and the cervical esophagus, in the area known as Killian triangle, a relatively weak area in the posterior hypopharynx between the inferior pharyngeal constrictors superiorly and the cricopharyngeus muscle inferiorly (Fig. 4-3).
      1. Etiology. The cause of Zenker diverticulum is not completely understood. Two potential causes are increased hyopharyngeal pressure accompanied by poor UES opening, or cricopharyngeal incoordination.

FIGURE
4-3   **Triangle of Killian, an area of weakness that allows Zenker's diverticulum to develop.**

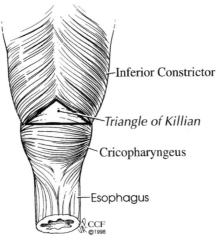

Inferior Constrictor

Triangle of Killian

Cricopharyngeus

Esophagus

CCF
©1998

(Reprinted, with permission, from Castell, Richeter. *Esophagus*, 4th ed. Lippincott Williams & Wilkins; 326.)

2. Clinical presentation. Patients with a Zenker diverticulum are usually advanced in age, and present with complaints of cervical dysphagia, regurgitation of food recently chewed, complaints of a "globus" sensation, and a left-sided neck mass. Aspiration and pneumonia are infrequent, and many small diverticula may be asymptomatic.

3. Diagnostic tests
   a. **Barium esophagram is the best test to identify the presence of a Zenker diverticulum. Diverticula almost always are demonstrated on the left side of the neck.**
   b. Esophagoscopy, in general, should be avoided because of its challenging nature, and for fear of the risk of perforation of the diverticulum. It is indicated only if an esophagram demonstrates findings consistent with neoplasia within the diverticulum, a rare finding.

4. Treatment involves surgery, as there is no effective medical therapy, with success rates ranging from 90% to 100%.
   a. Cricopharyngeal myotomy, with diverticulectomy or diverticulopexy, is classically performed through a left neck incision. The cricopharyngeus muscle is divided, and the diverticulum can either be resected or the fundus of the diverticulum can be sewn to the prevertebral fascia to facilitate its drainage.
   b. Endoscopic myotomy avoids an incision and shortens the hospitalization. An operating laryngoscope is used to expose the neck of the diverticulum, and a myotomy is performed using an endoscopic linear stapler. With this technique, the diverticulum becomes part of a common channel with the cervical esophagus.

B. Mid-esophageal diverticula may result from either traction or pulsion forces
   1. Traction (true) diverticula are formed when inflammatory or scar tissue adheres to the esophagus, pulling the wall away from its natural course.
   2. Pulsion diverticula arise in the mid-esophagus as result of esophageal motility disorders that lead to areas of high pressure and diverticular development, with the mucosa protruding through the esophageal wall.
   3. Clinical presentation. Many mid-esophageal diverticula are asymptomatic. Symptoms such as dysphagia and chest pain relate to an underlying motility disorder. Complications are rare.
   4. Diagnostic tests. Usually, diagnosis is made by a barium esophagram. However, flexible esophagoscopy may also be useful.
   5. Treatment. Most mid-esophageal diverticula are asymptomatic and do not require treatment. For those with symptoms and a mid-esophageal diverticulum, treatment consists of a myotomy and a diverticulectomy.

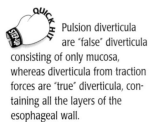

Pulsion diverticula are "false" diverticula consisting of only mucosa, whereas diverticula from traction forces are "true" diverticula, containing all the layers of the esophageal wall.

C. Epiphrenic diverticula are pulsion diverticula that are uncommon, and occur in the distal 4 to 10 cm of the thoracic esophagus.

1. Etiology. **Almost all epiphrenic diverticula are associated with an underlying motility disorder, such as achalasia or diffuse esophageal spasm.** Diverticula have also been seen above peptic strictures of the distal esophagus and in association with hiatal hernias.

2. Clinical presentation. Patients with epiphrenic diverticula may be asymptomatic, or may have symptoms related to the presence of an associated motility disorder. Dysphagia, regurgitation, and chest pain occur in variable degrees. Esophageal obstruction, perforation, and fistula formation tend to occur rarely.

3. Diagnostic tests
   a. A barium swallow is the best diagnostic test.
   b. Flexible esophagoscopy may be useful in identifying the presence of esophageal inflammation or stricture.
   c. Esophageal manometry is mandatory to rule out the presence of an underlying motility disorder.

4. Treatment. Therapy is directed at the associated motility disorder that is usually present, and any complication of the diverticulum.
   a. Small asymptomatic epiphrenic diverticula not associated with a motility disorder may be followed clinically.
   b. Complicated epiphrenic diverticula and those with an associated esophageal motility disorder usually require surgery.
      (1) Esophageal myotomy and diverticulectomy is the initial surgical option.
      (2) Nonsurgical options are reserved for patients with achalasia and an epiphrenic diverticulum. Both botulinum toxin injection and pneumatic balloon dilatation have been used.

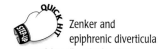
QUICK HIT Zenker and epiphrenic diverticula are pulsion diverticula whose cause is an underlying esophageal motility disorder. Primary therapy should be directed toward treating the motility disorder with treatment of the diverticula being a secondary concern.

VII. Tumors of the Esophagus

A. Benign tumors of the esophagus occur uncommonly and are usually asymptomatic.

1. Leiomyomas arise from the muscular layer of the esophagus, and are the most common benign esophageal tumor.
   a. Clinical presentation. Symptoms include dysphagia, chest pain, esophageal obstruction, and bleeding when the overlying mucosa becomes ulcerated.
   b. Diagnostic tests
      (1) On esophagram, these lesions appear as smooth filling defects in the esophageal lumen.
      (2) On endoscopy, the overlying mucosa appears normal, and the mass is firm and nodular.
      (3) On endoscopic ultrasound, the mass is hypoechoic, and confirms the layer of origin.
   c. Treatment. Therapy is through surgical resection by enucleation. Surgery is indicated for large (greater than 4 cm) tumors, lesions that are growing, or lesions that are symptomatic. Small asymptomatic lesions may be followed with interval imaging studies.

2. Fibrovascular polyps, or fibrolipomas originate from the mucosal layer and occur in the proximal cervical esophagus.
   a. Clinical presentation. Dysphagia, regurgitation, and respiratory problems are the main symptoms.
   b. Diagnostic tests. Diagnosis can be made with barium esophagram or endoscopic ultrasound.
   c. Treatment. Therapy is usually reserved for large or symptomatic polyps. Endoscopic resection or open resection via a cervical esophagotomy, or thoracic approach is the method of choice.

B. Malignant tumors. Adenocarcinoma and squamous cell carcinoma (SCC) are the two most common malignancies of the esophagus.

1. Adenocarcinoma of the esophagus is increasing in frequency, and is the most common malignant esophageal tumor in the United States.

a. Epidemiology. Adenocarcinoma commonly affects people in their sixth or seventh decade of life, men more than women (at a ratio of 5:1 to 7:1), and Caucasian men more than African-American men.

b. Etiology. Chronic GERD and Barrett esophagus are causative factors for esophageal adenocarcinoma.

c. Pathophysiology. Adenocarcinoma arises from the mucosal layer of the esophagus, and spreads by invasion through the wall of the esophagus to contiguous structures (aorta, trachea, and recurrent laryngeal nerve). Lymphatic metastasis occurs to periesophageal, cervical, mediastinal, and celiac lymph nodes. Distant metastasis is usually to the liver, lung, bone, adrenal gland, and brain.

2. Squamous cell carcinoma (SCC) is the most common malignant tumor of the esophagus worldwide.

a. Epidemiology. Like adenocarcinoma, SCC affects people in their sixth and seventh decades of life, and men more than women. However, SCC affects African-American men more than Caucasian men.

b. Etiology. Chronic exposure of the esophagus to noxious or caustic stimuli such as hot liquids or foods, lye, nitrosamines, alcohol, cigarette smoke, and previous radiation are thought to lead to dysplasia, and eventual neoplasia of the squamous-lined esophagus. Rare diseases such as tylosis, Plummer–Vinson syndrome, and achalasia are also linked to the development of SCC.

c. Pathophysiology. SCC arises from the squamous epithelium of the upper and mid-esophagus. Metastatic sites are similar to those of adenocarcinoma.

3. Clinical presentation. Symptoms are vague, and present late in the course of the disease process. They include dysphagia, weight loss, pain, and anemia due to ulceration of the tumor with resultant bleeding.

4. Diagnostic tests. Certain diagnostic tests are used to determine the stage of the tumor using the tumor-node-metastasis (TNM) system (Table 4-2 and Fig. 4-4).

TABLE 4-2 American Joint Committee on Cancer (AJCC) Staging of Esophageal Cancer

Primary Tumor (T Stage)	Description
Tis	Carcinoma *in situ;* tumor limited to the mucosa
T1	Tumor invades lamina propria or submucosa
T2	Tumor invades muscularis propria
T3	Tumor invades adventitia
T4	Tumor invades adjacent structures
Regional Lymph Nodes (N Stage)	
N0	No regional lymph node involvement
N1	Regional lymph node metastasis
Distant Metastasis (M Stage)	
M0	No distant metastasis
M1a	Upper thoracic esophagus metastatic to supraclavicular lymph nodes
	Lower thoracic esophagus metastatic to celiac lymph nodes
M1b	Upper thoracic esophagus metastatic to either distant lymph nodes or other distant sites
	Midthoracic esophagus metastatic to either distant lymph nodes or other distant sites
	Lower thoracic esophagus metastatic to either distant lymph nodes or other distant sites

FIGURE
4-4 **Esophageal Cancer Progression.**

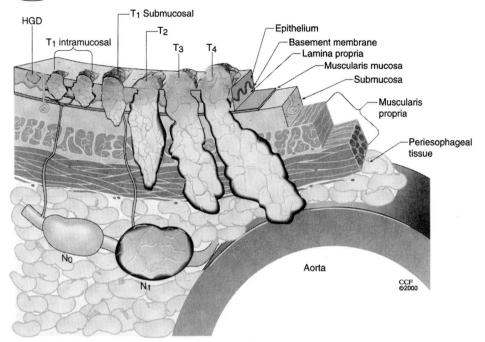

(Reprinted, with permission, from Castell, Richeter. *Esophagus*, 4th ed. Lippincott Williams & Wilkins; 292.)

a. Flexible esophagoscopy with biopsy for tissue diagnosis.
b. Barium esophagram is useful in the evaluation of obstructive symptoms, because it may identify a narrowing or stricture with the characteristic appearance of a tumor.
c. Endoscopic ultrasound is the most sensitive test to delineate the depth of tumor invasion through the esophageal wall ("T" of the TNM staging system). It may also identify enlarged periesophageal lymph nodes ("N" of TNM staging).
d. Computed tomography (CT) scanning is important for staging, because it is a sensitive method for detecting distant metastasis. It may also be useful for staging both the primary tumor and lymph nodes.
e. Fluroro-2-deoxy-D-glucose positron emission tomography (FDG PET) scanning may replace CT scans as the modality of choice for determining distant metastases.

5. Treatment. Therapy depends on the stage of the cancer (Table 4-3).
a. Surgical options consist of esophagectomy by a transhiatal (left cervical incision and laparotomy), or Ivor–Lewis (combined right thoracotomy and laparotomy) technique.
b. Chemotherapy and radiation therapy are used for unresectable cancers, and in combination with surgery in clinical trials of advanced stage cancers.
c. Endoscopic dilatation and stenting of the esophagus are palliative measures used for obstructing or near-obstructing tumors that are unresectable, or are receiving chemotherapy and radiation prior to resection.

VIII. Injury and Bleeding
A. Esophageal perforation is a highly lethal condition.
1. Etiology
a. **Iatrogenic perforation is now the cause of approximately 60%** of esophageal perforations, with esophagoscopy or endoscopic therapies being the most frequent antecedent interventions.
b. Other causes include spontaneous rupture or Boerhaave syndrome (postemetic rupture of the distal esophagus) 15%, foreign body ingestion 10% to 15%, trauma 10%, and tumor 1%.

QUICK HIT
Dysphagia is the most common symptom of esophageal cancer. Although not specific for the presence of cancer, dysphagia accompanied by weight loss should prompt evaluation with a barium esophagram and/or flexible esophagoscopy.

ESOPHAGUS AND STOMACH

TABLE 4-3	Treatment of Esophageal Cancer by Stage. American Joint Committee on Cancer (AJCC) Stage Grouping with Recommended Treatment Strategy and Predicted 5-Year Survival		
Stage	**TNM Designation**	**Recommended Treatment**	**5-Year Survival (%)**
0	Tis, N0, M0	Surgery	95
I	T1, N0, M0	Surgery	75
IIA	T2, N0, M0	Surgery	30
	T3, N0, M0		
IIB	T1, N1, M0	Surgery, or surgery with preoperative chemoradiation	20
	T2, N1, M0		
III	T3, N1, M0	T3 tumors: surgery, or surgery with preoperative chemoradiation	10–15
	T4, any N, M0	Palliation: chemotherapy, radiation therapy, stenting, or combination	
IVa	Any T, any N, M1a	Palliation: chemotherapy, radiation therapy, stenting, or combination	5
IVb	Any T, any N, M1b		1

TMN = tumor-node-metastasis.

2. Clinical presentation. This depends on the region of perforation and the length of time prior to discovery.
   a. Cervical esophageal perforations cause dysphagia, neck pain, and subcutaneous emphysema. Progression to mediastinitis and sepsis tends to be relatively slow.
   b. Intrathoracic perforations lead to direct mediastinal contamination and symptoms of chest pain, tachypnea, tachycardia, fever, and mediastinal emphysema. Progression to sepsis and shock is rapid.
   c. Intra-abdominal perforation of the esophagus causes peritonitis with symptoms of epigastric pain, back pain, tachypnea, tachycardia, and referred pain to the shoulders. Progression to sepsis is usually rapid.
3. Diagnostic tests. **A high index of suspicion and early diagnosis are key in effecting early therapy and decreasing mortality.** Diagnostic studies include:
   a. **Contrast esophagography is the study of choice to evaluate for esophageal perforation.** Barium, in general, is avoided because it may cause or worsen mediastinitis. If a water-soluble contrast swallow is negative and suspicion for perforation is high, the test should be repeated with barium, or a CT scan should be obtained.
   b. CT scanning of the chest and abdomen is useful for those who cannot undergo esophagography, or when the presentation is atypical.
   c. Flexible esophagoscopy is useful in the evaluation of perforations suspected from penetrating trauma and in cases of caustic ingestion.
4. Treatment. Management almost always involves surgery, with the type of surgery depending on the time course of the perforation.
   a. Initial therapy is directed toward volume resuscitation, and limiting mediastinal contamination with nasogastric decompression and intravenous antibiotics.
   b. Perforations of the cervical esophagus can be managed by drainage alone through a cervical incision, or by primary closure and drainage.
   c. Thoracic and abdominal esophageal perforations of less than 24 hours in duration are usually best managed by primary repair, buttressing of the repair with local vascularized tissue, and drainage of the chest and mediastinum.

d. Primary repair of perforations present for greater than 24 hours is usually not possible, because of the amount of contamination, inflammation, and necrosis. In this case, surgical therapy consists of either diversion of the esophagus above and below the perforation, with exclusion of the perforation from gastrointestinal secretions; or creation of a controlled fistula with T-tube drainage through the perforation along with wide drainage.

e. Esophagectomy is reserved for perforations due to cancer or untreatable obstructions.

f. Nonoperative therapy (antibiotics, cessation of oral intake, intravenous hydration) can be applied to a select group of patients with contained perforations secondary to instrumentation, who are clinically stable and have no signs of sepsis.

B. Bleeding from the esophagus can be a significant cause of upper gastrointestinal blood loss.

1. Esophagitis is usually secondary to GERD, and therapy is directed at decreasing gastric acid production and controlling duodenogastric reflux.

2. Esophageal varices are invariably due to portal hypertension, and carry a 20% to 30% mortality rate with each episode of bleeding.

a. Diagnosis is made by endoscopy.

b. Controlling hemorrhage can be accomplished via therapies directed at sites of hemorrhage, or by measures to decrease pressure in the portal system.

(1) Endoscopic control of bleeding consists of band ligation or sclerosis of individual varices. Efficacy is approximately 80%.

(2) Surgery is rarely performed for control of life-threatening variceal bleeding. Surgical options focus on decreasing portal venous pressures by shunting blood away from the portal circulation to the systemic circulation. Portocaval, mesocaval, and distal splenorenal shunts are examples of commonly used portosystemic shunts. Mortality for emergency shunting can be up to 20%.

(3) **Transjugular intrahepatic portosystemic shunting (TIPS) has largely replaced emergency surgical shunting** as the standard of therapy for bleeding, esophagogastric varices that are unresponsive to endoscopic and pharmacologic treatment.

(4) Temporary control of hemorrhage, when endoscopy, surgery, or TIPS are not available, can be accomplished by balloon tamponade of bleeding varices with the use of a Sengstaken–Blakemore tube. Definitive therapy is still needed, because bleeding recurs in 50% or more cases.

(5) Adjuncts to control hemorrhage include the use of the somatostatin analogue octreotide, which decreases bleeding by up to 50%, through splanchnic vasoconstriction.

3. Mallory–Weiss syndrome is massive upper gastrointestinal hemorrhage caused by a tear through the mucosa of the distal esophagus or gastroesophageal junction.

a. An acute increase in intra-abdominal pressure leading to the development of a pressure gradient across the gastroesophageal junction is thought to be the cause. Examples of causes are forceful retching or vomiting, paroxysms of coughing, blunt abdominal trauma, and straining during a bowel movement.

b. Hematemesis is the presenting symptom in 80% to 90%.

c. Upper endoscopy is diagnostic.

d. Bleeding stops spontaneously in greater than 90% of cases.

e. Endoscopic therapy is effective for those lesions that do not cease bleeding spontaneous. Endoscopic sclerotherapy, banding, hemoclipping, heater probe application, and multipolar electrocoagulation have all been used to control hemorrhage.

f. Surgery, which consists of suture ligation of the lesion, is rarely used to control bleeding.

STOMACH

I. Embryology

A. The stomach is derived from the embryonic foregut.

B. At the fifth gestational week, a caudal dilation of foregut becomes the future stomach.

C. Ventral mesentery becomes falciform ligament, lesser omentum, gastrohepatic, and hepatoduodenal mesenteries.

D. The celiac artery passes through the dorsal mesentery.

E. Dorsal mesentery forms the gastrocolic, gastrosplenic, and gastrophrenic ligaments.

F. In the six to seventh week of gestation, the left gastric wall (the greater curvature) growth is accelerated in comparison to the right gastric wall (the lesser curvature).

II. Anatomy

A. Anatomy of the stomach

  1. Gross anatomy

    a. The gastric cardia is the region just distal to the gastroesophageal junction.

    b. The gastric fundus is the region superior and to the left of the gastro-esophageal junction.

    c. The corpus (body) of the stomach encompasses the area between the fundus and antrum.

    d. The antrum compromises the distal stomach and ends at the pylorus.

  2. Vascularization

    a. Arterial supply

      (1) The left gastric artery is a branch of the celiac axis, and supplies a large portion of lesser curve and gastroesophageal junction.

      (2) The right gastric artery is a branch of the hepatic artery from the celiac axis, and supplies the distal lesser curve.

      (3) The short gastric and left gastroepiploic arteries are branches of the splenic artery, and supply the greater curvature and fundus.

      (4) The right gastroepiploic artery is a branch of the gastroduodenal artery, and supplies the distal greater curve of the stomach.

    b. Venous drainage of the stomach is to the portal system, and veins parallel the arterial supply.

  3. Innervation

    a. Parasympathetic/vagal

      (1) The vagal trunks pass through the esophageal hiatus along the anterior and posterior esophagus.

      (2) After the gastroesophageal junction, the anterior vagus nerve divides, and the hepatic branch sends fibers to the liver and gallbladder.

      (3) Distal to the hepatic branch, the anterior vagus becomes the nerve of Latarjet.

    b. Sympathetic

      (1) Sympathetic fibers originate from spinal nerve roots T5 to T10, and pass via gray rami communicantes to enter prevertebral ganglia.

      (2) Presynaptic fibers then follow the greater splanchnic nerves to the celiac plexus.

      (3) Postsynaptic fibers enter the stomach with the blood vessels.

  4. Lymphatic drainage

    a. The proximal stomach near the lesser curve initially drains lymph into the superior gastric lymph nodes that surround the left gastric artery.

    b. The distal stomach near the lesser curve drains into the suprapyloric nodes.

    c. The proximal greater curvature drains to the subpyloric and omental lymph nodes.

    d. Secondary drainage from these lymph node basins passes on to the celiac axis nodes.

QUICK HIT

Unequal growth at 6 to 7 weeks results in a rotation of the stomach placing the left vagal trunk anteriorly and the right vagal trunk posteriorly.

QUICK HIT

Although the distinction of the antrum from the corpus is not apparent externally, it is defined by a line from the incisura angularis on the lesser curve to a point on the greater curve one-fourth the distance from the pylorus to the gastroesophageal junction.

QUICK HIT

The stomach's blood supply is abundant, and it is protected from ischemia with its vast intramural and extramural collaterals. The viability of the stomach can be maintained by preserving only one primary vessel.

III. **Histology.** The gastric mucosa is composed of simple columnar epithelium with surface mucus cells.

  A. Oxyntic glands are located in fundus and body of stomach.

    1. Glands contain **parietal cells that are responsible for acid and intrinsic factor production.**

    2. They contain **chief cells that produce and secrete pepsinogen.**

    3. Mucus cells produce mucus and bicarbonate that protects the lining of the stomach from damage by luminal acid.

    4. Enterochromaffin-like cells (ECL) are also found in oxyntic glands. ECL cells produce histamine, and are a major regulator of gastric acid production.

  B. Antral glands are located in the distal stomach and pyloric channel.

    1. Most secrete mucus, but many also contain **G-cells that produce gastrin.**

    2. D-cells produce the inhibitory hormone somatostatin.

    3. Chief cells are also found in pyloric glands.

IV. **Physiology**

  A. Gastric peptides

    1. Gastrin

      a. Meals stimulate release of gastrin via intragastric breakdown of proteins.

      b. Gastric distension contributes to cholinergic activation, and subsequent gastrin release.

      c. Somatostatin decreases gastrin secretion.

      d. Acidification after a meal also inhibits gastrin release when luminal pH falls below 3.0.

    2. Somatostatin

      a. Inhibits acid secretion and gastrin release.

      b. A decreased intragastric pH stimulates its release, and an increased pH will inhibit its release.

    3. Ghrelin

      a. Ghrelin is produced by oxyntic glands.

      b. It is an orexigenic hormone, and it stimulates food intake.

    4. Pepsins are a group of proteolytic enzymes secreted by gastric chief cells.

      a. Cholinergic stimulus is the most important secretagogue.

      b. Pepsins initiate protein digestion.

    5. Intrinsic factor is secreted by parietal cells. It functions by binding cobalamin (vitamin B_{12}), which is subsequently absorbed in the ileum.

V. **Benign Disorders**

  A. Peptic ulcer disease (PUD)

    1. Epidemiology

      a. Peak incidence of PUD is in the sixth and seventh decades of life.

      b. PUD tends to occur in lower socioeconomic classes.

      c. Each year, approximately 300,000 to 500,000 new cases of PUD occur.

      d. Three to four million patients are self-medicating for symptoms of PUD, and 30,000 surgeries are performed annually for PUD.

    2. Etiology. Causes of ulceration are multifactorial. Predisposing conditions include:

      a. Age greater than 40

      b. Use of nonsteroidal anti-inflammatories

      c. Pepsin and acid secretion abnormalities

      d. Delayed gastric emptying

      e. Bile reflux

      f. Coexisting duodenal ulceration

      g. *Helicobacter pylori* infection

    3. Pathophysiology

      a. Mucosal *H. pylori* infection contributes to ulcer formation in most cases.

        (1) *H. pylori* is a helical gram-negative rod with flagella that resides beneath the mucus layer of stomach.

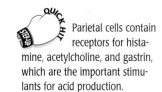

QUICK HIT Parietal cells contain receptors for histamine, acetylcholine, and gastrin, which are the important stimulants for acid production.

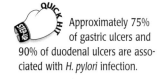

QUICK HIT A gastrectomy, either partial or total, that removes the oxyntic mucosa and parietal cell mass, or a gastric bypass, can lead to malabsorption of cobalamin and pernicious anemia.

QUICK HIT Approximately 75% of gastric ulcers and 90% of duodenal ulcers are associated with *H. pylori* infection.

TABLE 4-4	Types of Gastric Ulcers	
Type	**Location**	**Excessive Acid Secretion**
I	Lesser curve	No
II	Body and duodenum	Yes
III	Prepyloric	Yes
IV	Lesser curve near gastroesophageal junction	No
V	Anywhere, induced by nonsteroidal anti-inflammatory drug	No

(2) **Production of the enzyme urease allows *H. pylori* to survive in the acidic environment of the stomach.**
 b. There are five types of gastric ulcers (Table 4-4).
 c. The majority of ulcers are type I, and are not associated with excessive acid secretion.
 4. Clinical presentation
 a. PUD may occur intermittently, with relapsing episodes.
 b. Often, it is difficult to differentiate PUD from gastric carcinoma.
 c. Abdominal pain, bleeding, obstruction, and perforation are all symptoms of PUD.
 5. Diagnostic tests
 a. Physical examination often reveals epigastric abdominal pain. Peritoneal signs suggest perforation.
 b. Upright chest radiography is useful to evaluate for the presence of free intra-abdominal air, signaling perforation.
 c. Contrast radiography can diagnose PUD, but it may miss some malignant disease presenting as PUD.
 d. Flexible endoscopy is the mainstay in the diagnosis of PUD. Biopsy of all gastric ulcers is mandatory to rule out the presence of a gastric cancer presenting as PUD.
 e. Tests for *H. pylori* include serology, the urea breath test, and biopsy with rapid urease testing (CLO test), or histological analysis.
 6. Medical treatment
 a. Eradication of *H. pylori* with regimens that include a PPI in combination with two antibiotics for approximately 14 days
 b. Histamine receptor antagonists
 c. PPIs
 d. Sucralfate (an aluminum salt of sulfated sucrose that polymerizes, and becomes viscous to adhere to gastroduodenal mucosa and ulcer bed)
 e. Bismuth compounds for *H. pylori*
 7. Surgical treatment
 a. Indications include bleeding, perforation, obstruction, and intractable PUD resistant to medical therapy.
 b. Truncal vagotomy involves the division of vagal trunks at the esophageal hiatus, and is usually combined with a pyloroplasty (denervation results in delayed gastric emptying).
 c. Truncal vagotomy and antrectomy have the lowest recurrence rate for PUD.
 d. Proximal gastric vagotomy, where only the nerves to acid-secreting cells are divided. The hepatic and celiac branches, as well as fibers to the antrum and pylorus (nerves of Latarjet) are spared.
 e. Increasingly, treatments have involved addressing the acute problem, such as repairing a perforation, controlling the hemorrhage with nonresective surgical procedures, or managing the PUD medically with acid reduction and *H. pylori* eradication.

VI. Benign Tumors

A. Hyperplastic polyps
1. Polyps are usually small in size, and less than 2 cm in diameter.
2. Typically they arise in the setting of chronic atrophic gastritis.
3. Most resolve with *H. pylori* treatment.
4. Malignant transformation is unusual to rare, at 1% to 3%.
5. Endoscopic polypectomy is the treatment of choice.

B. Fundic gland polyps represent hyperplasia of normal fundic glands.
1. They can be associated with familial polyposis syndromes.
2. They harbor no malignant potential.

C. Adenomatous polyps
1. Polyps may be tubular, tubulovillous, or villous.
2. The risk of malignant transformation increases with larger size and villous type.
3. Gastric adenocarcinoma may be found in approximately 20% of cases.
4. Endoscopic polypectomy is effective if the entire polyp is removed, and no invasive carcinoma is found on review of the histologic specimen.
5. Surgical resection is indicated for sessile lesions greater than 2 cm, polyps with invasive tumors, or polyps causing symptoms such as bleeding or obstruction.

D. Ectopic pancreas or pancreatic rests
1. These occur during embryonic development while the dorsal and ventral fuse.
2. The majority of cases involve the stomach, duodenum, and jejunum.
3. Most patients are asymptomatic.
4. Symptoms include abdominal pain, discomfort, nausea, vomiting, and bleeding.
5. Diagnosis is made via endoscopy. Endoscopic ultrasound may helpful for location and biopsy.
6. Treatment of symptomatic lesions is by surgical resection.

VII. Other Gastric Lesions

A. Hypertrophic gastritis (Ménétrier disease) is an acquired rare premalignant disorder characterized by massive gastric folds involving the fundus and body.
1. On evaluation, the mucosa has a cobblestone appearance.
2. Histologic analysis reveals foveolar hyperplasia, and the absence of parietal cells.
3. Ménétrier disease is associated with protein loss from the stomach, excessive mucus production, and achlorhydria. It is linked with cytomegalovirus infection in children and *H. pylori* infection in adults.
4. Presenting symptoms are epigastric pain, weight loss, vomiting, and peripheral edema.
5. Medical treatment involves anticholinergics, acid suppression, octreotide, and *H. pylori* eradication.
6. Surgical treatment is via total gastrectomy, and is reserved for patients with massive protein loss despite adequate medical therapy, or for the development of dysplasia or carcinoma.

B. Dieulafoy gastric lesion
1. Pulsations of an abnormally large artery coursing through the submucosa lead to erosion of the mucosa, followed by exposure to gastric contents and hemorrhage. The vessel is usually located along the lesser curve within 6 cm of the gastroesophageal junction.
2. Peak incidence is in the fifth decade of life, and is more common in men.
3. Classic presentation is with sudden recurrent massive hematemesis and hypotension.
4. Endoscopy is used for diagnosis and treatment. Endoscopic control of hemorrhage may be therapeutic.
5. Treatment is surgical, and includes laparotomy, or laparoscopy with wedge resection that incorporates the offending vessel.

C. Gastric varices
1. These may occur with esophageal varices with portal hypertension, or secondary to sinistral hypertension from splenic vein thrombosis.
2. Treatment.
a. Splenectomy is the treatment of choice for splenic vein thrombosis.
b. Those associated with portal hypertension are treated in a similar manner as esophageal varices.
D. Gastric bezoars are collections of nondigestible substances within the lumen of the stomach.
1. Phytobezoars are made of cellulose from ingestion of vegetables.
a. Phytobezoars occur as a result of impaired gastric emptying.
b. Treatment is with enzymatic therapy with papain.
(1) Papain administration is followed by gastric lavage or endoscopic fragmentation.
(2) Failure of enzymatic digestion leads to surgical removal.
2. Trichobezoars are formed from the ingestion of hair.
a. Small lesions can be removed via endoscopy, lavage, or enzyme treatment.
b. Large casts require surgical removal.

VIII. Malignant Disease

A. Adenocarcinoma of the stomach
1. Epidemiology
a. The second most common cancer worldwide, adenocarcinoma of the stomach is the tenth most common cancer in the United States.
b. In the United States, it is more common in black males, and men are more likely to be affected than women, with a ratio of 2:1.
c. In Japan and in South America, incidence rates are higher.
d. The site of gastric cancers has shifted from the distal stomach to the more proximal gastric cardia.
2. Risk factors
a. Diet
(1) Salted meat or fish
(2) Nitrate consumption
(3) Complex carbohydrates
b. Medical
(1) *H. pylori* infection
(2) Adenomatous polyps
(3) Pernicious anemia
3. Clinical presentation
a. Symptoms include vague epigastric discomfort and indigestion.
b. More advanced disease is associated with anemia, anorexia, weight loss, fatigue, or vomiting.
B. Gastric lymphoma
1. Epidemiology
a. The stomach is the most common site for lymphoma in the gastrointestinal tract.
b. More than 50% of affected patients have anemia.
c. Peak incidence is in the sixth and seventh decades.
d. The disease is more common in males.
2. Mucosa-associated lymphoma tissue (MALT)
a. Gastric submucosa does not normally contain lymphoid tissue.
b. *H. pylori* infection is believed to be a causal factor for MALT.
c. Low-grade MALT resembles Peyer patches.
C. Gastrointestinal stromal tumors of the stomach
1. These account for 3% of gastric malignancies, because these tumors arise in the mesenchymal portion of the gastric wall.
2. Patients present at a mean age of 60, and after the sixth decade.

In the late stages of gastric adenocarcinoma, patients may have signs of advanced or metastatic disease. These include palpable masses or palpable lymph nodes.
- **Sister Mary Joseph nodes** are located in the periumbilical area.
- **Virchow nodes** are supraclavicular nodes.
- **Krukenberg tumor** is a palpable ovarian mass.
- **Blumer shelf** is peritoneal metastasis palpable by rectal examination.

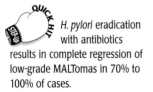

H. pylori eradication with antibiotics results in complete regression of low-grade MALTomas in 70% to 100% of cases.

3. Lesions with more than 5 to 10 mitoses per 10 high-powered fields demonstrate an increased potential for metastasis.
4. Metastasis occurs via the hematogenous route, and lymphatic involvement is rare.
5. Surgical resection is the treatment of choice.

D. Carcinoid
1. Gastric carcinoids are uncommon and account for only 3% to 5% of gastrointestinal carcinoids.
2. They appear as reddish-pink to yellow submucosal nodules.
3. Invasion is rare but occurs more frequently in tumors greater than 2 cm in size.
4. Curative resection is indicated in most cases.

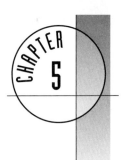
Small Bowel

Charles D. Goldman, MD
Jennifer Knight, MD

ANATOMY

I. Gross Anatomy

A. Duodenum: extends from the pylorus to the ligament of Treitz.

1. First portion (bulb): from pylorus to an area 5 cm distal, and most common site of peptic ulcers.

2. Second portion (descending): 10 cm in length with a retroperitoneal structure bounded by the pancreas medially and Gerota fascia posteriorly. The common bile duct is on the posterior-medial surface of the second portion, and the ampulla of Vater enters about 7 to 10 cm from the pylorus.

3. Third portion (transverse): almost completely retroperitoneal, except the distal segment.

   a. Attached to the uncinate process of the pancreas near L3.

   b. Directly posterior to the hepatic flexure of the colon, and passes between the superior mesenteric artery and aorta.

4. Fourth portion (ascending): short segment from the aorta to the ligament of Treitz.

B. Jejunum and ileum

1. No clear demarcation between the jejunum and ileum, and the total length ranges from 5 to 10 meters.

2. Jejunum has thicker mucosa than ileum, and more prominent plicae circulares (circular folds of the mucosa).

3. Ileal diameter decreases as it approaches the ileocecal valve.

   a. Ileocecal valve prevents reflux of fecal material from the colon into the small bowel, leading to different bacterial flora in the colon and terminal ileum.

   b. Distention of the terminal ileum causes relaxation of the ileocecal valve, and distention of the colon increases the tone.

II. Microscopic Anatomy. The small bowel wall has four distinct layers:

A. Mucosa: epithelial layer over lamina propria and muscularis mucosae (smooth muscle).

1. Cellular turnover of mucosa: 4 to 5 days.

2. Structural unit is villus, a finger-like projection of mucosa 0.5 to 1 mm high, covered in columnar epithelium.

   a. Contains a central lymphatic (lacteal), a small artery and vein, and capillary network.

   b. Columnar epithelial cells make up 90% of cell mass of the villus.

      (1) Apices of cells have microvilli—creating the brush border and increasing absorptive surface area.

      (2) Surface covered with glycocalyx—proteins and glycoproteins.

      (3) Maintenance of brush border is essential for absorption.

      (4) Tight junctions between cells—paracellular route with selective pores for ions and water versus transmembrane transport.

QUICK HIT

The gastroduodenal artery runs vertically behind the central portion of the bulb, and the common bile duct abuts the distal portion. The latter can be injured in attempts to ligate posterior bleeding ulcers.

SMALL BOWEL

TABLE 5-1 Endocrine Function of the Small Bowel

Enterohormone	Site of Production	Stimulus to Secretion	Actions
Cholecystokinin (CCK)	Jejunum	Fats, protein in lumen	Increases pancreatic enzyme output, GB contraction; trophic to pancreas and SB mucosa
Enteroglucagon	Ileum	Unknown	Decreases SB motility
Ghrelin	Uncertain	Unknown	Stimulates appetite, increases growth hormone release
Gastric inhibitory peptide (GIP)	Duodenum, jejunum	Fats, glucose	Potentiates insulin release from pancreas, decreases gastric secretion
Motilin	Jejunum	Unknown	Regulates baseline SB motility
Neurotensin	Ileum	Fats	Increases SB motility and pancreatic secretions, decreases gastric secretion, trophic to SB mucosa
Peptide YY	Terminal ileum, colon	Fats	Decreases motility and pan-SB secretions
Secretin	Duodenum, proximal jejunum	Acidification duodenum	Increases water and bicarbonate output from pancreas
Somatostatin	Stomach, entire small bowel, pancreas	Unknown	Inhibits all gastric, pancreatic, and enterohormone secretion; decreases gastric emptying and SB motility
Vasoactive intestinal peptide (VIP)	Small bowel	Unknown	Splanchnic vasodilatation; increases SB motility, pancreatic and intestinal secretion; decreases gastric acid output

GB, gallbladder; SB, small bowel.

3. Crypts of Lieberkühn. Contains anchored stem cells of four types:
   a. Absorptive enterocyte: migrates up to the villus tip in 3 to 7 days, and sheds shortly after it undergoes apoptosis.
   b. Goblet cell: mucus-secreting cell, which also migrates up the villus.
   c. Enteroendocrine cell; anchored in crypt, and produces enterohormones (including neurotensin, glucagons, motilin, and cholecystokinin). See Table 5-1.
   d. Paneth cell: remains in crypt, and is concentrate lysosomal host defense. Has 4-week lifespan.
B. Submucosa
   1. Dense fibroelastic connective tissue with rich blood supply, lymphatic drainage, and Meissner plexus.
   2. Strongest layer of the small bowel.
   3. Duodenal Brunner glands secrete protective mucus and bicarbonate.
   4. Ileal Peyer patches are collections of lymphoid follicles whose numbers diminish with age.
C. Muscularis: inner circular and outer longitudinal, between which resides the myenteric nervous plexus.
D. Serosa
   1. Thin layer of mesothelial cells over loose connective tissue constitutes visceral peritoneum.
   2. Heals by implantation of free-floating mesothelial cells, not by side-to-side reepithelialization (e.g., skin).

QUICK HIT The rapid turnover of the mucosal cells in the small bowel is a mixed blessing. It makes malignancy uncommon, but it also makes the mucosal lining acutely sensitive to degradation by infection, drug effects, or exposure to "allergens" such as gluten, as in celiac disease.

III. Vascular Anatomy

A. Duodenal bulb: arterial inflow from hepatic artery and gastroduodenal artery.

B. Second and third portion of duodenum: dual arterial supply from celiac via gastroduodenal artery (superior pancreaticoduodenal arteries), and from superior mesenteric (inferior pancreaticoduodenal arteries).

C. Fourth portion of duodenum distal: superior mesenteric artery branches.

D. Vasa recta are the most peripheral arterial branches of the superior mesenteric artery.
   1. Bifurcate as they reach the intestinal wall.
   2. Jejunal vasa recta are long and straight.
   3. Ileal ones are short, with extensive arborization.

E. Venous and lymphatic drainage parallels arterial anatomy.

IV. Innervation

A. Intrinsic nervous system consists of cell bodies in muscular wall.
   1. Mediates reflex activity independent of central nervous system control.
   2. Two major plexuses:
      a. Myenteric (Auerbach) controls motility and lies between the two muscle layers.
      b. Submucosal (Meissner) primarily is concerned with secretion and absorption.

B. Extrinsic control via vagus and splanchnic nerves
   1. Parasympathetic
      a. Pass through celiac and superior mesenteric ganglia.
      b. Postganglionic cell bodies in the enteric ganglia.
      c. Efferent fibers increase peristaltic activity and secretions.
      d. Afferents role uncertain, perhaps sensory.
      e. Mediates gastrocecal reflex, leading to discharge of ileum into cecum when there is food in the stomach.
   2. Sympathetic
      a. Efferent fibers travel in the splanchnic nerves, synapse with vagal fibers in the superior mesenteric ganglia, and inhibit motility and secretion.
      b. Afferent fibers transmit distension as pain.

PHYSIOLOGY

I. Motility

A. Basic electrical rhythm originates in the duodenal pacemaker.

B. Baseline rhythmic fluctuations from slow wave activity of smooth muscle.
   1. 11 to 13 times/minute in duodenum.
   2. 8 to 10 times/minute in ileum.

C. After a meal, two activity patterns ensue:
   1. Segmentation: circular muscle contraction divides bowel into segments, churning and circulating chyme to increase local mucosal contact.
   2. Peristalsis: wave-like propagation of contraction and relaxation propels chyme rapidly over larger surface area.

D. Mean transit time in small bowel is 221 ± 49 minutes.
   1. Meal composition affects transit time.
   2. Ileal transit time prolonged to aid absorption of bile salts and fat.

E. Fasting leads to cyclic pattern of migrating motor complexes (housekeeping motor activity).
   1. Starts proximal small bowel, and propagates to the terminal ileum with cycles every 90 to 120 minutes.
   2. Propels sloughed enterocytes, undigested food particles, and mucus into the colon.

3. Control is from the enteric nervous system, and enterohormone release from pancreas and elsewhere.
    a. In periods of stress, central and autonomic control may override.
    b. Cholecystokinin (CCK), gastrin, and motilin increase motility.
    c. Peptide YY and enteroglucagon decrease motility.

II. Digestion and Absorption

A. Water and electrolytes
   1. 8 to 10 L of fluid is presented to small bowel daily, the largest volume being from gastric secretion.
   2. 80% of water is absorbed in the small bowel, generally passively, via paracellular (proximal small bowel) or transcellular (distal small bowel and colon) routes.
   3. Sodium and chloride are absorbed either neutrally or by active transport. Sodium cotransporters aid in the absorption of glucose, amino acids, di- and tripeptides, and bile salts. Electroneutral absorption trades NaCl for H^+ and HCO_3^-.
   4. 85% of ingested K^+ is passively absorbed in the small bowel.

B. Carbohydrates
   1. Starch digestion starts with salivary amylase, and is completed by pancreatic amylase in the distal jejunum.
   2. Brush border enzymes cleave disaccharides (sucrose and lactose) to monosaccharides throughout the jejunum.
   3. Only monosaccharides (glucose, galactose, fructose) are absorbed by sodium-linked facilitated diffusion.

C. Protein
   1. Digestion initiated in the stomach by pepsin.
   2. Most proteolysis occurs in the small bowel, mediated by pancreatic proteases and peptidases (trypsin, chymotrypsin, elastase, carboxypeptidase A and B).
   3. Pancreas secretes inactive precursors, activated in duodenum by enterokinase in brush border.
   4. Jejunal enterocytes absorb dipeptides and tripeptides as well as single amino acids.

D. Lipids
   1. Entry of fat into the small bowel stimulates release of CCK from the duodenal mucosa, which in turn causes elaboration of lipase and cholesterol esterase from the pancreas.
   2. Fat products combine with bile salts to form water-soluble micelles, which also complex with fat-soluble vitamins.
   3. Micelles diffuse into terminal ileal cells to Golgi body, are packaged as chylomicrons, and then exit enterocyte by exocytosis into lymphatics.

E. Bile acids
   1. Enterohepatic circulation recovers 95% of secreted bile salts.
   2. A minor amount of reabsorption is passive throughout the small bowel. It is most active and sodium-dependent in the terminal ileum.
   3. Loss of terminal ileal function by resection or Crohn disease leads to increased cholelithiasis or bile acid diarrhea due to excess amount bile salts present in the colon.

F. Vitamins and minerals
   1. Fat-soluble vitamins (A, D, E, and K) are absorbed in micelles in the ileum.
   2. Water-soluble vitamins (B and C) are absorbed in the jejunum and ileum.
   3. Vitamin B_{12} absorption in terminal ileum requires intrinsic factor from gastric parietal cells.
   4. Calcium: the stomach solubilizes nonionic calcium salts.
       a. With low calcium intake, ionized calcium is actively absorbed in the duodenum.
       b. With normal or high calcium intake, ionized calcium is absorbed passively throughout the small bowel.

QUICK HIT Although bowel motility is a complex interaction of intrinsic myenteric activity, autonomic innervation and influences of enterohormones, it appears that the intrinsic activity is the most critical in almost all circumstances.

QUICK HIT Fat absorption is the most complex of the activities of the small bowel. Abnormalities present as either vitamin deficiencies (for example, coagulopathy from inability to absorb vitamin K or bone loss from vitamin D) or diarrhea.

SMALL BOWEL

    5. Magnesium: uptake is not calcium linked, and is marginal in all segments of the bowel.
    6. Iron
      a. Need gastric-secreted transfer factor
      b. Taken up in duodenum and proximal jejunum

IMMUNE FUNCTION

  I. Physical Defenses. These keep bacterial counts low in the upper gastrointestinal tract.
    A. Most important factor: acidification of the stomach
    B. Other factors that enhance host defense: mucin production, active peristalsis, rapid turnover of mucosal cells, and tight junctions between cells

  II. Gut-Associated Lymphoid Tissue
    A. Aggregated: lymph follicles, Peyer patches
    B. Nonaggregated

CROHN DISEASE

  I. Epidemiology
    A. Incidence: 4 cases per 100,000 per year
    B. Prevalence: 40 to 160 cases per 100,000 persons
    C. More common in North America and Europe
      1. Slightly more common in women
      2. Age of onset has bimodal peak: one peak at 15 to 25 years and another at 55 to 65 years
      3. In the United States, more common among whites, and three to four times more common among ethnic Jews. More common in persons of higher socioeconomic status

  II. Pathogenesis. Many theories have been advanced, but none have been validated. An altered immune response may be involved, although no specific defect has been identified.

  III. Pathology
    A. Features of Crohn disease are present anywhere from the mouth to the anus. The most common location is ileocolic (60%).
    B. The disease tends to be discontinuous and segmental.
    C. Transmural lymphocytic inflammation with noncaseating granulomata is the classic pathology in the bowel. The gross appearance of involved bowel is thickened mesentery with enlarged friable lymph nodes and "fat wrapping" of bowel.

  IV. Clinical Presentation
    A. Extraintestinal manifestations of Crohn disease may antedate the onset of the intestinal changes by months to years.
      1. One-third of patients demonstrate perianal fistulae.
      2. Other findings include oral aphthous ulceration, rashes such as erythema nodosum and pyoderma gangrenosum, uveitis, polyarthralgias or monoarthralgias, and sclerosing cholangitis.
    B. Symptoms of Crohn disease generally relate to bowel stricturing. Characteristic complaints include bloating, abdominal pain, abdominal distention, and post-obstructive diarrhea.
      1. Active disease or multiple strictures can result in a "failure to thrive" catabolic state.
      2. Diarrhea may indicate fistula of the proximal bowel to colon.

> **QUICK HIT**
> Crohn disease, which has a bimodal peak, should always be considered in the differential diagnosis of new-onset gastrointestinal obstructive symptoms in the late middle-aged patient.

> **QUICK HIT**
> Although ulcerative colitis has a more consistent association with sclerosing cholangitis, there remains a notable risk of the same change in patients with Crohn disease.

C. Bowel perforation and clinically evident bleeding are not frequently seen.

D. Other symptoms may result from fistulae to pelvic organs, such as bladder, or to skin, or retroperitoneal fibrosis causing ureteral obstruction.

E. Severe involvement of the terminal ileum leads to gallstone formation, and macrocytic anemia due to loss absorption of bile salts and vitamin B_{12}.

V. Diagnosis

A. Standard barium small bowel follow-through (or enteroclysis) is very helpful. It shows mucosal ulceration and nodularity, wall thickening, strictures, and fistulae.

B. Colonoscopy is useful in colonic Crohn disease, and intubation of the terminal ileum may confirm ileocolic disease.

C. Computed tomography (CT) scanning is not as specific as small bowel follow-through, but may better demonstrate complications of the disease (for example, obstruction, abscesses, or fistulae).

VI. Medical Treatment

A. Antibiotics, generally metronidazole, are of little value except in anorectal disease.

B. Mildly symptomatic disease should be treated with 5-aminosalicylic acid, especially ileocolic and colonic variants.

C. Moderately active disease mandates use of immunosuppressives.
   1. First-line therapy is corticosteroids, which are weaned quickly, if possible, to avoid the significant adverse effects of steroid administration.
   2. Steroid-resistant patients are offered azidothymidine or 6-mercaptopurine.
      a. Suppress helper T-cell and natural killer cell activity.
      b. Cause myelosuppression, hepatotoxicity, and pancreatitis.

D. Failure of immunosuppressive therapy may require a short course of an anti-tumor necrosis factor agent (infliximab).
   1. Chimeric human:mouse monoclonal antibody.
   2. Primary indication for use is fistula healing.
   3. Long-term use is not advisable, because of concerns about induction of non-Hodgkin lymphoma.
      a. Medical management should be continued for only as long as the patient with Crohn disease is symptomatic.
      b. There is no evidence for the prophylactic use of immunosuppressives to prevent recurrence of disease.

VII. Surgical Treatment

A. General principles
   1. Up to 90% of patients with Crohn disease eventually need surgery.
   2. Crohn disease is the second leading cause of surgically induced short bowel syndrome in adults, and **preserving bowel length is critical in surgery for Crohn disease.**
   3. Guidelines
      a. Do not look for normal bowel to use for anastomoses. Use thickened or fat-wrapped bowel, as long as it can be safely sutured or stapled.
      b. Do not use frozen sections to look for uninvolved margins. You will only waste useable bowel.
      c. Leave the enlarged nodes alone unless you think you are dealing with a Crohn disease-associated cancer. Resection of the mesentery causes devascularization of uninvolved bowel and further loss of bowel length.
      d. Avoid bypass of involved segments, because this leaves active disease in place, causing symptoms and extraintestinal manifestations to continue.
   4. Laparoscopic approaches to Crohn disease have been shown to be safe and effective, especially at the primary operation.
   5. Long side-to-side anastomoses are favored over end-to-end.

B. Indications for surgery
   1. Absolute indications include perforation, hemorrhage, suspicion of cancer, and nonresolving bowel obstruction.
   2. Relative indications are symptomatic fistula (for example, enterovesical fistula with recurrent infections), abscess, and "failure to thrive."
   3. Resecting the intestinal disease has little impact on most of the extraintestinal manifestations of Crohn disease, and therefore, resection should not be pursued for this reason.
C. Operative strategy in Crohn disease
   1. To save bowel length in small bowel disease, strictureplasty is favored over resection unless the strictures are all located in a short segment of bowel.
      a. Strictures less than 5 cm are best dealt with by the Heineke–Mikulicz approach of converting a longitudinal enterotomy to a transverse closure.
      b. Strictures up to 10 cm may require a Finney procedure.
      c. Longer strictures can be opened with a sliding type isoperistaltic strictureplasty.
   2. Ileocolic disease is generally resected with standard right hemicolectomy, creating a long side-to-side stapled ileocolostomy.
   3. Although segmental resection of colonic Crohn is generally pursued, some centers have reported much longer times to disease recurrence by using total abdominal colectomy if the rectum is uninvolved, or even total proctocolectomy with end ileostomy creation.
   4. Crohn bowel should not knowingly be used for the creation of pouches, such as the J-pouch for the ileoanal pull-through procedure.

VIII. Cancer Risk
   A. Risk of adenocarcinoma development in the Crohn segment is estimated at 15 to 100 times the risk of small bowel adenocarcinoma.
      1. The likelihood of malignant transformation begins after 10 years of active disease. If cancer develops, it is generally after 20 to 30 years of carrying the diagnosis.
      2. Experts are uncertain about whether patients with more symptomatic Crohn disease have a greater likelihood of undergoing malignant transformation than those with less symptomatic disease.
   B. The prognosis of Crohn-associated small bowel cancer is worse, **because of its late discovery** (symptoms of Crohn disease mimic those of a cancer), not inherent biological aggressiveness.

SMALL BOWEL OBSTRUCTION

I. Causes of Mechanical Obstruction
   A. Foreign body
   B. Gallstone ileus
      1. Generally seen in the elderly and debilitated
      2. Symptoms of "tumbling obstruction": pattern of sequential spontaneously resolving obstructions as gallstone alternately becomes lodged, and then passes more distal in small bowel.
      3. Cause is usually chronic cholecystitis, with fistula between gallbladder and second portion of duodenum, through which a large gallstone gains entry into the gastrointestinal tract.
      4. Stone eventually impacts itself in narrow terminal ileum, where complete bowel obstruction results.
      5. Abdominal films show high-grade distal small bowel obstruction, calcified gallstone outside the right upper quadrant (possibly), and pneumobilia.
      6. Treatment is to first rehydrate patient due to persistent vomiting. At exploration, milk the stone back into the dilated bowel, and extract through the

enterotomy. Make sure there are no other more proximal stones, and close the enterotomy. Due to tenuous patient condition, cholecystectomy and fistula closure is usually not pursued in the acute setting.

C. Intussusception
1. 5% to 15% of cases occur in adults, representing less than 1% of adult bowel obstruction.
2. 90% of cases are associated with a lead point such as a neoplasm (benign or malignant), diverticulum, old suture line, or adhesion.
3. Diagnosis usually made by contrast study or CT scan.
4. Barium column decompression, useful in children, is rarely used in adults.
   a. Presence of lead point makes radiologic reduction unlikely to be successful.
   b. Association with malignancy mandates surgery in most cases.
   c. The increasing risk of perforation and resultant malignant seeding of peritoneal cavity makes this practice questionable.
5. Surgery should be undertaken to decompress the intussusception and evaluate for cause.

D. Malignant obstruction
1. This condition rarely resolves with nonoperative measures.
2. A short trial of decompression may succeed. If this fails, resect or bypass.
3. If the obstruction cannot be reduced surgically, somatostatin may reduce cramping pain.

E. Crohn disease: trial of steroids or other immunosuppressants before exploration.

F. Radiation enteritis
1. Always consider in patients with history of radiation for gynecologic malignancy. It is less common after radiation therapy for colon or prostate cancer.
2. It usually occurs less than 10 years after radiation therapy.
3. Signs include obliterative vasculitis and muscular fibrosis.
4. Surgery is almost always needed, and can be daunting due to pelvic fibrosis. In some cases, bypass with venting stomas at the ends of the trapped pelvic bowel segment is all that is possible.

G. Adhesions
1. More than half of all small bowel obstructions are adhesions.
2. The vast majority of these occur postabdominal surgery, but occasionally congenital bands are encountered.
3. Up to 80% of adhesive small bowel obstructions resolve without need for operation.

H. Hernias
1. Hernias are the second most common cause of obstruction in Western countries, and first in the Third World.
2. In the United States, due to high rate of elective repair of inguinal and umbilical hernias, rare hernias such as femoral, obturator, bowel entrapment in the foramen of Winslow, or congenital defects of the omentum should be considered as causes of adhesions.
3. Also, consider the very dangerous Richter hernia, where only a portion of the bowel wall is fixed in the hernia sac, leading to a partial obstruction picture with high risk of bowel perforation.

II. Volvulus. Loop of bowel is twisted more than 180 degrees about its axis, and is caused by mismatch of bowel length to narrow area of attachment.
1. Ileocolic most frequent in small bowel, but can occur in small bowel alone.
2. Endoscopic decompression is generally not useful (unlike sigmoid volvulus).
3. Use laparotomy to decompress volvulus, and either perform cecopexy, or preferably, resect the involved segment.

III. Ileus. Motility alters without evidence of luminal obstruction.
A. Causes
1. Neurogenic (e.g., spinal cord injury)
2. Retroperitoneal process or surgery (e.g., ureteral colic)

The incidence of idiopathic intussusception rapidly decreases with increasing age. From adolescence onward, all intussusceptions should be considered to have a lead point such that most patients should have exploratory surgery.

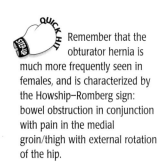
Remember that the obturator hernia is much more frequently seen in females, and is characterized by the Howship–Romberg sign: bowel obstruction in conjunction with pain in the medial groin/thigh with external rotation of the hip.

SMALL BOWEL

3. Opiates
4. Metabolic abnormalities, including hypokalemia, uremia, calcium or magnesium imbalance, hypothyroidism, and hyperglycemia
5. Intra-abdominal or distant infection
6. Drugs such as anticholinergics and antihistamines
   B. Normal return of small bowel function after abdominal surgery is 6 to 24 hours
   C. Ileus is less common after laparoscopic procedures compared with open surgeries

IV. Diagnosis of Small Bowel Obstruction

A. No reliable physical finding or serum laboratory test distinguishes ileus from mechanical obstruction, or rules out strangulated obstruction.
B. History is critical
   1. Prior abdominal surgery
   2. Signs of infection or peritonitis
   3. Prior history of obstructions
   4. History of malignancy or inflammatory bowel disease
   5. History of abdominal trauma
      a. Splenosis
      b. Diaphragmatic hernia
   6. History of endometriosis
C. Radiology of obstruction
   1. Plain films (3-way abdomen): said to be "diagnostic" in up to 80% of patients.
      a. Air–fluid levels may be present in both ileus and mechanical obstruction, although more common with latter.
      b. Assess for free air
   2. Contrast studies
      a. These studies may better delineate both nature and level of obstruction.
      b. Generally, these use water-soluble contrast unless closed loop obstruction is suspected. The hydrophilic activity of water-soluble contrast may cause swelling and perforation of the closed loop.
   3. CT scanning: most would consider this the preferred test for evaluating small bowel obstruction.
      a. Similar efficacy to contrast studies in terms of luminal findings.
      b. More sensitive to secondary signs in obstruction, such as presence of malignancy, mesenteric stranding, abscess, vascular compromise, intestinal wall thickening, and pneumatosis (air in the wall of the intestines).

V. Treatment of Small Bowel Obstruction

A. Obstructions with low likelihood of resolution with "conservative" measures such as malignancy-associated obstructions, high-grade obstructions, and hernias should be operated on promptly after fluid resuscitation.
B. If an ileus, assess for inciting factors (especially opiate use if fresh postoperative patient) and correct these if possible.
   1. CT is particularly helpful if the cause is uncertain, because it confirms the absence or presence of the transition zone associated with a mechanical obstruction, and allows assessment for other intra-abdominal processes, such as abscess.
   2. It may be necessary to try to administer an epidural with continuous local anesthesia (not opiates) to allow cessation of intravenous opiates.
   3. There is some evidence for vagal stimulation through limited oral intake or gum chewing, in order to reduce the duration of ileus.
C. Despite the adage that "the sun should not set on a bowel obstruction," what to do with the lower risk obstructions, such as the early postoperative adhesive obstruction, remains problematic.
   1. Most surgeons give a 24- to 48-hour trial of nasogastric decompression and bowel rest, with close observation of the patient's status and abdominal examination.
   2. There is some evidence for using the time it takes for oral contrast to enter the colon, as a predictor of the likelihood of resolution of partial small bowel obstructions.

MECKEL DIVERTICULUM

I. Epidemiology and Etiology

A. Meckel diverticulum is the most common congenital abnormality of the gastrointestinal tract.

B. It is found in 1% to 2% of the population, with slightly higher male incidence. More than 50% of symptomatic cases present in male children younger than 10 years of age. Complications occur disproportionately in males.

C. On average, the location is 60 cm proximal to the ileocecal valve, on the antimesenteric aspect.

D. Factors predictive of symptomatic Meckel diverticulum:
   1. Male sex (cause of male predominance unknown)
   2. Diverticular length less than 2 cm (increased length: orifice ratio inclines toward development of diverticulitis)
   3. Presence of ectopic tissue
   4. Presence of mesodiverticular or vitelloumbilical band

E. It results from failure of the omphalomesenteric (vitelline) duct to close. This should occur around the ninth gestational week.

F. Complete failure to involute results in the infrequently encountered enteroumbilical fistula.

II. Pathology

A. Meckel diverticulum is a true diverticulum of all layers of the intestinal wall.

B. Up to one-third of Meckel diverticula contain heterotropic tissue, with gastric and pancreatic the most frequently found.

C. The majority of symptomatic diverticula are lined with gastric mucosa.

III. Clinical Presentation

A. In children, bleeding from Meckel diverticula is usually occult, manifesting as unexplained anemia, although more brisk hemorrhage presenting as melena or even hematochezia has been seen. Bleeding due to peptic ulceration is the most common presentation, with occasional cases of peptic-induced perforation.

B. In adults, bowel obstruction is most frequent, caused by one of several mechanisms:
   1. Diverticulitis causing fibrous stricture.
   2. Ectopic tissue, usually pancreatic, or the diverticulum itself serving as lead point for intussusception.
   3. Internal herniation under a mesodiverticular band (remnant of the duct attaches the root of mesentery to diverticulum).
   4. Volvulus of ileum around vitelloumbilical band (bowel suspended from the base of the umbilicus).

C. Obstructive complaints may be partial intermittent type, especially with volvulus, or acute complete small bowel obstruction, as with intussusception.

IV. Diagnostic Workup

A. Rarely diagnosed preoperatively

B. Acute appendicitis is the most common preoperative diagnosis. Meckel diverticulitis is clinically indistinguishable from acute appendicitis.

C. CT scan and ultrasound have low sensitivity in this setting.

D. Barium small-bowel series is more sensitive, but generally is not used in the presence of acute abdomen because of concern for perforation.

E. Technetium scan is widely reported to have the highest sensitivity, but detects only Meckel diverticula that contain gastric mucosa.

V. Surgical Treatment

A. In the acute setting, limited resection of the ileal segment containing the diverticulum with primary anastomosis is indicated.

B. Controversy persists regarding indications for resection of the incidentally discovered Meckel diverticulum.
1. All incidentally discovered Meckel diverticula in children should be resected.
2. Some advocate the same strategy for adults, whereas others argue that one would have to resect almost 1,000 diverticula to save the life of one adult who would subsequently present with complications of the disease.
3. Factors favoring resection of the asymptomatic Meckel diverticula are palpable ectopic tissue (generally pancreatic, not gastric), diverticular length less than 2 cm, and the presence of an associated band.
    a. Vitelloumbilical bands can simply be divided without diverticulectomy.
    b. Mesodiverticular bands cannot be divided, because they are often the sole blood supply to the diverticulum; division of these bands necessitates concomitant diverticulectomy.
C. No incidental diverticulectomy should be pursued in the presence of peritonitis or in the medically unstable patient.

BENIGN SMALL BOWEL TUMORS

I. General Principles
A. These tumors represent about one-third of all small bowel neoplasms.
B. Growth pattern predicts associated symptoms and signs.
1. Infiltrative: bleeding
2. Intraluminal (for example, polypoid): obstruction either due to lesion or as lead point for intussusception; low-level bleeding
3. Serosal: pivot point for small bowel volvulus
C. Tend to be slow-growing with long duration, protean symptomatology.

II. Hyperplastic Polyps
A. Predilection for distal duodenum and small bowel
B. No malignant potential
C. Rarely symptomatic, except as lead point of intussusception

III. Gastrointestinal Stromal Tumor
A. Gastrointestinal stromal tumor (GIST) is the most common symptomatic small bowel lesion.
B. Benign leiomyomata tend to be smaller in size and firmer than GIST.
C. Differentiating leiomyoma from GIST is difficult, but is suggested by lack of cellularity on light microscopy, less than 2 mitoses per 10 high power fields, and absence of CD34 and CD117 staining on immunohistochemistry.
D. GIST presents with partial obstructive symptoms and minor bleeding from erosion of overlying mucosa.
E. Because intraoperative differentiation between leiomyoma and malignant GIST is difficult, treatment of all smooth muscle tumors of the small bowel is resection, **with at least a 2-cm margin** in all directions, and avoidance of tumor spillage or rupture.

IV. Lipoma
A. Benign submucosal tumors found anywhere in small bowel.
B. If large, may cause bowel obstruction and/or intussusception.
C. Occasional bleeding from mucosal erosion.
D. Require resection if symptomatic, and are highly amenable to laparoscopic resection.

V. Hemangiomata
A. These may comprise up to 10% of all small bowel lesions.
B. Cavernous variant is the most common.

TABLE 5-2 Unusual Small Bowel Benign Neoplasms

Neoplasm	Description
Amyloidosis	Infiltrative growth may cause obstruction, rarely bleeding.
Blue rubber bleb syndrome	Associated with intestinal hemangiomata.
Cowden syndrome	Germ-line mutation leads to hamartomas in all three germ layers. Increased risk of thyroid, breast, and endometrial cancer. Gastrointestinal polyps cause obstruction and bleeding.
Endometriosis	Serositis may cause fibrotic obstruction.
Ganglioneuroma	Associated with neurofibromatosis and MEN IIb/III.
Inflammatory fibroid polyp	Grossly resembles gastrointestinal stromal tumors but c-kit (−); obstruction/bleeding.
Inflammatory myofibroblastic tumor	Generally behaves as benign tumor; obstruction, and intussusception.
Myxoma	Very rare; may be part of Carney syndrome (myxomas of heart, skin, and breast, and pituitary adenomata), Cushing syndrome.

C. They are rarely large enough to cause obstruction unless intramural hematoma develops.

D. Bleeding, occasionally massive, is the most common presentation, followed by finding as lead point of intussusception.

E. They may be difficult to localize, even using arteriography. Intraoperative enteroscopy has much higher likelihood of success.

F. Arteriographic embolization can be tried for significant bleeding, otherwise, use surgical resection.

VI. Peutz–Jeghers Syndrome

A. This autosomal dominant disorder (mutation of 19p2.3 [*LKB1*] gene) is characterized by mucocutaneous pigmentation and myriad benign gastrointestinal hamartomas.

B. 90% of affected individuals have small bowel hamartomas.

C. No nuclear atypia are seen in polyps.

D. Hamartomas can cause abdominal pain, gastrointestinal bleeding, and obstruction from intussusception.

E. There is an increased rate of gastrointestinal cancers, but not from hamartomas. These arise in synchronous adenomatous lesions.

F. Surveillance recommendations include the following: starting at age 10, biannual esophagogastroduodenoscopy, colonoscopy, and barium small bowel follow-through due to cancer risk

G. Multiplicity of polyps makes localization of source of symptoms difficult (Table 5-2).

SMALL BOWEL MALIGNANCY

I. Epidemiology

A. Malignancy of the small bowel is very rare in industrialized Western countries (less than 2% of gastrointestinal cancers in the United States).

B. Several factors are implicated in low rate of small bowel cancer:
1. Rapid transit time
2. Sloughing of mucosal surface cells weekly
3. Low bacterial counts
4. Large volume of chyme dilutes carcinogen concentration
5. High levels of secretory immunoglobulin

C. Two-thirds of small bowel neoplasms are malignant. About 5,400 cases occur annually, with 40% of malignancies adenocarcinomas, followed by 30% carcinoids, 15% sarcomas, and 15% lymphomas.

D. The mean age of diagnosis is 60 years. Because of protean symptoms, the average delay in diagnosis from symptom onset is 6 months to 1 year.

II. Risk Factors

A. Polyposis syndromes
1. Patients with familial adenomatous polyposis and Gardner disease have a 300-fold increased risk of duodenal adenocarcinoma, but no apparent increase in other small bowel cancers.
2. Patients with hereditary nonpolyposis colorectal cancer have a 100-fold increased risk of small bowel adenocarcinoma, uniformly distributed throughout the small bowel.

B. Dietary factors. It is suggested that a high intake of animal fat, red meat, and cured foods is associated with a twofold to threefold increase in risk.

C. Crohn disease

D. Celiac disease
1. 300-fold increased risk of developing lymphoma, 95% of which are T-cell types.
2. 67-fold increased risk of small bowel adenocarcinoma.

E. Male sex (small bowel malignancy has a slight preponderance in men)

F. African-American race

III. Adenocarcinoma

A. Adenocarcinoma has a similar natural history to colorectal carcinoma, with a polyp as premalignant lesion.

B. Genetic changes parallel colon cancer, except the adenomatous polyposis coli mutation is rare in small bowel cancer, and SMAD4 tumor suppressor loss of heterozygosity is common.

C. Location: 50% duodenal, 30% jejunal, and 20% ileal.

D. Duodenal adenocarcinoma should be considered separately from more distal lesions, because it presents earlier, at a lower stage, and has a much higher 5-year disease-specific survival.

E. Except for tumors with limited or no nodal involvement, more extensive resection does not improve survival.

F. For less advanced tumors, resection with 5-cm luminal margins and modest lymph node resection is indicated.

G. For advanced stage III or IV disease, resection of primary tumors to avoid complications of hemorrhage, perforation, or obstruction as necessary. An extensive mesenteric resection should not be completed.

H. Adjuvant chemotherapy regimen parallels that of colon cancer, but number of small bowel cancers is so small that no sizeable study has been done to verify any benefit from chemotherapy following surgical resection.

IV. Sarcoma

A. Sarcoma is thought to be derived from the interstitial cells of Cajal.

B. Most of these tumors are not true sarcomas, because they do not express muscle-associated antigens such as smooth muscle actin.

C. These tumors are characterized by the generic term GIST.
1. About two-thirds of GISTs express a growth factor receptor with tyrosine kinase activity that is encoded for by the proto-oncogene *c-kit*.
2. **All suspected small bowel smooth muscle tumors should be tested for *c-kit* expression.**

D. The stomach is the primary location for GIST, with about 30% of the tumors occurring in the small bowel.
1. Small bowel sarcomas are believed to have a worse prognosis.
2. Due to their propensity for bleeding and perforation, all sarcomas should be resected, even in advanced-stage disease.

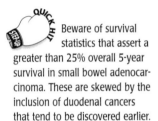

Beware of survival statistics that assert a greater than 25% overall 5-year survival in small bowel adenocarcinoma. These are skewed by the inclusion of duodenal cancers that tend to be discovered earlier.

SMALL BOWEL

3. As with most sarcomas, lymphatic involvement is rare, so only grossly involved nodes should be excised.
4. GIST tends to spread hematogenously to liver and lung.
5. Research is ongoing as to the utility of the tyrosine kinase inhibitor, as both an adjuvant drug after complete resection and as treatment for advanced disease.
6. Five year survival prior to the use of tyrosine kinase inhibitors was about 20%.

V. Lymphoma

A. The gastrointestinal tract is the most common site of extranodal non-Hodgkin lymphomas.
   1. These account for half of all extranodal lymphomas.
   2. Up to two-thirds of small intestinal lymphomas are diffuse large B-cell type.
   3. Small bowel lymphomas constitute about 25% of gastrointestinal lymphomas (gastric makes up about 50%).
B. Up to 50% of patients with gastrointestinal lymphomas present with an abdominal emergency.
C. In patients with disease limited to bowel (stage I) or nodal involvement that is infradiaphragmatic (including the spleen, but not the liver; stage II), there is benefit to resecting all disease, or debulking it.
   1. This includes mesenteric adenopathy that can be excised without sacrificing large amounts of bowel length.
   2. If the spleen is grossly abnormal, it should be removed.
   3. Nonadjacent adenopathy that cannot be easily resected should be biopsied, and marked with clips for possible radiotherapy to these nodal basins.
D. In stage III (involvement of nodal basins on both sides of the diaphragm) and stage IV (systemic disease including lung, liver, skin, and bone marrow) disease, no resection should be done unless laparotomy is mandated to deal with perforation of, or bleeding from, the primary tumor.
   1. Chemotherapy is the mainstay of treatment in these patients.
   2. Radiotherapy may be added to areas of bulky disease.

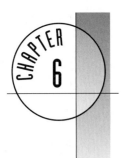
Colon, Rectum, and Appendix

Riaz Cassim, MD
Irfan Rizvi, MD

COLORECTAL AND ANAL DISORDERS

I. Lower Gastrointestinal Hemorrhage

A. Epidemiology. Lower gastrointestinal (GI) bleeding is a common clinical problem.

B. Etiology

1. Ischemic colitis, a mostly self-limiting disease, is characterized by the sudden onset of left-sided abdominal pain with bloody diarrhea. Associated conditions include renal failure requiring hemodialysis, hypertension, cardiovascular disease and vasoactive medication, and postaortic surgery. Colitis predominantly affects the mucosa.

   a. Diagnosis is by colonoscopy. A barium enema may outline mucosal ulcers, thereby showing a classic "thumbprinting" sign.

   b. Treatment includes active observation. Peritonitis with frank gangrene is indication for surgery.

2. Other causes: radiation proctitis, concealed intussusception (solitary rectal ulcer syndrome).

C. Diagnosis

1. Patients with brisk hemorrhage tend to pass bright red blood, whereas patients with slow or proximal colon bleeds tend to pass darker, altered blood mixed with feces.

2. Recognizing certain common patterns helps facilitate the correct diagnosis. The differential diagnosis includes:

   a. Hemorrhoids: bright red blood appears on the toilet paper or the bowl, and is rarely hemodynamically significant.

   b. Inflammatory bowel disease (IBD): patients with IBD tend to pass small amounts of blood mixed with mucus and feces.

   c. Tumors: the color of defecated blood becomes brighter from proximal to distal colon.

   d. Diverticular disease and angiodysplasia: bleeding is often sudden, brisk, but self-limiting.

      (1) Patients with recurrent or profuse bleeding pose a diagnostic dilemma, because the hemorrhage can be difficult to localize.

      (2) In colonic diverticulosis, bleeding occurs when a blood vessel breaks down as it passes through the weakened wall of a diverticulum. Although the disease is more common on the left side, at least half of the hemorrhages occur on the right side.

      (3) In colonic angiodysplasia, age-related degeneration of normal submucosal veins occurs. This condition predominantly affects the elderly. Most commonly present in cecum and ascending colon, it can be diagnosed either by colonoscopy or selective mesenteric angiography.

   e. Ischemic colitis: patients are usually elderly and present with left-sided abdominal pain.

 Passage of bright red blood per rectum may indicate brisk upper GI bleeding. Whether the source is from the upper or lower GI tract can be easily resolved by passing a nasogastric tube. If clear bilious fluid is aspirated, in most cases the bleeding source is distal to the ligament of Treitz.

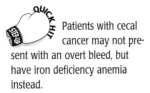 Patients with cecal cancer may not present with an overt bleed, but have iron deficiency anemia instead.

The classical angiographic finding is a slow emptying, dilated, tortuous vein seen in more than 90% of the cases of AVM.

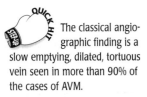 Ninety percent of patients with recurrent or profuse bleeding have either diverticular disease or colonic angiodysplasia.

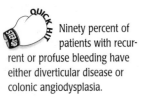

D. Management of minor bleeding
1. History and physical examination
2. Anorectal examination
3. Anoscopy, proctosigmoidoscopy
4. Colonoscopy
5. Treatment of the cause
E. Management of major bleeding. Regardless of the cause, the initial management in all patients with severe lower GI bleeding is identical.
1. Resuscitation
2. History
3. Anorectal examination
4. Colonoscopy
5. If the source of the hemorrhage is not revealed by colonoscopy, then consider:
   a. Technetium-99m sulphur colloid isotope red cell scan
      (1) Most sensitive
      (2) Shows extravasation onto the gut with bleeding, to the order of 0.05 to 0.1 mL/min
      (3) May not precisely localize the site
   b. Selective visceral arteriography
      (1) Localizes bleeding more precisely
      (2) Can be used therapeutically for embolization
      (3) However, it is an invasive test and requires a higher rate of bleeding (0.5 to 1 mL/min) to be diagnostically useful.
6. Laparotomy
   a. Consider performing concomitant endoscopy to localize bleeding source.
   b. If bleeding continues, and cannot be controlled endoscopically, surgery is indicated.
   c. Indicated for patients who require more than 6 units of red blood cells in 24 hours (hemodynamic instability).
7. Resection
   a. A segmental resection involving the bleeding segment is ideal.
   b. Uncontrolled, nonlocalized bleeding may necessitate a total abdominal colectomy with ileorectal anastomosis.
8. In colonic diverticulosis:
   a. Because 90% of the patients stop bleeding, nonoperative management is reasonable.
   b. Supportive care in the form of fluid resuscitation and transfusion of blood and blood products is indicated.
   c. Patients who rebleed ultimately need resection of the involved colonic segment.

II. Large Bowel Volvulus

A. General principles
1. In volvulus, the bowel twists on its own mesenteric axis, leading to bowel obstruction.
2. Venous congestion may lead to bowel infarction.
B. Sigmoid volvulus
1. Epidemiology and etiology
   a. Sigmoid volvulus accounts for about 5% of all cases of large bowel obstruction in developed countries. The incidence is higher in the Third World, which has been attributed to fiber-rich diets.
   b. The narrow mesenteri base of the sigmoid colon, along with an elongated floppy loop, makes it particularly susceptible to twisting on its axis.
   c. This condition is seen mostly in elderly, institutionalized patients with chronic medical and neuropsychiatric conditions.
   d. It is postulated that psychotropic drugs affect colonic motility, thus predisposing to volvulus.

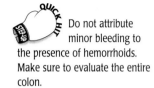

QUICK HIT

Do not attribute minor bleeding to the presence of hemorrhoids. Make sure to evaluate the entire colon.

QUICK HIT

The most common site for volvulus in the large bowel is sigmoid colon (approximately 75% of all cases of volvulus), followed by the cecum and (rarely) the transverse colon.

2. Clinical features
   a. Patients present with colicky abdominal pain, constipation, nausea, vomiting, and an inability to pass flatus.
   b. The air is able to enter the sigmoid loop but unable to exit. This leads to progressive distention of the sigmoid loop.
   c. The abdomen is usually markedly distended, and tympanic on percussion. Severe pain with peritoneal signs is an indicator of underlying bowel ischemia and/or impending perforation.

3. Diagnosis
   a. In most patients, the diagnosis can be made on the combination of history, physical examination, and plain abdominal radiography.
   b. The rectal vault is usually empty on examination.
   c. Plain radiographs show a markedly distended sigmoid loop, which assumes a bent inner tube or inverted U-shaped appearance, with the limbs of the sigmoid loop directed toward the pelvis.
   d. Single-contrast barium enema examination is useful, because it demonstrates that the barium readily enters the empty rectum and usually encounters a stenosis, likened to a beak, the so-called *bird beak* or bird-of-prey sign.

4. Management
   a. Patients may be dehydrated, and should be fluid resuscitated.
   b. Rigid proctoscopy should be performed at the bedside. The instrument may pass into the obstructed segment. If this maneuver succeeds, there is a sudden, dramatic gush of fluid and feces. It is recommended that a well-lubricated rectal tube be used to prevent early relapse and facilitate continued drainage.
   c. A full colonoscopy should be performed after bowel preparation to rule out an associated neoplasm.
   d. Volvulus can recur in up to 50% of patients; therefore, elective sigmoid resection should be offered to all good-risk surgical patients.
   e. Occasionally, it is not possible to decompress the bowel endoscopically. Alternatively, proctoscopy may reveal mucosal ischemia suggesting sigmoid necrosis. Such a patient should be emergently taken to the operating room.

C. Cecal volvulus
   1. Cecal volvulus is uncommon, and presents with abdominal pain and distention.
   2. Colonoscopic decompression has a high failure rate. Risk of gangrene of the involved bowel segment is also high; therefore appropriate treatment is right hemicolectomy.
   3. A much more common condition is a *cecal bascule*, in which a mobile cecum folds cephalad on a fixed ascending colon. This results in intermittent bowel obstruction.

D. Pseudo-obstruction
   1. This condition is characterized by pronounced abdominal distention, suggestive of a mechanical large bowel obstruction, in the absence of an obstructing lesion.
   2. Commonly seen in hospitalized patients with chronic medical conditions.
   3. The abdomen is distended, tympanic with bowel sounds. There is minimal pain or vomiting.
   4. It is important to exclude a mechanical obstruction by water-soluble contrast enema.
   5. Management
      a. Nasogastric decompression, and correction of fluid and electrolyte abnormalities, especially hypokalemia.
      b. All medications that inhibit bowel motility like opiates should be stopped.
      c. Serial abdominal exams and radiographs are performed.
   6. Colonoscopic decompression may be necessary in patients with marked colonic dilation, and impending cecal perforation.

 The distended cecum comes to lie in the left upper quadrant in most cases, and appears on the abdominal radiograph like a "bean" or a "comma."

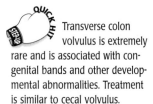 Transverse colon volvulus is extremely rare and is associated with congenital bands and other developmental abnormalities. Treatment is similar to cecal volvulus.

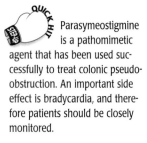 Parasymeostigmine is a pathomimetic agent that has been used successfully to treat colonic pseudo-obstruction. An important side effect is bradycardia, and therefore patients should be closely monitored.

III. Diverticular Disease
A. General principles
  1. Colonic diverticula are mucosal outpouchings through the submucosa and the muscular layer of the colon.
  2. They occur most commonly in the sigmoid colon, and up to 10% involve the entire colon.
  3. They arise between antimesenteric taenia and the mesenteric taenia, at the site of entry of the blood vessels.
B. Epidemiology and etiology
  1. Diverticular disease of the colon is an acquired condition.
  2. This condition is a disorder of modern civilization, and is associated with consumption of refined food products. It is rare in rural African and Asian populations where dietary fiber is high.
C. Clinical features. Most patients are asymptomatic. Occasionally diverticulosis is associated with lower abdominal colicky pain.
D. Diagnosis of diverticular disease
  1. A history of chronic intermittent lower abdominal pain, and presence of diverticula on barium enema or colonoscopy are indicative of this condition.
  2. In acute diverticulitis, computed tomography (CT) may help distinguish a phlegmon from an abscess.
  3. Sigmoidoscopy and colonoscopy should be avoided in acute flare-ups of the disease, because the risk of perforation is high.
E. Management
  1. In acute diverticulitis/phlegmon, intravenous (IV) fluids, antibiotics, and bowel rest are necessary.
  2. Abscesses should be drained.
  3. Fecal peritonitis necessitates exploratory laparotomy. The most commonly performed operation is the *Hartmann procedure,* in which the sigmoid colon is resected, the proximal colon is exteriorized as a stoma, and the rectal stump is oversewn.
  4. Patients with strictures may need an elective sigmoid colectomy and primary anastomosis.
  5. Fistulae are a complex problem. The patient's nutrition should be optimized, and infection should be controlled before surgical repair is attempted.
F. Complications
  1. Acute diverticulitis. A diverticulum may become inflamed when a fecalith obstructs its neck. Patients present with left lower quadrant abdominal pain, fever, and leukocytosis.
  2. Diverticular abscess. Acute diverticulitis may result in a peridiverticular abscess. Patients experience severe pain, high fever, and white blood cell elevation. A CT scan can identify the collection, and guide percutaneous drainage.
  3. Diverticular phlegmon. The local response to the diverticular inflammation may lead to formation of an inflammatory mass or phlegmon. Such patients need bowel rest and IV antibiotics.
  4. Diverticular stricture. Recurrent episodes of inflammation may lead to fibrosis, resulting in luminal narrowing. Patients may present with acute large bowel obstruction.
  5. Fecal peritonitis. Perforation of diverticula may lead to fecal peritonitis, which has a mortality rate of about 50%. Patients need emergency exploratory laparotomy.
  6. Hemorrhage. Erosion of a peridiverticular vessel can lead to significant bleeding.
  7. Fistula. Peridiverticular abscess may erode into adjacent viscera, forming a fistula.

IV. Ulcerative Colitis. This nonspecific IBD affects the mucosa of the colon and rectum.
A. Epidemiology and etiology
  1. New cases of ulcerative colitis are seen each year at the rate of 1 to 15 new cases per 100,000 population. The disease has a *bimodal distribution,* with

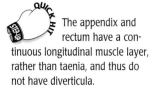
Because colonic diverticula do not possess all layers of the bowel wall, they are "false" or "pseudo-diverticula."

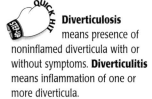
The appendix and rectum have a continuous longitudinal muscle layer, rather than taenia, and thus do not have diverticula.

Diverticulosis means presence of noninflamed diverticula with or without symptoms. **Diverticulitis** means inflammation of one or more diverticula.

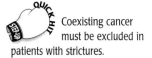
Coexisting cancer must be excluded in patients with strictures.

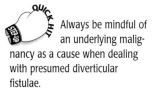
Always be mindful of an underlying malignancy as a cause when dealing with presumed diverticular fistulae.

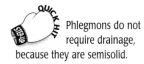
Phlegmons do not require drainage, because they are semisolid.

most cases occurring in the teen years followed by a second peak in the forties.

2. A positive family history is seen in about 10% of patients.

3. Etiology is uncertain. Changes in fecal flora, a history of nonsmoking, appendectomy, milk allergy, and certain genes (12q13, MHC class2 genes) have all been considered important in the etiology.

B. Pathology. The primary pathological process remains unknown.

1. Macroscopic appearance

a. The disease is limited to the mucosa and submucosa.

b. The rectum is always involved. The proximal colon may be the site of variable disease.

c. The mucosal surface is ulcerated with areas of heaped regenerating mucosa called *pseudopolyps*.

2. Microscopic appearance: *crypt abscesses* form at the base of the mucosa.

C. Clinical features

1. Clinical severity is extremely variable.

2. For most patients, frequent passage of blood-stained stools that contain mucus is the most common initial presentation.

3. Some patients complain of mild lower abdominal pain, fever and tenesmus, but have little in the way of weight loss.

4. In 80% of patients, the disease affects the distal colon.

5. Abdominal examination is usually unremarkable. Rectal examination reveals blood and, on sigmoidoscopy, there is evidence of proctitis.

6. Biopsy of the rectal mucosa is performed to confirm the diagnosis histologically.

7. A minority (20%) of patients with ulcerative colitis present either initially, or subsequently, with a severe attack usually with *pancolitis*.

a. Such patients have unremitting bloody diarrhea (10 to 24 times a day), colicky lower abdominal pain, and weight loss.

b. On examination, they look pale and ill, and they have tachycardia, fever, and a tender lower abdomen.

D. Extraintestinal features

1. Dermatologic

a. Pyoderma gangrenosum: ulcerated pretibial lesions.

b. Erythema nodosum: symmetric, red, tender papules on extensor surface of limbs.

c. Clubbing

2. Ocular

a. Iritis

b. Uveitis

c. Scleritis

3. Rheumatologic

a. Ankylosing spondylitis

b. Sacroiliitis

c. Peripheral arthritis

4. Hepatobiliary

a. Sclerosing cholangitis

b. Fatty liver

c. Cirrhosis

5. Vascular

a. Thromboembolism

b. Coagulopathy

E. Diagnosis

1. History should be taken, and a physical examination performed to exclude an infectious cause for diarrhea. Send a stool culture for *Shigella, Salmonella, Campylobacter, Giardia, Escherichia coli,* and *Clostridium difficile.*

2. Colonoscopy is a definitive imaging technique. A full examination to the cecum is performed. Attempt ileal intubation to rule out Crohn disease.

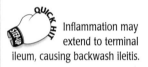
Inflammation may extend to terminal ileum, causing backwash ileitis.

3. In many patients, the macroscopic distribution of the colitis is confined to the rectum and part of the sigmoid colon in continuity.

4. Systemic biopsies throughout the colon enable diagnosis, definition of distribution, and identification of dysplasia.

5. A barium enema is used less frequently in the imaging of ulcerative colitis, but can be used in identifying its characteristic distribution.

6. In up to 10% of patients, the differentiation between ulcerative colitis and Crohn disease may not be complete, and the colitis is thus labeled *indeterminate*.

F. **Management.** The treatment of all patients with IBD is the management of symptoms. This requires an integrated medical and surgical approach that delivers the appropriate therapy consistent with symptom relief.

1. Medical management of the stable patient consists of drug therapy at a minimum dose that is compatible with good health and fewest side effects. Such a patient may be maintained for months or years on minimal medication, with occasional periods of high-dose steroid therapy for exacerbations.

   a. Steroids. These drugs remain the mainstay of treatment for moderate to severe ulcerative colitis, or for patients who have failed aminosalicylate treatment. Their main use is to control symptoms and not to maintain remission.

   b. Aminosalicylic acid compounds. 5-Aminosalicylic acid is the active compound in different formulations available in the market. As 5-ASA is disintegrated in the stomach by gastric juices, it is linked to a "stabilizing" compound, which facilitates its release at a higher pH in the colon. This drug induces remission and prevents recurrence, and is the mainstay of medical treatment.

   c. Antidiarrheal drugs may be used to reduce bowel frequency, but do not affect the course of the disease. Bowel rest and TPN are indicated in severe colitis.

   d. Immunomodulators

      (1) Calcineurin inhibitors, such as cyclosporin or tacrolimus, are used for refractory colitis.

      (2) The purine antimetabolites (azathioprine and 6-mercaptopurine) are used to facilitate remission induced by cyclosporine. Bone marrow suppression is a serious complication.

   e. Biological agents

      (1) The antitumor necrosis factor (TNF) antibody infliximab has not seen the same efficacy as it has in Crohn disease.

      (2) The anti-interleukin-2 receptor antibody and the anti-CD3 antibodies have recently shown promise.

2. Surgical management

   a. Indications for surgery

      (1) The most common indication is intractability of disease and failure of medical management to control symptoms.

      (2) A long history of colitis, and a pancolitic distribution of disease, are both associated with the potential for malignant change in the colonic mucosa. Mucosal biopsies that show high-grade dysplasia or carcinoma *in situ* indicate the need for surgical removal of the colon. Colonoscopic surveillance once every 3 years for evidence of mucosal dysplasia is usually started 10 years after diagnosis.

      (3) Other indications for surgical intervention include bleeding, perforation, toxic colonic dilatation, and infection.

   b. Acute severe colitis

      (1) A few patients present with, or develop, an acute exacerbation of colic symptoms that fails to respond to oral high-dose steroids. They require treatment in the hospital.

      (2) IV fluids and hydrocortisone, with bed rest, are the main treatment.

      (3) Combined surgical and medical management from admission is critical, because failure to respond quickly to medical measures is an indication for abdominal colectomy.

      (4) Once it is clear that medical therapy has not controlled symptoms within 72 hours of admission, the patient must be apprised of the

QUICK HIT On barium examination, loss of haustra with a flat mucosa and narrow caliber (lead-pipe colon) are indicative of chronic ulcerative colitis.

COLON, RECTUM, AND APPENDIX

need for a colectomy. In the acutely ill patient, this comprises abdominal colectomy and ileostomy.

(5) Subsequent removal of the rectum is necessary in most patients for surgical cure of ulcerative colitis.

c. From resection to restoration: the pouch.

(1) The elimination of ulcerative colitis and risk of cancer can be done through removal of all colonic mucosa. For many years, total procto-colectomy was the "gold standard" for curing ulcerative colitis.

(2) *Total proctocolectomy* involves excising all colon, rectum, and anus with closure of perineal wound. A permanent right lower quadrant spouted (*Brooke*) ileostomy is created.

(3) The ileal pouch (J, W, or S pouch), or the construction or a new reservoir or neorectum to replace diseased rectum, offers the chance of surgical cure without the need for a permanent ileostomy.

(4) An important aspect of this surgery is the need to discuss with the patient what the pouch procedure does and does not offer. The ileal pouch does not offer patient "normal" bowel function.

(5) The ileal reservoir most commonly used is the J pouch. Frequency of pouch evacuation usually settles at 4 to 5 times daily with good continence.

(6) Long-term sequelae of restorative proctocolectomy include pouchitis, anastomotic stricture, pouch failure, and sexual dysfunction.

G. Complications. The extraintestinal features complicate 25% to 30% of cases.

1. Although most respond to treatment of the primary condition, articular and hepatic manifestations do not resolve.

2. Primary sclerosing cholangitis (PSC) increases the risk of cholangiocarcinoma.

3. Liver failure secondary to PSC may necessitate a transplant.

V. Crohn Disease

A. Epidemiology and etiology

1. Crohn disease is a transmural IBD that can affect any part of the GI tract—from the mouth to the anus.

2. The incidence is about 3 new cases for every 100,000 people, with a prevalence of about 30 cases for every 100,000 people.

3. Both genetic and environmental factors are implicated.

a. About 10% of patients give positive family history of IBD. The IBD1 locus on chromosome 16 is strongly associated with Crohn disease.

b. Infective agents, about which there is speculation, include the measles virus and *Mycobacterium paratuberculosis*.

4. The etiologic factor that could provide a preventative or curative strategy remains elusive.

B. Clinical features. (Crohn disease in the small bowel is discussed elsewhere in this text. The following description is confined to the large bowel.)

1. Three distinct patterns of disease are seen: inflammatory, stricturing, and perforating.

2. Patients are usually young (peak 15 to 35 years) and present with abdominal pain, weight loss, and diarrhea.

3. Abdominal pain is colicky. A minority of patients present with the symptoms of colitis: frequent bloody stools with mucus. These patients are indistinguishable from those with ulcerative colitis, including the occasional development of toxic colitis.

4. Extraintestinal manifestations of Crohn disease include erythema nodosum, pyoderma gangrenosum, uveitis and sacroiliitis, large joint involvement, and clubbing.

5. Perianal Crohn disease (PCD; see below), which is often associated with colonic disease, affects about 33% of patients. Perianal pain and suppuration are main symptoms. Rectal examination reveals evidence of ulceration, edematous skin tags, perianal abscess and/or fistulation, and stricture.

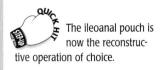
QUICK HIT
The ileoanal pouch is now the reconstructive operation of choice.

C. Diagnosis and imaging
  1. Colonic disease is best diagnosed by colonoscopy. The distribution of colitis is discontinuous with rectal sparing. Often terminal ileum can be visualized and biopsied to confirm small bowel disease. Barium enema examination also demonstrates Crohn's colitis, and reflux of barium into the terminal ileum can be used to diagnose disease at this site. White cell scans using technetium-labeled white cells can also be useful in delineating distribution of IBD.
  2. Definitive imaging of perianal disease may require examination under anesthetic with endoscopy of the rectum. Other techniques that might help in defining perianal lesions include transrectal ultrasonography and magnetic resonance imaging of the anal canal.

D. Medical management
  1. Aim is symptom relief and maintenance of well-being with minimum side effects.
  2. It is important for the patient to have a well-balanced diet and maintain weight.
  3. An acute flare-up of obstructive symptoms can be managed with a short high-dose regimen of oral steroids.
     a. In a patient in whom oral steroids cannot be reduced below acceptable levels without symptom reactivation, azathioprine may allow maintenance at a lower steroid dosage.
     b. Budesonide is an enteric-coated steroid that is released into the terminal ileum. It offers means of treating the small bowel without the systemic side effects of oral steroids.
  4. Disease activity can be monitored through measurement of hemoglobin, platelet count, erythrocyte sedimentation rate, C-reactive protein, and orosomucoids. In a patient with quiescent colonic disease, sulfasalazine derivatives may also be used (for example, mesalazine or Pentasa).
  5. PCD. Treatment is conservative, because repeated surgical procedures may damage the sphincters.
     a. Effective medical therapies include antibiotics such as ciprofloxacin and metronidazole. Immune suppressants such as azathioprine and cyclosporine have been shown to be effective.
     b. The anti-TNF antibody infliximab has been shown to promote healing in complex cases of PCD.

E. Surgical management
  1. Integrated medical and surgical management is required to achieve correct use of surgical resection as treatment.
  2. Surgery is used when drug therapy cannot achieve optimal relief of symptoms with acceptable level of side effects. The presence of a mass in association with the disease is an absolute indication for operation.
  3. Ileocecal disease
     a. The management of ileocecal disease is similar to the management of disease limited to the terminal ileum.
     b. The best option is resection to grossly normal bowel with primary anastomosis. Recurrence tends to occur at the anastomosis and preanastomosis proximal bowel.
  4. Extensive colitis with rectal sparing
     a. Patients with Crohn colitis come to surgery, because of chronic ill health, but can present acutely with colitis requiring urgent colectomy.
     b. Tendency of Crohn colitis to spare the rectum means that ileorectal anastomosis is the preferred option for subsequent reconstruction.
  5. Segmental Crohn colitis also lends itself to segmental resection and reanastomosis.
  6. Rectal Crohn disease
     a. Many patients with Crohn colitis require panproctocolectomy to eliminate their colonic symptoms.
     b. The ileal pouch is not a generally accepted option after colectomy for Crohn colitis, because of the tendency of Crohn disease to affect the pouch, leading to its failure.

VI. Colorectal Polyps
A. General principles
  1. A polyp is a discrete growth that protrudes into the lumen of the colon or rectum.
  2. Polyps are found throughout the colon and rectum.
B. Epidemiology and etiology
  1. Most commonly arise from the mucosa, but may be submucosal.
  2. Mucosal polyps are divided into neoplastic or non-neoplastic.
  3. Prevalence parallels that of colorectal cancer, being more common in the developed Western countries such as the United States.
  4. From 20% to 40% of asymptomatic patients older than 50 years may have adenomatous polyps, in studies using colonoscopy.
  5. Adenoma prevalence increases with age in all populations.
  6. From 30% to 50% of patients with one adenoma have a synchronous adenoma elsewhere in the colon.
  7. Adenomas precede carcinomas in a given population by 5 to 10 years. Relatively few adenomas progress to carcinomas.
C. Submucosal polyps
  1. Any submucosal growth can expand and push the mucosa into the bowel lumen, and appear as a polypoid lesion.
  2. Lipomas.
    a. Benign fatty tumors mostly seen in the cecum near the ileocecal valve, but can be found throughout the colon or rectum.
    b. Smooth yellowish appearing polyps that are easily deformable.
  3. Carcinoid tumors (see section on Colorectal Cancer, below).
D. Neoplastic mucosal polyps
  1. These are more commonly called adenomatous polyps.
  2. Most colorectal cancers arise in preexisting adenomatous polyps.
  3. Cancer risk is proportional to the following factors:
    a. The number of adenomas present, synchronously or metachronously.
    b. The degree of dysplasia or atypia. The degree of dysplasia correlates with the size of the polyp and degree of villous architecture.
    c. The size of the lesion. Polyps greater than 2 cm have a 30% to 40% risk of harboring a malignancy, whereas polyps less than 1 cm have a risk of 1% to 2%.
    d. The degree of villous component in the polyp.
  4. Removal of adenomatous polyps during surveillance proctosigmoidoscopy decreases the risk of subsequent death from colorectal cancer.
  5. Adenomatous polyps are characterized according to the following:
    a. Physical structure: sessile, with a broad-based attachment to the colon wall or pedunculated, being attached to the colon wall by a fibrovascular stalk.
    b. Glandular structure.
      (1) Tubular adenoma characterized by a complex network of branching adenomatous glands (75% of all adenomatous polyps).
      (2) Villous adenomas gland that extends straight down from the surface to the base of the polyp (10% of all adenomatous polyps).
      (3) Mixed tubulovillous adenomas (15% of all adenomatous polyps).
E. Non-neoplastic mucosal polyps
  1. Hyperplastic polyps
    a. Small sessile lesions frequently are seen in the distal colon and rectum.
    b. Indistinguishable from small adenomas, they have no malignant potential.
    c. These are found in one-third of the population older than 50 years of age.
  2. Juvenile polyps
    a. These growths are also known as retention polyps.
    b. They can occur sporadically or as part of a familial polyposis syndrome (FAP).

    c. Approximately 75% of these polyps occur in children less than 10 years of age, and are seen in about 2% of asymptomatic children.

    d. Presenting symptoms include hematochezia. Rectal prolapse and autoamputation may occur with distal lesions, and intussusception may be precipitated by proximal juvenile polyps.

    e. Individually, the polyps have no malignant potential.

  3. Inflammatory polyps: seen in idiopathic IBD or severe chronic inflammation of any kind (tuberculosis, amebiasis, schistosomiasis).

  4. Peutz–Jeghers hamartomas (see GI polyposis syndromes).

F. Clinical features

  1. Most polyps are asymptomatic and are discovered on routine screening colonoscopy.

  2. Overt bleeding may be seen as hematochezia, with larger polyps located distally. More commonly blood loss is clinically occult.

  3. Very large polyps may be associated with alterations in bowel habits.

  4. Secretory diarrhea with accompanying hypokalemia and hypochlorhydria is associated with large villous adenomas of the rectum and distal colon.

G. Management

  1. Polyps must be removed, once detected. This can be easily accomplished for pedunculated and small polyps, endoscopically using a biopsy forceps or a snare.

  2. Colonoscopy is the most accurate means of detecting polyps, and allows biopsy and removal of suspicious lesions.

  3. If the polyps cannot be removed via the endoscope, then segmental colon resection is required.

  4. Endoscopic polypectomy is adequate for polyps with carcinoma *in situ* (not invading the basement membrane), and confined to the head of the polyp.

  5. There is a 30% to 40% cumulative recurrence rate after index polypectomy in patients over 60 years of age, for multiple adenomas, and for large polyps.

H. Gastrointestinal polyposis syndromes

  1. Familial adenomatous polyposis (FAP)

    a. General principles. FAP is characterized by the development of multiple adenomatous polyps throughout the colon and rectum. Polyps first appear in adolescence (mean age about 16 years). If the polyps go untreated, 100% of affected patients will develop colorectal carcinoma by the third decade of life.

    b. Epidemiology and etiology. This is an autosomal disease with 100% penetrance.

      (1) A germ-line mutation in the adenomatous polyposis coli (APC) gene is located on chromosome 5q.

      (2) Each first-degree relative of an affected individual has a 50% likelihood of inheriting the mutation, and 25% of patients have a germ-line mutation in the APC gene that is not present in either parent.

      (3) The incidence of FAP in the United States is 1 in 10,000 persons.

    c. Pathophysiology. Polyps develop in the stomach and small bowel in 90% of patients. Gastric polyps are primarily fundic gland hyperplasia and not premalignant.

      (1) Small intestinal neoplasia: periampullary region of the duodenum.

      (2) Periampullary neoplasia: 90% of patients with FAP develop adenomas in the duodenum close to the ampulla of Vater. With time, carcinoma develops in 5% of these patients; this area needs surveillance. Adenomas and carcinomas rarely occur in the jejunum and ileum.

    d. Extraintestinal features. These include osteomas of the mandible, skull, and long bones, as well as soft-tissue tumors such as lipomas and fibromas.

    e. Desmoid tumors. These develop in 10% to 15% of patients with FAP. Benign but aggressive tumors of mesenteric fibroblasts, they can obstruct the GI tract, vessels, or ureters.

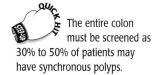 The entire colon must be screened as 30% to 50% of patients may have synchronous polyps.

f. Attenuated FAP
   (1) Less than 100 polyps
   (2) Later development of polyps and cancer
g. Diagnosis and management
   (1) At-risk relatives of patients with known FAP should undergo surveillance sigmoidoscopy on an annual basis, beginning after puberty. It is prudent to wait until patient reaches full maturity before planning surgery.
   (2) Goal of treatment is to remove entire large bowel mucosa, which is at risk for developing colorectal carcinoma.
   (3) This is accomplished by total proctocolectomy, with end ileostomy or total proctocolectomy, with ileoanal pouch anastomosis.
   (4) Esophagogastroduodenoscopy is performed every 2 to 3 years for surveillance and removal of gastric and duodenal mucosal polyps.
   (5) Surgical management of desmoid tumors is avoided, unless simple local excision of abdominal wall or localized lesions is possible. Postoperative recurrences are common. A combination of sulindac and tamoxifen has been successful in some patients.
2. Peutz–Jeghers syndrome
   a. Autosomal dominant familial syndrome. The gene that causes this syndrome has not yet been identified.
   b. Multiple GI polyps are seen in the stomach, small intestine and colon. Polyps are non-neoplastic hamartomas consisting of a supportive framework of smooth muscle tissue covered by hyperplastic epithelium. No inflammatory cell infiltrate is present.
   c. Rectal bleeding is the most common presentation. Intussusception may also occur. Characteristic skin pigmentation is seen from birth as dark, macular lesions on the mouth (skin and buccal mucosa), nose, lips, hands, feet, genitalia, and anus. This becomes less obvious by puberty.
   d. There is no increased risk of colorectal cancer. However, affected individuals are at increased risk of other GI tumors, gonadal tumors (ovarian cysts and sex cord tumors in females, and Sertoli cell testicular tumors in males), breast, and pancreatic and biliary cancers.
   e. Management consists of endoscopic polyp removal. Patients presenting with intussusception caused by small bowel polyps require bowel resection.
3. Juvenile polyposis
   a. These polyps are the most commonly solitary lesions seen in the rectum of children. They can be multiple in the entire GI tract.
   b. Manifestations can vary but are limited to bleeding, obstruction, and intussusception.
   c. Patients are at risk for colorectal cancer if they harbor mixed juvenile and adenomatous polyps. When mixed lesions are found, regular colonoscopic surveillance is recommended.
4. Cowden syndrome
   a. In these multiple GI hamartomas, polyps are usually asymptomatic, and may be hyperplastic or ganglioneuromas of the colon.
   b. There is an increased risk of development of breast, benign and malignant tumors of the thyroid gland.
   c. No therapy needs to be directed toward the polyps.
   d. This condition is complicated by lesions of the face that arise from follicular epithelium (pathologically trichilemmomas).

VII. Colorectal Cancer

A. Epidemiology and etiology
   1. Colorectal cancer is the second most common malignancy in the United States, with more the 155,000 new cases diagnosed annually. Incidence is highest in industrialized countries and is age specific, increasing steadily from the second to the ninth decades.

2. It is the second leading cause of all cancer-related deaths.

3. Rates of colon and rectal cancer are the same in men and women.

4. Animal fats play an etiologic role. They cause an increase in total fecal bile acids that stimulate the generation of reactive oxygen metabolites, enhancing conversion of unsaturated fatty acids to compounds that promote cellular proliferation.

5. Fiber (cereal products, vegetables, and fruits) plays a protective role. Its exact role is not known, but binding to carcinogens and thus reducing their contact with colonic epithelium and increasing their transit time may be important.

6. Increased calcium intake inhibits colonic proliferation, and is associated with decreased risk of colorectal cancer.

7. Clinical risk factors
   a. Familial
      (1) FAP accounts for less than 1% of all colorectal cancers.
      (2) Hereditary nonpolyposis colorectal cancer (HNPCC) accounts for 5% to 10% of all cancers.
      (3) IBD: risk of chronic ulcerative colitis increases after 10 years of active disease by 1% cumulative /year. It is less in Crohn colitis.
      (4) Adenomatous polyps
   b. General: age greater than 40 years
      (1) Family history of colon cancer
      (2) Personal history of colon polyps or cancer (three-fold increase)
      (3) Pelvic radiation for gynecologic cancer (two- to three-fold increase)

B. Pathogenesis

1. Development is a multistep process wherein carcinomas arise from benign adenomas.

2. The mucosal epithelium progresses through a series of molecular and cellular events that lead to altered proliferation, cellular accumulation, and glandular disarray leading to the formation of adenomatous polyps. Further genetic alteration results in higher degrees of cellular atypia and glandular disorganization (dysplasia), which may evolve to a carcinoma.

3. The adenoma-to-carcinoma sequence is always associated with genetic changes, even in sporadic colon cancers. Sporadic polyps and cancers are associated with multiple somatic mutations contributed by environmental insults.

4. Genetic changes that lead to development of adenomas include:
   a. Alteration in proto-oncogenes.
   b. Loss of tumor suppressor gene. In more than 75% of cases, stepwise tumor progression is associated with loss of tumor suppressor gene designated DCC (deleted in colorectal cancer) on chromosome 18q– (maintains normal cell–cell adhesive interactions).
   c. Deletions of chromosome 17p involving the p-53 tumor suppressor gene.
   d. Abnormalities of genes involved in DNA repair.

C. Clinical features

1. Patients may have intermittent abdominal pain, bleeding, nausea, vomiting, and iron deficiency anemia.

2. Changes in bowel habits such as constipation and decreased stool caliber are found in constricting rectal cancers. With locally advanced rectal cancers symptoms of tenesmus, urgency, and perineal pain can occur.

D. Diagnosis

1. Presence of nonspecific symptoms

2. In fecal occult blood test in the asymptomatic population, results are positive in 2.5% of patients, and among those only 10% to 15% have colorectal cancer. The test is not specific, because not all polyp and tumors bleed or may bleed intermittently. False-positive results may occur with high-peroxidase diets with rare beef. False-negative results may occur with oral intake of iron, cimetidine, antacids, and ascorbic acids.

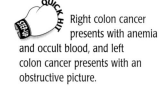
Right colon cancer presents with anemia and occult blood, and left colon cancer presents with an obstructive picture.

3. Screening is necessary in the following instances:
    a. Every 5 to 10 years in asymptomatic individuals starting at age 50.
    b. Yearly, in first-degree relatives of individuals with known hereditary colon cancer syndromes starting at age 20.
    c. Yearly, in patients who have had an adenomatous polyp removed, until no polyps are apparent, and then every 3 to 5 years.
    d. 8 to 10 years after disease activity in patients who have had chronic ulcerative colitis, and then yearly.
E. Staging
    1. 95% percent of all colorectal cancers are adenocarcinomas.
    2. 10% to 20% of adenocarcinomas are described as mucinous, or colloid based on abundant production of mucin. These tumors are associated with a poorer 5-year survival.
    3. Staging is based on the tumor-node-metastasis (TNM) classification.
F. Modes of spread
    1. Colorectal cancer spreads by direct invasion, lymphatic spread, and hematogenous spread. Most commonly, the cancer spreads to the liver, lungs, and bone.
    2. Another mode of spread is via intraluminal or extraluminal exfoliation of tumor cells with subsequent implantation, which may occur during surgical resection with tumor spillage, leading to recurrences in bowel anastomosis, abdominal incisions, or other intra-abdominal sites. Tumors penetrating the intestinal wall can shed cells intraperitoneally and cause carcinomatosis.
G. Management
    1. Surgical therapy is the mainstay of treatment. If colorectal cancer is diagnosed in the early stages, it is curable by surgery.
    2. Surgical goal is resection of the primary colorectal cancer with adequate normal proximal and distal margin (2 cm, tumors rarely spread more than 2 cm intramurally, distally), lateral margin, and regional lymph nodes.
    3. Evaluation for metastasis is important. Careful physical examination is essential, looking for hepatomegaly, ascites, or adenopathy. For rectal tumors, assessing the distance of the tumor from the anal verge and mobility are important in determining resectability, and the type of operation required.
    4. Laboratory studies should include a complete blood count, liver function tests (LFTs), and a carcinoembryonic antigen (CEA) assay. A CT scan helps delineate distal metastases. Colonoscopy is essential to look for synchronous lesions.
    5. Adjuvant radiation therapy is used for rectal tumors in which the incidence of local recurrence is significant, including those extending though the bowel wall or with lymph node involvement. Radiation can be given preoperatively or postoperatively. Preoperative therapy prevents radiation to the small bowel and neorectum, and it improves survival.
    6. Adjuvant chemotherapy. Despite local-regional control, patients who die from colon cancer, die from disseminated disease: 25% of patients with stage II disease, and 50% with stage III disease die from growth of micrometastatic disease present at the time of primary resection. Chemotherapy is offered to patients with stage III colon cancer to improve survival, as well as to patients with stages II and III rectal cancer.
H. Follow-up
    1. A subset of colon cancer patients can be cured. Comprehensive follow-up program in patients is appropriate.
    2. Recurrences are likely, with 50% evident within 18 months of surgery, and 90% evident by 3 years. Metachronous primary tumors develop in 5% of patients.
    3. CEA is not helpful as a screening or diagnostic test, but as a tumor marker. Concentrations are elevated in 90% of patients with disseminated disease and 20% with localized disease. In two-thirds of patients with recurrence, an increased CEA level is the first marker of disease.
    4. Follow-up with periodic physical examinations, CEA assay, LFTs, CT yearly, endoscopy, and chest x-ray.

5. Hepatic metastasis is the most common site of spread. A subset is resectable.

6. Pulmonary metastasis: 10% of patients with colorectal cancer usually have widespread metastatic disease. If the pulmonary metastasis is solitary, it can be resected with a 20% 5-year survival rate.

7. Prognostic factors

   a. Patients younger than 40 years of age present with more advanced stages than do symptomatic patients.

   b. Prognosis is poorer when obstruction and perforation are present.

   c. Exophytic tumors are associated with less advanced stage compared with ulcerative tumors.

   d. Prognosis is poorer when blood vessel invasion, lymphatic vessel invasion, perineural invasion, and aneuploid tumors are present.

I. Other types of colorectal cancer

1. Hereditary nonpolyposis colorectal cancer (HNPCC)

   a. HNPCC is also known as Lynch syndrome I. Lynch syndrome II is the same as Lynch syndrome I but with a predisposition to other cancers (for example, endometrial, ovary, and stomach).

   b. It is responsible for approximately 4% to 6% of all colorectal carcinomas.

   c. It is inherited in an autosomal dominance pattern. The genetic mutation is seen in the DNA mismatch repair genes (hMSH2, hMLH1, hPMS1).

   d. Cancers arise in adenomas, but polyposis does not occur. Adenomas and carcinomas occur at an early age (adenomas in the 20- to 30-year range, and carcinomas in the 40- to 45-year range). Tumors are often proximal and multiple.

   e. HNPCC is defined by the Amsterdam criteria:

      (1) Three relatives with colorectal cancer, one of whom is a first-degree relative of the other two.

      (2) Colorectal cancer must involve at least two generations.

      (3) At least one cancer must occur before the age of 50 years.

2. Carcinoid tumors

   a. Most GI carcinoids are found in the ileum. The remainder of tumors are found in the appendix, rectum, and colon.

   b. Most rectal tumors are less than 2 cm, submucosal, yellow-gray nodules. Patients are asymptomatic but may present with hematochezia.

   c. The majority are less than 1 cm in diameter, and can be removed by local excision. Transanal local excision is the treatment of choice because small tumors rarely metastasize.

   d. Tumor size is a prognostic factor. Lesions greater than 2 cm are more commonly malignant, but seldom give rise to metastases.

   e. Carcinoid tumors do not give rise to carcinoid syndrome.

3. Lymphomas

   a. These rare tumors account for less than 0.5% of all colorectal malignancies.

   b. In most cases, widespread disease is documented.

   c. Treatment is chemotherapy and radiation therapy.

VIII. Anal Cancer

A. General principles

1. Anal cancer is uncommon and accounts for 2% of large bowel cancers.

B. Carcinoma of the anal margin

1. Squamous cell carcinoma (SCC)

   a. SCC grows slowly, and has rolled edges with central ulceration.

   b. It is usually well differentiated, and diagnosis is delayed.

   c. All anal ulcers should be biopsied to disprove SCC.

   d. Lymphatic drainage is to the inguinal lymph nodes. SCC is slow-growing and late to metastasize. Surgical therapy involves local excision. If the cancer has invaded the underlying sphincter muscle, metastases can occur proximally along the superior and middle rectal nodes.

   e. Overall 5-year survival is 34% to 82% depending on stage.

QUICK HIT The anal canal above and below the dentate line has different lymphatic drainage. Thus, the anal canal is divided into the area above the dentate line, called the anal canal, and below the dentate line, called the anal margin.

2. Basal cell carcinoma
   a. This rare cancer occurs three times more frequently in men than women.
   b. Lesions are centrally ulcerated and irregular with raised edges.
   c. Local excision is treatment of choice.
   d. Overall 5-year survival is 73%.
C. Bowen disease
   1. In this rare, slow growing intraepidermal, squamous cell carcinoma, lesions are scaly or crusted plaque. Biopsy is confirmatory.
   2. From 70% to 80% of patients eventually develop primary internal malignancy or skin cancer.
   3. Wide local excision is the treatment of choice.
D. Perianal Paget disease
   1. Perianal Paget disease is a rare malignant neoplasm of the intraepidermal portion of apocrine glands, with or without dermal involvement. Lesions are erythematous, scaly, or eczematoid and plaque-like.
   2. It has a long preinvasive course, but invasive adenocarcinoma may develop.
   3. The disease occurs in more women than men, with the highest incidence in the seventh decade.
   4. 80% of patients develop second primary carcinoma (e.g., breast or rectum).
   5. Biopsy reveals Paget cells—large pale, vacuolated cells with hyperchromatic eccentric nuclei.
   6. Wide local excision is the treatment of choice.
   7. Metastasis to the inguinal nodes, pelvic lymph nodes, liver, bone, lung, brain, or bladder may occur. Once metastasis has occurred, prognosis is poor.

IX. Carcinoma of the Anal Canal

A. General principles
   1. The carcinomas arise from the ducts of the anal glands.
   2. They present with pain, bleeding, and a perianal mass.
   3. Diagnosis is usually made at an advanced stage, when disease has spread beyond hope for cure.
   4. Abdominoperineal resection is the treatment of choice. There is no role for radiation therapy.
   5. This includes SCC, basaloid (cloacogenic arising from the anal transition zone), and mucoepidermoid carcinoma.
   6. Metastasis may occur, with 40% of tumors metastasizing to the superior rectal nodes, and 33% to the inguinal nodes.
   7. Overall 5-year survival is 50%.
B. Management
   1. Local excision: reserved for small well-differentiated lesions that involve the submucosa only, or poor-risk patients.
   2. Recurrence rates are high after local excision.
   3. Abdominoperineal resection: 5-year survival averages 50%, with 25% to 30% local recurrence after surgery.
   4. Combination chemoradiation therapy. If the lesion disappears grossly and is microscopically absent, no further therapy is needed. If there is residual disease or recurrence, than proceed to surgery.
   5. Cure rates are between 70% and 90%.

ANORECTAL DISORDERS

I. Hemorrhoids

A. General principles
   1. In the upper anal canal, there are three cushions of submucosal tissue composed of connective tissue containing venules and smooth muscle fibers. Usually there are three cushions: left lateral, right anterior, and right posterior.

2. Their function is to aid anal continence. During defecation, they become engorged with blood and cushion the anal canal, and support the lining of the canal.

3. Muscles that arise partly from the internal sphincter and partly from the conjoint longitudinal muscle support the anal cushions.

4. Hemorrhoid is the term used to describe the downward displacement of the anal cushions, causing dilatation of the contained venules, and they develop when the supportive tissues of the anal cushions deteriorate.

B. Classification
1. External hemorrhoids are dilated venules of the inferior hemorrhoidal plexuses below the dentate line. Thrombosed external hemorrhoids are intravascular clots in the venules.

2. Internal hemorrhoids are the anal cushions located above the dentate line that have become prolapsed. These are graded according to the degree of prolapse.
   a. First-degree: the anal cushions slide down beyond the dentate line on straining.
   b. Second-degree: the anal cushions prolapse through the anus on straining but spontaneously reduce.
   c. Third-degree: the anal cushions prolapse through the anus on straining or exertion, and require manual replacement into the anal canal.
   d. Fourth-degree: the prolapse is not manually reducible.

C. Clinical features
1. The most common manifestation is painless, bright red rectal bleeding associated with bowel movements.

2. The common complaints of burning, itching, swelling, and pain are usually not from hemorrhoids but from pruritus ani, anal abrasion, fissure, thrombosed external hemorrhoids, or prolapsed anal papilla. Patients with thrombosed external hemorrhoids present with abrupt onset of a mass and pain. The pain usually becomes minimal after the fourth day.

3. Patients may also have a feeling of incomplete evacuation. Most patients with thrombosed external hemorrhoids do not give a history of straining, physical exertion, or hemorrhoids.

4. In chronic prolapse, exposed rectal mucosa often causes perianal irritation and mucous staining on the underwear.

5. Congestion of external hemorrhoids or skin tags can cause pain. Symptoms are aggravated by diarrhea or constipation.

D. Diagnosis
1. Diagnosis of hemorrhoids is by careful examination.
2. Internal hemorrhoids cannot be palpated.
3. Anoscopy is used to look for vascular engorgement.

E. Management
1. According to modern concepts, prolapse of the anal cushions is initiated by the shearing effect of the passage of a large hard stool, or by the precipitous act of defecation, as in urgent diarrhea. If prolapse of the vascular cushion can be prevented, the anal cushions return to their normal state, and symptoms are ameliorated.

2. A high-fiber diet is ideal for first-degree and second-degree hemorrhoids.

3. Rubber band ligation is suitable for first-degree and second-degree hemorrhoids that do not respond to bulk-forming agents. This technique is also suitable for some third-degree hemorrhoids.

4. Infrared photocoagulation coagulates tissue protein, or evaporates water in the cells. This technique is used for first-degree and second-degree hemorrhoids.

5. Hemorrhoidectomy is considered when hemorrhoids are severely prolapsed requiring manual reduction, or when they are complicated by associated pathology such as ulceration, fissures, fistulas, large hypertrophied papilla, or excessive skin tags.

6. Treatment of thrombosed external hemorrhoids is aimed at prevention of recurrent clot, relief of severe pain, and prevention of residual skin tags. It involves excision of the hemorrhoid or evacuation of the clot.

7. If pain is subsiding, conservative treatment is with sitz baths, proper anal hygiene, and bulk-forming agents.

8. If strangulated hemorrhoids are untreated, they progress to ulceration and necrosis. Pain is severe, and urinary retention is common. Proper treatment requires urgent or emergent hemorrhoidectomy.

II. Anal Fissure

A. General principles
1. An anal fissure is an ulcer in the lower portion of the anal canal.
2. It may be acute or chronic.
3. The primary fissure occurs without association with other local or systemic diseases.
4. The secondary fissure occurs in association with Crohn disease, leukemia, or aplastic anemia.
5. Most tears of the anal canal can be traced to the passage of large, hard stool or explosive diarrhea, trauma to the anus, or a tear during vaginal delivery.
6. In men, almost all fissures are located in the posterior midline, whereas in women, 10% are in the anterior midline.

B. Clinical features
1. Patients have increased resting anal resting pressure, caused by the increased tone of the internal sphincter muscle.
2. Anal pain during and after defecation is the most prominent symptom. The pain is described as burning, throbbing, or dull aching.
3. Bleeding is common and stains the toilet paper.

C. Diagnosis. Physical examination confirms the diagnosis. Chronic fissures have a triad of a fissure, sentinel skin tag, and hypertrophied anal papilla. The sentinel skin tag is the fibrotic or edematous skin adjacent to the fissure.

D. Management
1. Initial treatment of acute anal fissure is pain relief with proper anal hygiene, and warm sitz baths to relax the anal canal. Bulk-forming agents are used to relieve constipation. Nitroglycerin ointment or calcium-channel blockers applied topically help. Anal fissures usually heal within 6 weeks.
2. Surgery is not usually required unless the fissure fails conservative therapy.
3. Lateral internal sphincterotomy is the surgical procedure of choice.
4. Fissures or ulcers in Crohn disease are larger and deeper than primary anal fissures. The surrounding skin is macerated and edematous. Treatment consists of proper anal hygiene and treatment of the underlying inflammatory disease.

III. Anorectal Abscesses

A. Etiology
1. In the wall of the anal canal, a variable number of anal glands (4 to 10) lined by stratified columnar epithelium have direct openings into the anal crypts at the dentate line.
2. Infection of the glands leads to perianal abscess.
3. Because the glands lie between the internal and external sphincter, an intersphincteric abscess is formed. Infection then spreads to various spaces: perianal, ischiorectal, intersphincteric, and supralevator.
4. Supralevator abscesses, which are uncommon, can arise from upward extension of an intersphincteric abscess.

B. Clinical features
1. Presenting features include pain and fever. Depending on the location, a swollen mass may be felt.
2. Intersphincteric abscesses do not present with overt perianal swelling.

C. Diagnosis
1. An anorectal abscess is suspected when anorectal pain is so severe that rectal examination is not possible.
2. A supralevator abscess is difficult to diagnose. Examination reveals a bulging tender mass on either side of the lower rectum, or posteriorly above the anorectal ring.

D. Management
1. Treatment is primary incision and drainage. Antibiotics after drainage are given to patients with cardiac valvular abnormalities, or to patients who are immunodeficient.
2. Perianal abscesses are the most superficial and easiest to treat. A cruciate incision is made on the most prominent part of the skin subcutaneous tissue overlying the abscess cavity.
3. Ischiorectal abscess causes diffuse swelling of the ischioanal fossa. Drainage is the same as in perianal abscess.

IV. Fistula-in-Ano

A. Etiology. In this chronic form of perianal abscess, the abscess cavity does not heal completely, but becomes an inflammatory tract with the primary internal opening in the anal crypt at the dentate line, and the secondary opening in the perianal skin.

B. Classification. The four main types are based on the relation of the fistula to the sphincter muscle:
1. Intersphincteric: fistula tract traverses through the internal sphincter.
2. Transsphincteric: fistula tract traverses through the external sphincter.
3. Suprasphincteric: fistula starts in the intersphincteric plane, and then passes upward to a point above the puborectalis muscle, and then laterally over this muscle, and downward between the puborectal and levator muscles into the ischiorectal fossa.
4. Extrasphincteric: the fistula passes from the perineal skin through the ischiorectal fossa, and levator ani muscle, and finally penetrates the rectal wall. This may arise from trauma, foreign body, pelvic abscess, or cryptoglandular abscess.

C. Clinical features
1. Most patients have a history of anorectal abscess subsequently associated with subsequent drainage.
2. Low rectal or anal canal carcinomas may present as fistulas.
3. A superficial tract may be palpable. The external opening is usually visible as a red elevation of granulation tissue, with purulent or serosanguineous drainage.

D. Management. Principles of fistula surgery include unroofing the fistula, elimination of the primary opening, and establishing adequate drainage. Open the entire fistula tract with a guide in place.

V. Pilonidal Sinus

A. Epidemiology and etiology
1. Pilonidal sinus is more likely to occur in hirsute patients.
2. Incidence is highest in the second and third decades of life.
3. The cause is an infected hair follicle in the sacrococcygeal area.

B. Clinical features
1. Pilonidal sinus may present with an acute abscess that ruptures spontaneously, leaving unhealed sinuses with chronic drainage.
2. Most sinus tracts run cephalad (93%).

C. Diagnosis
1. Physical examination may reveal pits in the intergluteal folds.
2. The differential diagnosis includes furuncles of the skin, anal fistula, syphilitic or tuberculous granulomas, and osteomyelitis with multiple draining sinuses.

D. Management. Drainage of an acute abscess may be performed under local anesthesia. There may be tufts of hair in the abscess cavity that must be removed.

VI. **Rectal Prolapse**
   A. Epidemiology and etiology
      1. Procidentia is an uncommon condition, in which the full thickness of the rectal wall turns inside out into or through the anal canal. The extruded rectum is seen as concentric rings of mucosa. The cause is poorly understood, and the disorder is a form of intussusception. Most patients have a history of straining with intractable constipation or chronic diarrhea. High incidence in patients with mental retardation. Patients have impaired resting and voluntary sphincter activity, and impaired continence.
      2. Predominates in females with a female:male ratio of 5:1 to 6:1.
      3. Classification
         a. Partial: prolapse of rectal mucosa only.
         b. Complete: first-degree with an occult prolapse. Several anatomic defects are constantly demonstrated in patients with chronic rectal prolapse.
         c. Complete: second-degree; prolapse to, but not through the anus.
         d. Complete; third-degree; protrusion through the anus for a variable distance.
   B. Clinical features. Early symptoms include anorectal discomfort during defecation. Feeling of incomplete evacuation is common. In overt prolapse, protrusion occurs only during or after defecation. As the problem becomes more pronounced, the prolapse may be precipitated by coughing, walking, and exertion. Bleeding from ulcerated mucosa.
   C. Diagnosis. Demonstrated on clinical exam by asking the patient to strain, or in the bathroom asking the patient to defecate. Occult prolapse by defecography.
   D. Management
      1. The goal is to repair the prolapse, and prevent intussusception from recurring.
      2. The most reliable repair is via the abdomen involving anterior resection with rectopexy.
      3. For elderly or unfit patients, a transperineal rectosigmoidectomy is more appropriate.
      4. Incontinence is due to mechanical stretch of the sphincter, as well as pudendal nerve dysfunction. 50% of patients improve after repair.

APPENDIX AND APPENDICITIS

I. **Appendicitis**
   A. Etiology. The cause of appendicitis is unclear.
      1. However, luminal obstruction resulting from lymphoid hyperplasia, secondary to bacterial (*Salmonella, Shigella*) or viral (infectious mononucleosis) has been postulated.
      2. Fecaliths (literally fecal stones, or hard stool pellets) can also cause luminal obstruction, and may be responsible for up to 30% of cases.
   B. Clinical features
      1. Typically, patients present with vague periumbilical pain, fever, anorexia, nausea and/or vomiting, right lower quadrant pain, and tenderness.
      2. Occasionally, patients present with urinary or other complaints.
   C. Diagnosis
      1. Dunphy sign: increased pain with coughing or other movement.
      2. Rovsing sign: left lower quadrant palpation induces right lower quadrant pain.
      3. Obturator sign: pain on internal rotation of the right hip.
      4. Psoas sign: pain on extension of the right hip.
   D. Laboratory
      1. Leukocytosis, with a moderate elevation in white blood cell count, less than 20,000/mL is seen.
      2. Pyuria (white blood cells in the urine) may be present.

E. Radiology
  1. Plain film may show a calcified fecalith.
  2. Ultrasound shows thick-walled, noncompressible luminal lesion (target lesion). This image may be helpful in ruling out other pathologies.
  3. CT allows for prompt diagnosis, and obviate the need and consequent costs of in-hospital observation.
F. Management: open or laparoscopic appendectomy.
G. Unusual presentations
  1. Variants in certain patient populations.
    a. Children: higher perforation rates may occur. CT is helpful.
    b. Elderly: higher perforation rates may occur. Be sure to rule out cecal neoplasia.
    c. Immunocompromised patients: cytomegalovirus-related bowel perforation and neutropenic colitis may masquerade as appendicitis.
    d. Pregnant women: confusion may arise due to normal elevations in white blood cell counts, and the presence of nausea and vomiting. Be aggressive, because perforated appendix has a high fetal mortality rate (greater than 30%).
  2. Appendiceal masses: form an average of 5 days after symptom onset, and usually represent a phlegmon or abscess. These should be managed nonoperatively, with percutaneous drainage with or without IV antibiotics.
H. Appendiceal neoplasms
  1. Carcinoids
    a. 50% of GI carcinoids arise in the appendix. They have a firm yellow appearance.
    b. Most are found incidentally.
    c. Size is prognostic. Neoplasms less than 1.5 cm are curative by appendectomy, and those 2 cm or greater require right hemicolectomy.
  2. Mucoceles
    a. These neoplasms are either cystadenomas or cystadenocarcinomas.
    b. Cystadenomas: appendectomy is curative.
    c. Cystadenocarcinomas: an association with peritoneal implantation leads to pseudomyxoma peritonei, which has no effective cure, and may need several debulking operations.
  3. Adenocarcinoma
    a. These neoplasms are rare.
    b. T1 lesions are cured by appendectomy, and more advanced lesions require right hemicolectomy.
    c. There is a high incidence of secondary GI tumors.
I. Appendiceal cancer
  1. This form of cancer is rare (1.3% of all appendectomy specimens).
  2. Carcinoids
    a. Appendiceal carcinoids represent two-thirds of all appendiceal neoplasms. Half of all GI carcinoids are in the appendix.
    b. These are usually seen as an incidental finding after an appendectomy. The mean age of patients is 41.
    c. The majority are small, less than 2 cm, and have minimal metastatic potential. Those greater than 2 cm have metastatic potential. Appendectomy is sufficient. If larger lesion, or close to the base, need right hemicolectomy.
    d. Overall, 5-year survival is 99%.
  3. Appendectomy for benign disease is sufficient, even if in cases of perforation that result in mucinous ascites.
  4. In the malignant form of the disease, the neoplastic mucosa invades the wall of the appendix, and may implant in the peritoneum, causing pseudomyxoma peritonei. The 5-year survival is 50%.

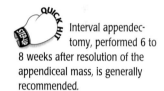

QUICK HIT

Interval appendectomy, performed 6 to 8 weeks after resolution of the appendiceal mass, is generally recommended.

CHAPTER 7

Hepatobiliary System

Santosh Shenoy, MD
Magesh Sundaram, MD

HEPATIC SYSTEM

I. General Principles

A. Anatomy
1. The portal vein and hepatic artery are the vascular inflow to the liver. The hepatic veins are the venous outflow from the liver.
2. The liver is divided into the right and left lobes by an imaginary plane, running from the gallbladder to the left side of the inferior vena cava (IVC), known as the portal fissure or Cantlie line.
3. The functional anatomy of the liver is eight segments, each supplied by a single portal triad (portal vein, hepatic artery, and bile duct). These segments are further organized into four sectors separated by the scissurae containing the three main hepatic veins, which drain into the IVC.
4. Hepatic artery
   a. The common hepatic artery arises from the celiac axis, and runs adjacent to the superior border of the pancreas to the porta hepatis or hepatoduodenal ligament. It becomes the proper hepatic artery after giving off the gastroduodenal artery. The proper hepatic artery then splits into the right and left hepatic arteries, which enter the liver.
   b. The hepatic artery provides approximately 25% of the hepatic blood flow, and 30% to 50% of its oxygenation. In the liver, the right hepatic artery branches to the right anterior and right posterior segments, and the left hepatic artery branches to the left lateral and left medial segments.
   c. The most common variant of hepatic artery anatomy is the right hepatic artery arising from the superior mesenteric artery. The left hepatic artery may arise from the left gastric artery in 25% of individuals as well.
5. Portal vein
   a. The portal vein provides about 75% of the hepatic inflow, and due to this large volume of circulation, it also provides 75% more oxygenated blood to the liver than the hepatic artery.
   b. The portal vein forms behind the neck of the pancreas at the confluence of the superior mesenteric vein and the splenic vein. It is posterior to the bile duct and the hepatic artery in the hepatoduodenal ligament. The portal vein divides into the right and left portal branches as it enters the liver.
   c. There are a number of potential connections between the portal venous system and the systemic venous system. Under conditions of high portal venous pressure, these portosystemic connections may enlarge, and clinically manifest portal hypertension. The more significant locations are:
      (1) The coronary vein, draining the stomach and the distal esophagus.
      (2) Umbilical and abdominal wall veins, which recanalize from flow through the umbilical vein in the ligamentum teres, resulting in caput medusae.

> **QUICK HIT**
> The portal vein carries the venous drainage from the entire capillary system of the small and large intestine, pancreas, and spleen to the liver for further digestive processing.

      (3) The superior hemorrhoidal plexus, which receives portal flow from the inferior mesenteric vein tributaries, and may cause large hemorrhoids.

      (4) Retroperitoneal collaterals, ultimately leading back to the vena cava.

  6. Hepatic veins

    a. The three main hepatic veins entering the suprahepatic IVC are the right, middle, and left hepatic veins.

    b. The caudate lobe of the liver sits directly above the IVC, and has three or four small but prominent branches draining it directly into the IVC, not to the three main hepatic veins.

  7. Nerves and lymphatics

    a. Lymphatic channels in the liver may be deep and found adjacent to the portal and hepatic veins, or superficial and found along the liver capsule. The superficial lymphatic channels drain the liver to the coronary and falciform ligaments, to the diaphragm, and to periesophageal nodes. The deep lymphatic channels drain to nodes at the hepatic hilum, in the porta hepatis, and adjacent to the IVC.

    b. The liver has a rich parasympathetic and sympathetic innervation.

      (1) Vagal innervation adjacent to the bile ducts stimulates the digestive metabolism functions of the liver, as well as increases glycogen synthesis in the liver.

      (2) Sympathetic innervation from the lower thoracic and celiac ganglia to the liver run adjacent to the hepatic arteries and monitor intrahepatic sinusoidal pressure. Afferent nerves to the liver register pain when the liver capsule is distended.

B. Physiology

  1. Bile formation and secretion

    a. The formation and secretion of bile are major functions of the liver. Bile secretion is initiated at the hepatocytes, by the driving force of osmotic filtration across the sinusoids.

    b. Bile is a clear yellow aqueous solution composed of bile salts, electrolytes, lipids, and amino acids. The primary bile salts are chenodeoxycholic acid and cholic acid, which are produced from cholesterol, and then conjugated with glycine and taurine within the hepatocytes. The primary bile acids, when exposed to intestinal bacteria, are converted to the secondary bile acids, deoxycholic acid and lithocolic acid.

    c. Bile is used to direct cholesterol metabolism, excrete potentially toxic lipophilic substances such as drugs and heavy metals, and promote absorption of lipids and lipid-soluble vitamins. Bile, which also contains IgA, prevents the systemic manifestation of enteric infections.

  2. Bilirubin metabolism

    a. Bilirubin is derived from heme in the breakdown process of red blood cells.

    b. It is initially bound to serum albumin, and circulates as the bilirubin-albumin complex. This complex then enters the hepatic circulation, where it is dissociated. Here, the bilirubin is conjugated to glucoronic acid, is secreted in the bile and passes into the gastrointestinal (GI) tract.

    c. Enteric bacteria then deconjugate the bilirubin to urobilinogens. Most of this urobilinogen is further oxidized and reabsorbed into the enterohepatic circulation. A small portion is excreted into the urine and excreted into the stool, which imparts the yellow color to the urine, and the brown color to the stool.

  3. Carbohydrate metabolism

    a. After meals, the absorbed carbohydrates are circulated systemically and reach the liver, where most of them are converted to the storage form of glycogen.

    b. During fasting for more than 48 to 72 hours, the glycogen is converted to glucose, and provides energy to glucose-dependent tissues. The liver then

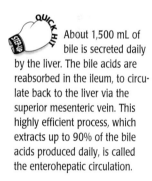

QUICK HIT
The coronary vein drains the lesser curvature of the stomach and the distal esophagus. In portal hypertension, this important tributary of the portal vein enlarges and leads to esophageal varices.

QUICK HIT
About 1,500 mL of bile is secreted daily by the liver. The bile acids are reabsorbed in the ileum, to circulate back to the liver via the superior mesenteric vein. This highly efficient process, which extracts up to 90% of the bile acids produced daily, is called the enterohepatic circulation.

assumes the role of gluconeogenesis from amino acids, mainly from alanine derived from muscle breakdown.

4. Lipid metabolism
   a. Fatty acids are synthesized in the liver during states of glucose excess, when the ability of the liver to store glycogen has been exceeded.
   b. Excess fatty deposition leads to steatosis, or diffuse fatty infiltration of the liver.

5. Protein metabolism
   a. Ingested protein is broken down into the amino acids and circulated throughout the body. Here, they are used as the building blocks for proteins, enzymes, hormones, and nucleotides.
   b. Excess amino acids are transported to the liver to be converted to glucose, ketone bodies, or fats.
   c. The end product of amino acid catabolism is ammonia, which is converted into urea by the liver.

6. Protein synthesis. The liver is the main site of synthesis of various other proteins, such as the coagulation factors, iron-binding proteins, alpha 1-antitrypsin, ceruloplasmin, albumin, and acute-phase proteins.

7. Vitamin metabolism. The liver is responsible for the metabolism of the fat-soluble vitamins A, D, E, and K. Bile is a cofactor in the intestinal absorption of these lipophilic vitamins.
   a. Vitamin A is stored solely in the liver.
   b. Vitamin K is a cofactor in the posttranslational carboxylation of the synthesized coagulation factors 2, 7, 9, 10, protein C, and protein S.

II. Evaluation of the Liver

A. History and physical examination for evaluation of liver disease
   1. Jaundice and icterus refer to the yellow appearance to the skin and the eyes as a result of retention and systemic deposition of bile pigments. Jaundice or icterus is a reflection of liver disease, including obstruction of the biliary tract, acute hepatic injury from drugs and toxins, and the chronic loss of hepatic reserve from cirrhosis due to alcohol, the hepatitis virus, iron or copper, and parasitic infection.
   2. The triad of splenomegaly, ascites, and caput medusae (dilated abdominal wall veins) indicates portal hypertension.
   3. A history of pruritus suggests cholestasis, either intrahepatic or extrahepatic. Causes may be at the hepatocellular level (viral hepatitis), canalicular level (drugs, total parenteral nutrition, amyloidosis), or biliary ductal level (PBC, PSC).

B. Diagnostic liver enzymes
   1. Bilirubin total and fractionated, conjugated (direct), and unconjugated (indirect) are affected in a number of disease processes and are related to the metabolism of the bilirubin.
      a. Unconjugated bilirubin is generally elevated in hemolysis, drug hepatotoxicity, inherited enzymatic disorders, and the physiologic disorders of the newborn.
      b. Conjugated bilirubin is usually elevated in hepatocellular diseases, cholestasis, or biliary obstruction.
   2. The serum transaminases alanine aminotransferase (ALT) and aspartate aminotransferase (AST) are nonspecific indicators of acute hepatocellular injury. However, an AST/ALT ratio greater than 2:1 is more suggestive of alcoholic liver disease.
   3. Alkaline phosphatase can be used as a marker of cholestasis. Alkaline phosphatase is released by damaged hepatocytes as a consequence of cholestasis, but other organ and tissue production of alkaline phosphatase (for example, bone, placenta, kidneys, and leukocytes) make it a nonspecific indicator in

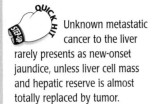

QUICK HIT

Unknown metastatic cancer to the liver rarely presents as new-onset jaundice, unless liver cell mass and hepatic reserve is almost totally replaced by tumor.

the evaluation of liver disease. The heat-stable fraction of alkaline phosphatase is more suggestive of liver pathology.

4. The synthetic function of the liver is measured by the serum albumin level and the prothrombin time (PT). Albumin is produced solely by the liver, and is reflective of the protein metabolism function, as well as the digestive K-dependent coagulation factors 2, 7, 9, and 10. The most sensitive indicator of deficiency of hepatic synthetic function is an abnormal (prolonged) PT. No improvement in the PT despite vitamin K administration reflects severe hepatic functional loss.

C. Imaging and diagnostic tests
1. Ultrasound
   a. This quick, easy to perform, noninvasive test involves no radiation.
   b. It is the primary modality to identify cholelithiasis. Focal and diffuse liver disease can be identified.
   c. Doppler ultrasound allows for evaluation of vascular anatomy and pressures.
2. Computed tomography (CT) scan
   a. To evaluate the liver for tumors and other pathology, a CT scan with constrast should be obtained.
   b. It demonstrates hepatic segmental anatomy, focal disease such as tumors, or diffuse liver disease such as cirrhosis or steatosis.
3. HIDA scan shows excretion of tracer along the biliary tract and thus, is useful for detecting bile leaks or obstruction.
4. Magnetic resonance imaging (MRI) scan
   a. MRI provides exquisite detail of hepatic parenchyma, and finer detail of tumors to differentiate benign (hemangiomas) from malignant.
   b. Reconstruction of the biliary tree with great detail is possible, including recognition of ductal stone disease, biliary damage, or tumors, through magnetic resonance cholangiopancreatography (MRCP).

III. Benign Disorders

A. Infection
1. Pyogenic abscesses
   a. Most pyogenic hepatic abscesses are caused by infection originating from the GI tract or the biliary tract.
      (1) In the preantibiotic era, the most common cause of pyogenic liver abscess was appendicitis.
      (2) Now, the more common causes are related to malignancy, or stone disease.
   b. The potential routes of hepatic exposure to bacteria are the biliary tree, portal vein, and hepatic artery, direct extension from nearby foci of infection (gallbladder, kidney), and trauma.
   c. Common intra-abdominal sources of pyogenic abscesses include appendicitis, diverticulitis, cholecystitis, infected pancreatitis/pancreatic abscess, and perinephric abscess.
   d. Pyogenic abscesses with no identifiable primary infection are called cryptogenic hepatic abscesses.
   e. Signs and symptoms may include fever (90%), malaise, rigors, and right upper quadrant (RUQ) pain. Chills and weight loss may be seen in 50% of patients. Symptom duration is typically less than 2 weeks. Jaundice is uncommon, unless biliary tract obstruction is also present. At the time of presentation, 50% of patients have positive blood cultures.
   f. Diagnosis is made most commonly with CT scan (93% accurate).
   g. Organisms cultured include gram-negative aerobes, which are found 68% of the time. *Escherichia coli* and *Klebsiella* species are most commonly isolated. Aerobic *Streptococcus* and *Staphylococcus* are seen in 20% and 12% of pyogenic abscesses, respectively. Increased use of indwelling biliary stents

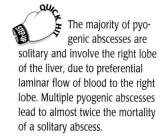

The majority of pyogenic abscesses are solitary and involve the right lobe of the liver, due to preferential laminar flow of blood to the right lobe. Multiple pyogenic abscesses lead to almost twice the mortality of a solitary abscess.

and broad-spectrum antibiotics has led to an increased prevalence of *Pseudomonas*, anaerobic *Streptococcus*, and fungi.

    h. Management
- (1) Percutaneous abscess aspiration and drainage, and selective antibiotics.
- (2) Treatment of the primary intra-abdominal source of infection is mandatory (e.g., surgical management of appendicitis, diverticulitis). Surgical co-drainage of hepatic abscess during laparotomy is still required in up to one-third of patients.

    i. Changing trends involve increased incidence, decreased mortality, better identification (CT), etiology (more likely caused by biliary tract manipulation, such as stents, or malignant biliary obstruction), and better treatment (percutaneous drainage, selective antibiotics).

2. Amebic liver abscess
    a. Amebic liver abscess is the most frequent complication of invasive amebiasis.
    b. *Entamoeba histolytica* is the causative agent of dysentery, colitis, and amebic liver abscess. Infection is endemic in the tropics and in poor communities with inadequate sanitation. The greatest risk is from healthy carriers, who may eliminate up to 1.5×10^9 cysts daily in stools.
    c. Positive serology to *E. histolytica* is indicative of tissue invasion. Higher antibody titers are seen in initial stages of disease, but elevated levels are seen up to 3 years after infection occurred.
    d. Parasitic trophozites penetrate the bowel, and progress to the liver via the portal vein. Solitary space-occupying echogenic lesion or abscess is seen most commonly in the right lobe of the liver.
    e. Liver parenchyma is replaced by necrotic yellowish material with ring of congested liver tissue, often 5 to 15 cm in size.
    f. Treatment is oral metronidazole up to 1 gram PO bid for 10 days in adults. Drainage of abscess is not part of initial therapy, but may be needed if a rapid response does not occur (antibiotic therapy fails).
    g. Complications include extension of the amebic abscess to the peritoneum, pericardium, diaphragm, abdominal organs, great vessels (IVC, aorta), and rupture into pleural space with amebic empyema.

3. Parasitic infections of the liver are called hydatid cysts.
    a. Hydatid cysts are caused by echinococcal tapeworms. Tapeworms are commonly found in sheep-herding dogs, and transferred to humans in contact with the dogs. This infection has a worldwide distribution, but species (*Echinococcus vogelii*) that cause human polycystic hydatid disease are limited to Central and South America.
    b. The cysts are often asymptomatic, fluid-filled structures in the liver, which are associated with daughter cysts. This infection is the most common cystic lesion of the liver outside the United States. Cyst wall calcification is seen on a CT scan along with compression and fibrous reaction of adjacent liver tissue.
    c. The most common presenting symptom is RUQ pain and palpable hepatomegaly. Eosinophilia and positive serology with indirect hemagglutination or enzyme-linked immunosorbent assay is positive in 90% of cases. Casoni skin test is 85% sensitive. Parasitic eggs are not seen in human stool.
    d. Management
- (1) The cysts should not be aspirated to avoid spillage of the organisms and development of new cysts.
- (2) Antihelminthic therapy with mebendazole, praziquantel, or albendazole is given three times daily for up to 16 weeks. Toxicity is alopecia, leukopenia, and elevated transaminases.
- (3) Surgical therapy includes isolation of the cyst from the rest of abdomen with packs, careful cyst fluid aspiration, and instillation of hypertonic

QUICK HIT

Classic features of amebic liver abscess are residence or travel in endemic areas, symptoms of 2-week duration, RUQ pain, abrupt onset of fever (38 to 40°C), tender hepatomegaly, solitary hypoechoic or mixed echogenic liver lesion, leukocytosis with greater than 15,000/μL, and positive serology.

saline to kill the parasitic scolices. This is followed by simple cyst excision from the liver.

B. Benign tumors and cysts

1. General principles. Solid tumors of the liver can be incidentally found on imaging of asymptomatic patients, or for symptoms of abdominal pain. A single imaging study is often nondiagnostic, leading to other studies and even biopsy to confirm the diagnosis. However, biopsy of vascular liver lesions may have serious consequences.

2. Cavernous hemangioma

   a. Cavernous hemangioma is the most common benign mesenchymal tumor. Size of these tumors varies from 1 to 20 cm, and if they are greater than 4 cm, they are called giant hemangiomas. From 60% to 80% are found in women in the third to fifth decade of life. If greater than 10 cm, 90% present with symptoms of liver capsule distension and pain.

   b. MRI is the most accurate noninvasive test, with sensitivity greater than 90%. Hemangiomas have a low T1 signal and a high T2 signal. Technetium pertechnate liver scans are also useful in identifying hemangiomas. Percutaneous biopsy is potentially dangerous, inaccurate, and not recommended.

   c. Hemangiomas do not require treatment and may be left alone. 90% of patients with hemangiomas greater than 10 cm present with symptoms of liver capsule distension and pain. Spontaneous rupture of even giant hemangiomas is very rare, even in pregnancy. Surgical enucleation of the hemangioma is preferred to surgical resection, yielding less blood loss and fewer transfusion requirements.

3. Hepatic adenoma

   a. Hepatic adenomas are uncommon solid lesions seen in women of child-bearing age, usually with antecedent use of oral contraceptives with high doses of estrogen, and used for more than 5 years. 93% of adenomas occur in this segment of the population.

   b. Grossly, adenomas are soft fleshy tumors with smooth surfaces, and microscopically, they consist of monotonous sheets of hepatocytes containing glycogen. The portal triads are absent. Kupffer cells are usually absent in hepatic adenomas, and thus these tumors will be found to be "cold" spots on nuclear liver scan with 99Tm-sulfur colloid, an agent that selectively demonstrates Kupffer cell distribution in the liver.

   c. Most patients (52%) present with right upper abdominal pain due to local compression, but they rarely hemorrhage into the tumor, or rupture leads to an acute presentation with hypotension and shock from bleeding.

   d. Management

      (1) Spontaneous regression is observed in smaller adenomas with withdrawal of oral contraceptives. Asymptomatic smaller adenomas may also be observed.

      (2) Asymptomatic larger lesion (greater than 5 cm), increasing alpha-fetoprotein (AFP), an enlarging mass, or one with irregular borders should prompt surgical resection, because malignant transformation is associated with these characteristics in hepatic adenomas.

      (3) If the larger hepatic adenoma is not resected, pregnancy should be avoided due to an increased risk of tumor growth, hemorrhage, or rupture during pregnancy.

4. Focal nodular hyperplasia (FNH)

   a. FNH is the second most common benign solid tumor of the liver. Seen in all ages and both sexes, it is slightly more common in women from age 20 to 50. The incidence of FNH is not increased with prolonged oral contraceptive use; however, it tends to be seen slightly more frequently in women who take oral contraceptives.

   b. FNH are non-neoplastic solid tumors characterized by a central fibrous scar with radiating septa, often lobulated, and sharply demarcated from

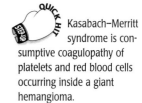

Kasabach–Merritt syndrome is consumptive coagulopathy of platelets and red blood cells occurring inside a giant hemangioma.

HEPATOBILIARY SYSTEM

adjacent liver, without a capsule. The central scar often contains a large artery that branches out in a spoke wheel pattern. These tumors arise as a hyperplastic, hepatocellular response to either hyperperfusion, or vascular injury from the anomalous central artery in the lesion, which is not accompanied by a portal vein or bile duct branch. Their average size is 5 cm, and they rarely exceed 10 cm.

c. Regenerative nodules resembling FNH tumors may be seen in chronic advanced liver disease. These nodules have the hallmark of vascular inflow reduction, liver cell atrophy centrally in the nodule, and regeneration around the intrahepatic portal triads.

d. Patients with FNH are usually asymptomatic, but those who do present with pain are more commonly women who take oral contraceptives.

e. Physical examination and liver function tests are normal. Liver nuclear scan with 99-Tc sulfur colloid shows FNH tumors to be "hot" with increased presence of Kupffer cells. Both CT and MRI may accurately demonstrate the classic central scar in a solid liver tumor as the characteristic finding of an FNH tumor.

f. Management. Because rupture and malignant transformation are not seen with FNH tumors, they may be left alone. Rarely, the enlarging FNH tumor or a patient with severe pain from liver capsule distension should be taken for surgical resection.

5. Cystic diseases of the liver
   a. Specific types
      (1) Simple hepatic (nonparasitic) cysts
      (2) Adult polycystic disease
      (3) Congenital hepatic fibrosis is the malformation of the ductal plate leading to dense fibrous bands of tissue interposed in the hepatic lobules.
      (4) Caroli disease is a congenital intrahepatic biliary dilatation, and a congenital segmental saccular dilatation of the intrahepatic bile ducts without other hepatic abnormalities.
         (a) This disease is usually accompanied by autosomal recessive polycystic kidney disease.
         (b) It presents with cholangitis and septicemia from episodes of focal bile sludging.
         (c) Antibiotic therapy is indicated for cholangitis episodes. Liver transplantation may be necessary, but only if no evidence of persistence of cholangitis infections.
      (5) Caroli syndrome is a combination of Caroli disease and cholangitic congenital hepatic fibrosis.
      (6) Choledochal cyst is a dilation of the common bile duct or biliary tree. Possible causes include anomalous pancreaticobiliary ductal system, allowing for the reflux of pancreatic enzymes into the developing biliary tract.
   b. Management
      (1) Radical complete excision of all cystic parts of the biliary tract with hepaticojejunostomy is essential. Anastomosis of any part of the cystic biliary tree leads to complications of cholangitis and stricturing.
      (2) Carcinoma is a risk of untreated or incompletely excised choledochal cysts.

C. Portal hypertension
   1. Portal hypertension is the most common and lethal complication of chronic liver disease. It is the result of increases in both the vascular resistance to portal flow and the blood flow entering the portal system.
   2. Classification is based on the site of increased resistance to hepatic vascular inflow (presinusoidal or postsinusoidal).
      a. Presinusoidal obstruction
         (1) Extrahepatic

Portal hypertension is defined as free portal vein pressure above the normal of 5 to 10 mm Hg. However, direct portal pressure measurement is difficult. Hepatic vein catheterization with measurement of wedged and free pressures is the simplest and safest indirect means of estimating portal pressure. Complications develop with pressures greater than 12 mm Hg.

       (a) Splenic vein thrombosis

       (b) Portal vein thrombosis

       (c) Splenomegaly

       (d) Hypercoagulable states (polycythemia vera, oral contraceptive use, thrombocytosis)

       (e) Mechanical obstruction (tumors, lymphadenopathy, pancreatitis)

    (2) Intrahepatic

       (a) Congenital hepatic fibrosis

       (b) Schistosomiasis

       (c) Primary portal hypertension (hepatoportal sclerosis)

       (d) Sarcoidosis and Gaucher disease

       (e) Arsenic toxicity

       (f) Primary biliary cirrhosis

    (3) Sinusoidal obstruction

       (a) Wilson disease

       (b) Toxic hepatitis

  b. Postsinusoidal obstruction

    (1) Intrahepatic

       (a) Cirrhosis (alcoholic, secondary biliary)

       (b) Hemochromatosis

       (c) Alcoholic hepatitis

       (d) Intrahepatic Budd–Chiari syndrome

    (2) Extrahepatic

       (a) Budd–Chiari syndrome

       (b) Hepatic neoplasms

       (c) Trauma and sepsis

       (d) Chronic congestive heart failure

3. Management

  a. Acute hemorrhage from esophageal varices should be managed with fluid and/or blood resuscitation, endoscopic identification followed by sclerotherapy or balloon tamponade, and pharmacotherapy. Pharmacotherapy is directed at reducing portal pressure with vasoconstrictors, or reducing intrahepatic vascular resistance with vasodilators.

    (1) Vasopressin causes splanchnic vasoconstriction, reducing portal pressure. Toxic effects include reduction of cardiac output.

    (2) Octreotide is the synthetic analogue of somatostatin. It selectively reduces splanchnic blood flow without producing the systemic cardiac effects of vasopressin.

    (3) Propranolol is a nonselective beta blocker that reduces the portal pressure. It limits portal venous inflow by dual effect of reducing cardiac output and splanchnic vasoconstriction. It is used for the prevention of the first variceal hemorrhage.

  b. Emergency endoscopic therapy

    (1) Injection sclerotherapy

    (2) Endoscopic banding ligation

    (3) Variceal obturation

  c. Balloon tamponade

    (1) The Sengstaken–Blakemore tube is a large triple-lumen tube with esophageal and gastric balloon and is used to provide temporary mechanical occlusion against the bleeding varix.

    (2) This tube has no role in long-term control of bleeding, but is used when endoscopic or pharmacotherapy is unable to control bleeding. It should not be used for more than 24 hours, because of risks such as esophageal rupture, gastric necrosis, and aspiration pneumonia.

  d. Transjugular intrahepatic portosystemic shunt (TIPS)

    (1) TIPS can provide definitive control of bleeding varices by reducing portal pressures at the intrahepatic level.

(2) Interventional radiology access of the right hepatic vein is via the jugular approach, with deployment of an expansile metal stent across liver parenchyma from a hepatic vein branch to a portal vein branch.

e. Surgical shunts
   (1) All surgical shunts—total, partial, or selective—are designed to control variceal bleeding in up to 90% of patients. However, these shunts are not effective in cases of extensive portal vein thrombosis.
   (2) Existing liver failure and reduction/loss of portal inflow in shunt procedures determines the consequences of encephalopathy and fulminant hepatic failure.
   (3) Total portal systemic shunts decompress all portal hypertension.
      (a) End-to-side portocaval shunt.
      (b) Side-to-side portocaval shunt.
   (4) Partial portal systemic shunts are designed to reduce portal hypertension to less than 12 mm Hg.
   (5) Selective shunts are designed to decompress esophageal varices, but not treat the underlying portal hypertension.
      (a) The distal splenorenal shunt (DSRS) is the most widely used surgical shunt worldwide over the past 15 years.
      (b) It is used by surgeons to treat the episode of variceal bleeding, but also to preserve central venous anatomy of the liver in hopes of a potential liver transplant.

f. Devascularization procedures
   (1) This surgical procedure involves splenectomy, gastric and esophageal devascularization, and occasionally, esophageal in-line transection/anastomosis.
   (2) It may control variceal bleeding in patients who are not candidates for surgical shunts.
   (3) Current management algorithm of bleeding esophageal varices from portal hypertension include:
      (a) Beta blockade
      (b) Endoscopic sclerotherapy and pharmacotherapy
      (c) Temporary balloon tamponade
      (d) TIPS
      (e) DSRS or Sugiura procedure, if still bleeding despite (b) and (c) and TIPS not available
      (f) Also, consider 8-mm partial portocaval H-shunt as a bridge to liver transplant
      (g) Liver transplant

g. Liver transplantation
   (1) Liver transplants are one therapy that significantly improves survival in Childs Class C patients with bleeding varices.
   (2) It removes the cirrhotic liver, replacing it with a normal, low-resistance liver, and ultimate shunt treatment for portal hypertension.
   (3) The initial 6-month mortality is 10% to 15%, with a long-term risk of major morbidity or mortality of 2% to 5% per year.
   (4) Major complications include rejection, recurrent viral hepatitis in transplant liver leading to failure, immunosuppression-related infections, and malignancies.

h. Long-term management
   (1) Patients surviving an episode of variceal hemorrhage are at high risk of rebleeding in the following 6 months, with a progressive rise in episodic mortality.
   (2) Long-term management of portal hypertension in such patients includes:
      (a) Selective devascularization surgical procedures
      (b) Surgical shunts

          (c) Liver transplant, which has significantly improved the survival of Childs Class C patients with history of variceal bleeding.

    i. Complications

      (1) Portal-systemic collateral formation is a main consequence of portal hypertension.

          (a) The most clinically significant of these collaterals is gastroesophageal varices. These collaterals develop between the coronary vein; a tributary to the portal, and the short gastric, periesophageal, and azygos veins.

          (b) Anorectal varices, or hemorrhoids, are seen when collaterals develop between the superior hemorrhoidal vein of the portal system, and the middle and inferior hemorrhoidal veins of the caval system. The umbilical vein may dilate and allow portal decompression to the abdominal wall, draining through the epigastric veins. The characteristic finding is caput medusae.

      (2) Esophageal variceal hemorrhage is the most lethal complication of portal hypertension. Risk of bleeding increases with variceal size, but can be prevented if the portal pressure is reduced below 12 mm Hg.

IV. Malignant Disorders

A. Hepatocellular carcinoma (HCC)

  1. HCC is one of the most common malignancies worldwide, and is the number one cause of cancer mortality worldwide. One of the few cancers that can be clearly traced to an antecedent etiology, HCC is almost always linked to the background state of chronic liver disease.

  2. Etiology

    a. Any process that causes chronic liver damage, or cirrhosis, may eventually result in HCC, but the most notable conditions are chronic viral hepatitis, alcoholism, hemochromatosis, intrinsic liver diseases, and parasitic diseases.

    b. In the Far East and Africa, HCC is more commonly associated with chronic hepatitis B virus (HBV), and appears in the third or fourth decade of life. In the West, HCC is more often associated with hepatitis C virus (HCV), and appears later in life. Worldwide, chronic HBV is the most common etiologic cause of HCC.

    c. Chronic HBV infection leads to repeated liver injury through episodes of inflammation, regeneration, and fibrosis. Although HCV alone can lead to HCC, synergistic risk is created when alcoholism, HBV coinfection, and porphyria cutanea tarda are also present. The mechanism underlying the development of HCC from chronic HCV infection is not as clearly understood as is that from chronic HBV disease.

    d. Other etiologic factors include smoking, exposure to thorium dioxide (Thorotrast), aflatoxin, estrogens, and androgens. Aflatoxin is a fungal mycotoxin released by *Aspergillus* species that typically contaminates damp, warm foods such as corn and peanuts.

    e. Premalignant lesions that lead to HCC include dysplastic nodules that are seen in the regenerative phase of cirrhosis as well as hepatic adenomas.

  3. Presentation includes weight loss, abdominal swelling, and RUQ abdominal pain may be evident. In a patient known to have stable cirrhosis, sudden hepatic decompensation may be an indicator of HCC development. HCC may also present with paraneoplastic syndromes caused by ectopic hormonal production (sexual changes, hypercalcemia, carcinoid-like syndrome), metabolic changes (hypoglycemia, hypercholesterolemia, acute porphyria), skin changes (vitiligo, pityriasis, thrombophlebitis migrans), as well as fever, leukocytosis, and cachexia.

4. Diagnosis
   a. Imaging (ultrasound, CT [arterial phase of CT shows HCC lesion to be hypervascular], and MRI) is used for diagnosis. Because of abnormal appearance of the cirrhotic liver on imaging, diagnostic tissue biopsy confirming HCC may sometimes be required.
   b. Serum AFP is elevated in the majority of patients, but may be normal. It may also be elevated by benign causes such as chronic active hepatitis, cirrhosis, and pregnancy. An AFP level greater than 400 ng/mL is considered diagnostic for HCC.
5. Management. One of the keys to treatment of HCC is prevention, because the reduction or improvement of chronic liver damage by treatment of the underlying etiology reduces the risk of HCC development. For example, HBV infection can be prevented by vaccination. Screening in the Far East has been successful in identifying HCC earlier, by screening patients with cirrhosis, a family history of HCC, chronic active hepatitis with elevated viral loads, or increasing AFP.
   a. Optimal therapy for HCC is surgical resection (or liver transplant). However, cirrhosis and poor hepatic reserve greatly limit the extent of surgical resection possible without causing postoperative fulminant hepatic failure. Limited surgical resection, even enucleation of the cancer, may sometimes be defined by the severity of liver function abnormality. Despite successful resections, there is a high tumor recurrence rate of up to 25% per year.
   b. Liver transplant is now a more widely accepted alternative for curative intent of HCC when the tumors are small (less than 3 cm), and few in number (less than 3). Survival after transplantation in the presence of HCC is up to 50% at 3 years. Contraindications to liver transplant in HCC include tumor greater than 5 cm, tumor with associated satellite nodules, major vessel invasion by HCC, extrahepatic metastases, multifocal tumor greater than 3, or vascular tumor thrombus.
   c. Local ablative therapy designed to provide disease control for palliative purposes or as a bridge for those awaiting transplant include radiofrequency ablation and cryoablation as well as chemoembolization of the HCC. Older techniques include percutaneous injection of absolute alcohol into the HCC tumor, causing local destruction of the cancer.
   d. Palliative chemotherapy alone (for example, without surgical resection or ablative therapies) has not been shown to improve survival in HCC.
   e. Radiation has no role in treatment of HCC.
6. Unusual forms of HCC include the fibrolamellar variant of HCC. This variant is rarely associated with cirrhosis, and presents in young adults (ages 20 to 30) in the Western population. There is no association with HBV or HCV infection. AFP levels are rarely elevated. Fibrolamellar HCC usually carries a better prognosis than regular HCC, because the patients are younger and do not usually have liver dysfunction.

B. Metastatic cancer in the liver
   1. The liver is the most common site of metastatic disease for a variety of cancers.
      a. Isolated liver metastases are more commonly seen in association with colorectal cancer, neuroendocrine tumors of the GI tract, stromal tumors of the GI tract, and ocular melanomas.
      b. Hepatic metastases from colorectal cancer are often asymptomatic, and rarely yield jaundice or liver function derangement at presentation.
   2. Management
      a. In selected patients, surgical resection of colorectal hepatic metastases offers 5-year survival rates of up to 25% to 46%.
      b. Systemic multidrug chemotherapy regimens show promising ability to completely clear hepatic metastases, significantly reduce tumor volume, or prevent spread of extrahepatic disease.

c. Colorectal metastases preferentially grow off oxygenated blood from the hepatic arteries. Therefore, chemotherapy administration selectively through hepatic artery infusion (by either percutaneous or surgically placed arterial pump) can target the metastatic disease, while preserving hepatic function and preventing systemic toxicity.

d. Management of hepatic metastases from neuroendocrine tumors, ocular melanomas, and specific GI tract stromal tumors is individualized based on the patient's clinical course, extent of disease, and symptoms.

e. Local tumor ablation with cryoablation or radiofrequency ablation achieves local destruction of active cancer tissue, and is useful in palliative disease control, but does not improve overall survival.

f. Aggressive surgical or ablative management of liver metastases from gastric, pancreatic, small intestine adenocarcinomas, soft-tissue sarcomas, and skin melanomas has no oncologic benefit. Patients should be managed with palliative systemic chemotherapy.

BILIARY SYSTEM

I. General Principles
A. Anatomy
1. Hepatic ducts
   a. The left hepatic duct is formed from the union of the three segmental ducts draining segments 2, 3, and 4.
   b. The right hepatic duct is formed from the union of segmental ducts draining 5, 6, 7, and 8.
   c. Segment 1, the caudate lobe, drains most commonly into both the right and left hepatic ducts.
   d. Both the right and left hepatic ducts join to form the common hepatic duct.
2. Gallbladder
   a. The gallbladder is a pear-shaped distensible reservoir structure with an average capacity of 30 to 50 mL.
   b. The inferior and lateral surface is covered by peritoneum, and the superior surface is associated with the hepatic fossa.
   d. This organ has four anatomic portions: the fundus, body, infundibulum, and neck.
   e. It is supplied by the cystic artery, which is most commonly a branch of the right hepatic artery.
3. Cystic duct
   a. This arises from the gallbladder and drains into the common hepatic duct to form the common bile duct.
   b. Its average length is 2 to 4 cm.
4. Common bile duct (CBD)
   a. The CBD is formed by the union of the cystic duct and the common hepatic duct.
   b. It is approximately 8 cm in length, with an average diameter of 4 to 9 mm in adults, and 3 to 5 mm in children. After cholecystectomy, it may dilate an additional 2 to 3 mm in size, and not be considered significant.
   c. It most commonly joins the pancreatic duct, to open into the second portion of the duodenum at the ampulla of Vater. The opening is regulated by the sphincter of Oddi.
5. Triangle of Calot. This region is bordered by the common hepatic duct medially, the cystic duct laterally, and the liver edge superiorly.
6. Sphincter of Oddi
   a. Located at the ampulla of Vater
   b. Length of 4 to 6 mm
   c. The basal resting pressure is 13 mm Hg

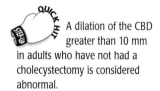

A dilation of the CBD greater than 10 mm in adults who have not had a cholecystectomy is considered abnormal.

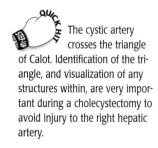

The cystic artery crosses the triangle of Calot. Identification of the triangle, and visualization of any structures within, are very important during a cholecystectomy to avoid injury to the right hepatic artery.

    d. Regulates the flow of bile and pancreatic juice

    e. Relaxation occurs with cholecystokinin and vagal stimulation. Sympathetic stimulation causes increased pressure and sphincter constriction.

B. Physiology

    1. The gallbladder absorbs water and solute from bile, thereby concentrating the solute components.

    2. It acts as a storage organ for bile.

    3. In addition, it secretes mucus and glycoproteins.

    4. Gallbladder contractility is controlled by enteric hormones and autonomic nervous system. Primarily, these stimulants are cholecystokinin and vagal firing.

II. Gallstone Disease

A. Types. Gallstones are classified according to their cholesterol content as either pigment or cholesterol stones. Most of the gallstones are mixed, containing calcium salts in their center.

    1. Pure cholesterol stones constitute only 10% of all gallstones. However, 70% to 80% of the gallstones are considered to be cholesterol stones.

    2. Approximately 20% to 30% gallstones are pigment stones.

B. Pathogenesis. A combination of the following factors favor the development of the stones:

    1. Cholesterol supersaturation in the bile.

    2. Crystal nucleation due to aggregation, and precipitation of the cholesterol-rich vesicles.

    3. Gallbladder dysmotility.

    4. Gallbladder absorptive dysfunction.

    5. Percentages of saturation of three elements in bile leads to precipitation and cholesterol stone formation. These three elements are lecithin, cholesterol, and bile salt.

C. Pigment gallstones

    1. There are two types of pigment gallstones: black stones and brown stones.

    2. Black stones consist of calcium bilirubinate and calcium palmitate. They are frequently small and multiple, and tend to occur almost exclusively in the gallbladder. Risk factors for black stones are hemolytic anemia and cirrhosis.

    3. Brown stones are more common in the Asian population, in the setting of biliary dysmotility and chronic bacterial and parasitic infections. These may also occur as primary common bile duct stones.

D. Clinical presentation

    1. Asymptomatic

        a. The vast majority of patients with gallstones are asymptomatic.

        b. 20% of these patients become symptomatic in 20 years.

        c. Of this group of patients, 1% to 2% develop serious symptoms or complications related to their gallstones.

    2. Symptomatic

        a. Biliary colic

            (1) This condition is due to intermittent obstruction of the cystic duct with passage of small stones.

            (2) There is intermittent, spasmodic RUQ pain that occurs most commonly after a fatty meal, and may last for a few hours. It is associated with nausea, vomiting, and bloating.

        b. Acute cholecystitis

            (1) This condition is due to occlusion of the cystic duct, and this incites an inflammatory response. Bile may become infected with gram-negative bacteria, most commonly *E. coli*.

            (2) Patients present with RUQ pain, which is usually longer lasting, and they may have constitutional signs of fever and tachycardia. Abdominal examination usually reveals RUQ tenderness.

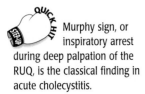
Murphy sign, or inspiratory arrest during deep palpation of the RUQ, is the classical finding in acute cholecystitis.

(3) Laboratory findings include an elevated white blood cell count and mild hyperbilirubinemia.

E. Diagnosis

1. RUQ ultrasound is the most useful diagnostic test. Ultrasound has 85% specificity and 95% sensitivity in diagnosing acute cholecystitis. Findings suggestive of acute cholecystitis are:

   a. Presence of gallstones.

   b. Thickening of the gallbladder wall greater than 4 mm.

   c. Pericholecystic fluid.

2. Radionucleotide scanning, or a HIDA scan, may also be helpful.

   a. The radionucleotide is administered intravenously, and the patient is scanned in 30 minutes.

   b. Nonfilling of the gallbladder with the radiotracer, but filling of the CBD and the duodenum indicates an obstructed cystic duct and acute cholecystitis.

   c. Highly sensitive and specific, about 95% for each, for acute cholecystitis.

F. Management of symptomatic gallstones. Medical management of severe acute cholecystitis includes hospital admission, no oral intake, intravenous fluids, and use of broad-spectrum antibiotics.

1. Surgical management

   a. Early cholecystectomy, within 3 days of presentation is advocated by some authors, and may be accomplished before onset of second phase of acute inflammatory response. Initial phase often includes pericholecystic fluid or tissue edema which makes surgical removal easier.

   b. Relative indications for prophylactic cholecystectomy are:

      (1) Pediatric gallstone disease.

      (2) Congenital hemolytic anemias (for example, sickle-cell disease).

      (3) Gallstones greater than 2.5 cm, which increases the incidence of cancer of gallbladder and acute cholecystitis.

      (4) Porcelain gallbladder, which increases the incidence of gallbladder cancer.

      (5) Bariatric surgery.

      (6) Note: Asymptomatic gallstone disease in diabetics is no longer considered an indication for prophylactic cholecystectomy.

   c. If patients present later than 3 days into their symptoms, it may be prudent to treat the gallbladder disease conservatively (medical management as described above), and perform cholecystectomy electively in 4 to 6 weeks.

   d. In certain high-risk patients, or in severely ill patients in the intensive care unit whose conditions do not permit cholecystectomy, percutaneous cholecystostomy may be performed to relieve obstruction, and decompress the gallbladder.

   e. Cholecystectomy could be performed either with the laparoscope, or in an open fashion. Laparoscopic cholecystectomy has the advantage of short hospital stay and less morbidity associated due to smaller wounds.

G. Complications

1. Empyema

2. Emphysematous cholecystitis. This is more commonly seen in patients with diabetes mellitus. Patients present with RUQ pain and sepsis. Abdominal films or CT scan may show air in the gallbladder wall or lumen. Infection generally due *E. coli, Enterococcus, Klebsiella,* or *Clostridia* species.

3. Gangrene and perforation

4. Cholecystenteric fistula. This is seen in up to 2% of patients with acute cholecystitis.

5. Small bowel obstruction

   a. The gallbladder may perforate into adjacent viscera such as the duodenum, and hepatic flexure of the colon (two most common sites). Chronic erosion of the gallbladder wall by a 2 cm or larger gallstone can also form the cholecystenteric fistula.

b. Following fistula formation, the large stone may tumble through the GI tract until it reaches the ileum, with the narrowest luminal size. Here, the stone may cause small bowel obstruction, which is termed gallstone ileus. This occurs in up to 15% of patients with cholecystenteric fistulas.

c. The obstruction is described as episodic and recurrent, because the impacted stone temporarily impacts in the gut lumen, and then dislodges and moves forward. This is known as tumbling obstruction. Abdominal imaging may show evidence of small bowel obstruction and presence of pneumobilia.

6. Surgical management includes proximal enterotomy with stone removal. Takedown of the biliary enteric fistula and cholecystectomy prevent recurrent obstruction, cholangitis, and gallbladder cancer.

H. Acute cholangitis
1. Acute cholangitis is a bacterial infection of the biliary ductal system, due to ductal obstruction and significant bacterial concentration in the bile. The most common causes of biliary obstruction are choledocholithiasis, benign strictures, and tumors.

2. Patient may present with fever, RUQ pain, and jaundice (Charcot triad), combined with mental status changes and hypotension (Reynolds pentad). Initial management is resuscitative, with intravenous antibiotics, fluids, and systemic support. Urgent clearance of the infected and obstructed biliary tract is better achieved by percutaneous transhepatic cholangiography, or endoscopic retrograde cholangiopancreatography (ERCP), and not by surgical intervention. Once the patient is stabilized, surgical removal of the gallbladder (during the same hospitalization) is recommended to prevent recurrent obstructions and episodes of cholangitis.

I. Inflammatory lesions of biliary tract
1. Primary Sclerosing Cholangitis (PSC).
a. PSC is a chronic progressive cholestatic disease, in which the inflammatory process involves the bile ducts, resulting in intrahepatic or extrahepatic strictures.

b. This autoimmune disease is associated with other inflammatory bowel disease, with 85% of the patients having ulcerative colitis, and 15% patients having Crohn disease. Males are more commonly affected than females, and PSC tends to present in the fourth decade of life. Prevalence is 10 per 100,000 population.

c. Patients present with signs and symptoms of biliary obstruction, jaundice, pruritus, weight loss, and fatigue.

d. Diagnosis is based on liver biopsy, which may show presence of cholestasis and cirrhosis. ERCP or MRCP show the characteristic beaded appearance of the ductal system from the areas of the stricture and dilatation.

e. Management. The only definitive cure is liver transplant. Medical management with immunosuppressives and bile acids, such as ursodeoxycholic acid has shown some temporary benefit.

f. Complications may be secondary to:
(1) Choledocholithiasis
(2) Postoperative biliary strictures
(3) Infections, such as ascending cholangitis and parasitic infections
(4) Iatrogenic operative ischemia of the bile ducts
(5) Drugs, chemotherapy with intra-arterial 5-fluorouracil
(6) AIDS-associated cholangiopathy

J. Malignant biliary disease
1. Gallbladder cancer
a. Incidence
(1) Women are affected more than men, in part due to their higher incidence of gallstones. The overall incidence of cancer is 2.5 cases per a population of 100,000.
(2) The disease is more common in Native Americans.

(3) The highest incidence occurs in residents of Chile.

b. Etiology

(1) Risk factors include gallstones greater than 2.5 cm, porcelain gallbladder, choledochal cysts, primary sclerosing cholangitis, and cholecystenteric fistula.

(2) Approximately 1% of all elective cholecystectomies performed for cholelithiasis harbor an occult gallbladder cancer.

c. Pathology

(1) 90% of the cancers of the gallbladder are adenocarcinoma.

(2) At diagnosis, 25% of the cancers are localized to the gallbladder wall, 35% have associated metastases to the regional lymph nodes or extension into adjacent organs, and 40% have already metastasized to distant sites.

d. Presentation

(1) Most often, patients present with RUQ abdominal pain, often mimicking other common biliary and nonbiliary disease.

(2) Other symptoms may include weight loss, jaundice, and abdominal mass.

e. Diagnosis. Ultrasound or CT usually demonstrates a mass in the gallbladder. In addition, a CT scan shows the extension into the surrounding structures and the vascular anatomy.

f. Management

(1) Patients with a preoperatively suspected cancer of the gallbladder, should undergo open cholecystectomy to minimize the chance of bile spillage and tumor dissemination.

(2) If cancer of the gallbladder is diagnosed after a cholecystectomy, and on pathologic examination of the specimen, lesions are confined to the mucosa, submucosa, or the muscularis (T1), the cholecystectomy is adequate therapy. These patients have an 85% to 100% 5-year survival rate.

(3) Cancer of the gallbladder with invasion beyond the muscularis is associated with an increasing incidence of regional lymph node metastases, and needs an extended cholecystectomy with a 2-cm margin of the adjacent liver tissue with lymphadenectomy .

(4) Palliative care

(a) In patients with an unresectable tumor, the obstructive jaundice can be managed with biliary decompression, through percutaneous or endoscopically placed biliary stents.

(b) Pain should be aggressively treated.

2. Cholangiocarcinoma

a. This uncommon cancer is located commonly at the hepatic duct bifurcation.

b. Incidence

(1) Each year, 2,500 to 3,000 new cases are diagnosed.

(2) The carcinoma occurs with equal frequency in men and women, and the incidence increases with age.

c. Etiology

(1) Risk factors include primary sclerosing cholangitis, choledochal cysts, hepatolithiasis, and previous biliary enteric anastomosis. Other risk factors include parasitic disease, liver flukes, dietary nitrosamines, dioxin, and thorium dioxide (Thorotrast).

(2) Common factors in all cases are bile stasis, infection, stones, and chronic inflammation.

d. Classification consists of three broad groups:

(1) Intrahepatic: 6%

(2) Perihilar: 67%

(3) Distal: 27%

e. Clinical presentation. 90% of patients present with jaundice, pruritus, fever, and abdominal pain. In addition, they may present with acute cholangitis.

    f. Diagnosis
       (1) CT is the initial diagnostic test of choice. This reveals dilated bile ducts, lymph nodes, and vascular anatomy.
       (2) A cholangiogram obtained through either the percutaneous transhepatic route, or the endoscopic retrograde route further defines the biliary anatomy.
    g. Management
       (1) For the intrahepatic group, a partial hepatectomy is indicated.
       (2) For the perihilar group, a resection and hepaticojejunostomies is indicated.
       (3) For the distal group, a pancreaticoduodenectomy is indicated.

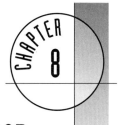

Pancreas and Spleen

Irfan A. Rizvi, MD
David McFadden, MD, FACS

PANCREAS

I. Anatomy and Physiology (Color Fig. 8-1)

A. Two endodermal buds form the pancreas.
1. The **dorsal bud** forms the bulk of the gland.
2. The **ventral bud** rotates dorsally along with the bile duct, and forms the inferior part of the pancreatic head and uncinate process.

B. The main pancreatic duct (of **Wirsung**) is formed by the distal part of the dorsal pancreatic duct, and the entire ventral duct. It joins the common bile duct, and opens in a globular cavity (**ampulla of Vater**) in the posteromedial wall of the second part of the duodenum. Sphincteric muscles surround this ampulla, and the ends of the two ducts. The entire complex is called the **sphincter of Oddi.**

C. The ampulla drains into the duodenal lumen through a nipple-shaped orifice called the **major duodenal papilla.**
1. The proximal part of the dorsal pancreatic duct (of **Santorini**) drains into the duodenum through a minor papilla that opens approximately 2 cm proximal to the major papilla.
2. Successful cannulation of the major papilla allows an endoscopist to perform an endoscopic retrograde cholangiopancreatography (ERCP) (Color Fig. 8-2).

D. In **pancreas divisum**, the pancreatic duct systems fail to fuse. Some experts believe that this predisposes to acute pancreatitis. This occurs in approximately 10% of cases.

E. In **annular pancreas**, an aberrant migration of the ventral bud results in the second part of the duodenum being encircled by a band of normal pancreatic tissue. Complete duodenal obstruction may result. Treatment is bypass, not resection (Color Fig. 8-3).

F. The pancreas derives its blood supply from branches of the celiac and superior mesenteric arteries. The superior mesenteric vessels lie posterior to the neck of the pancreas (portal vein forms behind the neck). Invasion of pancreatic head cancer into these vessels is the single most important factor precluding a successful resection (Color Fig. 8-4).

G. Physiology of the exocrine pancreas
1. The pancreas releases approximately 2 L of pancreatic juice into the duodenum. Daily secretion of pancreatic juice is under control of the vagus nerve, and the two enteric hormones cholecystokinin (CCK) and secretin.
   a. Secretin stimulates the pancreas to secrete a high volume bicarbonate rich juice in response to acid in the duodenum.
   b. Cholecystokinin is stimulated by dietary fat, and increases the enzyme content of pancreatic juice (Color Fig. 8-5).

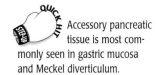
Accessory pancreatic tissue is most commonly seen in gastric mucosa and Meckel diverticulum.

FIGURE
8-1   Relation of the pancreas to the duodenum and extrahepatic biliary system.

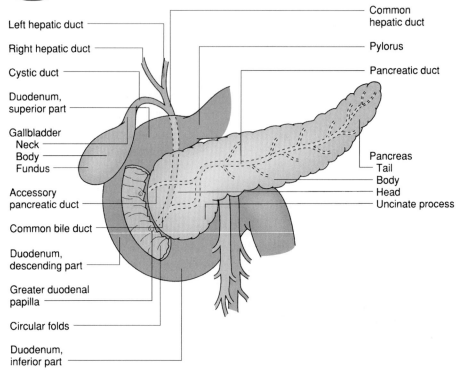

(After Woodburne RT. *Essentials of Human Anatomy.* New York: Oxford University Press; 1973.)

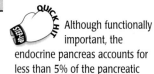 Although functionally important, the endocrine pancreas accounts for less than 5% of the pancreatic mass.

2. The proteolytic enzymes are secreted as inactive precursors trypsinogen and chymotrypsinogen, which are activated to trypsin and chymotrypsin in the duodenum by enterokinase.

3. Pancreatic amylase and lipase break down carbohydrate and lipids respectively, and their serum levels are also useful clinical tools in the diagnosis of pancreatitis.

H. Physiology of the endocrine pancreas: the islets of Langerhans develop in the third month of fetal life. The following types of cells have been described. Their percentage and products are listed below:

1. Alpha cells (15%): glucagon
2. Beta cells (65%): insulin
3. Delta cells (5%): somatostatin
4. PP cells (15%): pancreatic polypeptide
5. Others: D2 cells (vasoactive intestinal peptide), EC cells (substance P and serotonin)

II. Acute Pancreatitis

A. General principles

1. Acute pancreatitis (AP) encompasses a wide spectrum of clinical presentations, ranging from a mild and self-limited entity in 80% to 85% of patients, to a serious illness complicated by shock, sepsis, and multisystem organ failure in the remaining 15% to 20%.

2. AP is a disorder whose pathogenesis remains obscure, and for which treatment is largely supportive.

3. Clinically, the overall mortality for AP is approximately 10%, but in its most severe form, which is characterized by pancreatic hemorrhage and necrosis, it induces a systemic inflammatory response whose severity can increase the mortality to 20% to 30%.

FIGURE

8-2 Anatomic configuration of the intrapancreatic ductal system. A lack of communication between the two ducts, which occurs in 10% of cases, is referred to as
pancreas divisum.

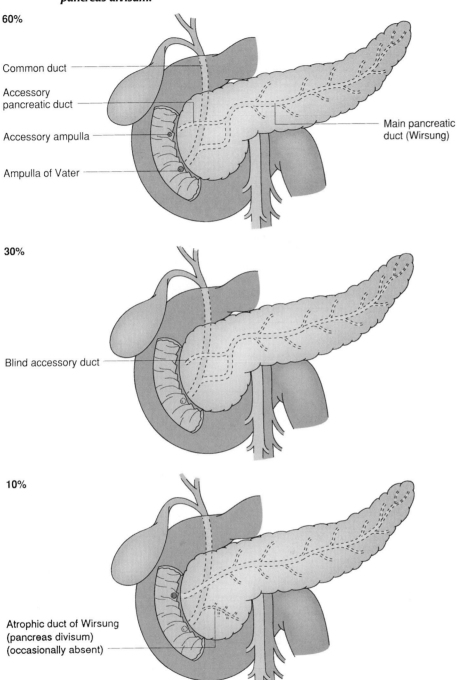

60%

Common duct

Accessory
pancreatic duct

Accessory ampulla

Ampulla of Vater

Main pancreatic
duct (Wirsung)

30%

Blind accessory duct

10%

Atrophic duct of Wirsung
(pancreas divisum)
(occasionally absent)

(After Silen W. Surgical anatomy of the pancreas. *Surg Clin North Am.* 1964;44:1253.)

B. Etiology (Table 8-1)
1. Common causes include gallstones and alcohol, which are implicated in
80% to 90% of the cases of AP. The **"common channel-reflux"** mechanism is
a popular explanation, implicating gallstones as the precipitator of AP. It
suggests migration of either gallstones or sludge through the distal bile duct.
This results in damage to the common "biliary-pancreatic channel" with
resultant edema and blockage of the pancreatic duct. This leads to the pool-
ing of enzymes, and their activation within the gland (Color Fig. 8-6).

FIGURE 8-3 The ring of pancreatic tissue contains a large duct and may be heavily fixed to the duodenal musculature. The duodenum beneath the annulus is often stenosed. Thus, cutting the ring may not provide relief from symptoms of obstruction. There is also the danger of creating a pancreatic fistula or duodenal perforation. Duodenojejunostomy bypassing the annulus is the accepted procedure. Annular pancreas usually produces symptoms in the first year of life, but where the stenosis is mild or absent, it may remain silent for many years.

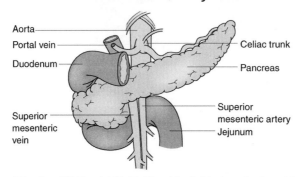

(After Gray SW, Skandalakis JE. *Atlas of Surgical Anatomy for General Surgeons.* Baltimore: Williams & Wilkins; 1985.)

FIGURE 8-4 Cross-sectional relation of the pancreas to other abdominal structures in an oblique plane through the long axis of the pancreas extending from the level of L2 on the right to T10 on the left.

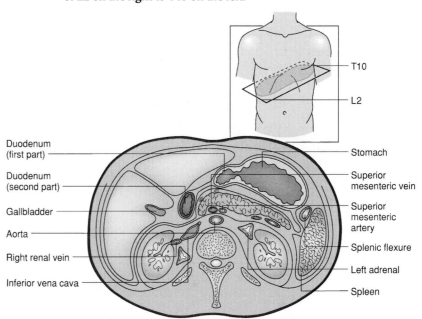

(After Mackie CR, Moossa AR. Surgical anatomy of the pancreas. In: Moossa AR, ed. *Tumors of the Pancreas.* Baltimore: Williams & Wilkins; 1980.)

FIGURE 8-5 Relation of pancreatic secretion and concentration of electrolytes.

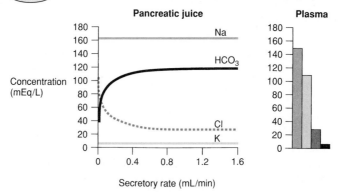

(Reprinted, with permission, from Bro-Rasmussen F, Kilman SA, Thaysen JH. The composition of pancreatic juice as compared to sweat, parotid saliva, and tears. *Acta Physiol Scand.* 1956;37:39.)

TABLE 8-1	Etiology of Acute Pancreatitis
Gallstones	
Ethanol	
Iatrogenic causes 　ERCP 　Abdominal and nonabdominal operations 　Cardiopulmonary bypass	
Trauma	
Neoplasms (e.g., pancreatic cancer)	
Pancreas divisum	
Sphincter of Oddi spasm	
Medications	
Toxins 　Parathion 　Scorpion venom	
Hyperlipidemia	
Hypercalcemia	
Infectious agents 　Viruses (e.g., mumps and Coxsackie B viruses; HIV) 　Bacteria (e.g., *Salmonella* and *Shigella* species; hemorrhagic *Escherichia coli*) 　Biliary parasites (e.g., *Ascaris lumbricoides*)	
Genetic causes 　Hereditary pancreatitis 　Cystic fibrosis	
Vasculitis (e.g., systemic lupus erythematosus and polyarteritis nodosa)	
Ischemia	
Pregnancy	

ERCP, endoscopic retrograde cholangiopancreatography.
(Reprinted, with permission, from Mulholland MW, Lillemoe KD, Doherty GM, et al. Acute pancreatitis. In: *Greenfield's Surgery*, 4th ed. Baltimore: Lippincott Williams & Wilkins; 2006:841.)

PANCREAS AND SPLEEN

2. Rare causes include trauma, hypercalcemia, hyperlipidemia (Fredrickson types 1 and 5), infections (viral and parasitic), drugs (more than 100 drugs, including Imuran, valproate, steroids), hereditary (locus 7q35), and scorpion venom. About 5% to 10% of the time, AP is idiopathic.

3. Only 3% to 8% of symptomatic gallstone disease results in AP. However, the incidence increases to 30% when microlithiasis is involved.

C. Clinical presentation

1. Abdominal pain is by far the most common complaint. Typically it is epigastric, with radiation to the back.

2. Vomiting and retching are prominent associated symptoms.

3. Because the signs and symptoms of AP mimic many acute intra-abdominal and extra-abdominal pathologies, a thorough history and physical examination are extremely important.

a. Depending on the etiology of the AP, patients may give a history of an inciting factor (e.g., recent ingestion of a fatty meal or alcohol, trauma to the abdomen).

b. A complete drug and family history is mandatory, as this may give vital clues to the etiology.

FIGURE
8-6   Illustration of the common channel concept. A gallstone lodged at the ampulla of Vater can cause reflux of bile into the pancreatic duct.

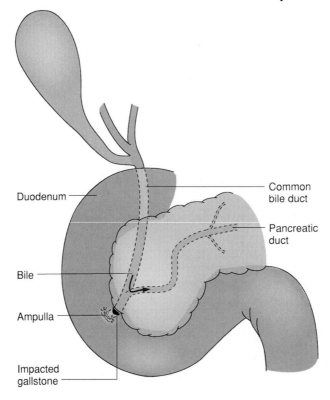

Duodenum

Common bile duct

Pancreatic duct

Bile

Ampulla

Impacted gallstone

4. Patients with severe AP may present in shock, multisystem organ failure, or coma.
   a. On physical examination, these patients are usually tachycardic and may have a fever.
   b. Signs of dehydration from vomiting and excessive fluid sequestration in the abdomen are evident. The abdomen is markedly tender, and may have obvious guarding and distention.
   c. Severe AP with resultant bleeding in the retroperitoneum and abdominal cavity may reveal ecchymosis in the flanks called Grey–Turner sign, and in the periumbilical region called Cullen sign, respectively.
D. Laboratory findings
   1. Serum amylase and lipase are the most commonly accepted blood tests for diagnosing AP.
      a. Serum amylase has a sensitivity of 75% to 90%, but falls short in specificity (20–60%), because virtually any intra-abdominal pathology can elevate its level in the blood. Perforated duodenal ulcers, mesenteric ischemia, intestinal obstruction, salivary gland pathology, and renal failure can all give false-positive results.
      b. Serum lipase levels are more specific (50–99%) and sensitive (80–100%) for AP. Studies have shown that serum lipase levels preferentially rise higher in alcoholic AP. Therefore, the lipase:amylase ratio is higher in AP secondary to alcohol than gallstones.
   2. If available, serum trypsin levels are the most sensitive and specific.
   3. C-reactive protein is directly correlated with disease severity, but values may not become significantly elevated until 48 hours post-onset of inflammation.
E. Radiology
   1. A plain chest radiograph rules out pneumonia as a possible etiology for the acute abdomen. It also may show signs of acute respiratory distress syndrome (ARDS) in severe AP.

FIGURE
8-7 Computed tomography scan of acute interstitial pancreatitis.

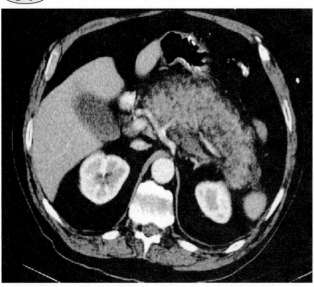

2. A dilated loop of duodenum (sentinel loop), or transverse colon (colon cutoff sign), secondary to a localized ileus from the inflammatory process in the neighboring pancreas may be evident on plain abdominal films.

3. Ultrasound is good for imaging the edematous pancreas. However, its sensitivity is marred (60%) if intraluminal gas obscures the view. Ultrasound remains the imaging modality of choice for visualizing the gallbladder and biliary system.

4. Computed tomography (CT) scan with intravenous contrast remains the gold standard for diagnosing AP and its complications. It reaches a sensitivity of greater than 90% in diagnosing pancreatitis, and is excellent in showing pancreatic necrosis by nonenhancement of the affected area. A sensitivity of 100% is attained if more than 30% of the gland is involved. It also has the added advantage of ruling out other potential causes of acute abdominal presentation, and a means of guidance for sampling pancreatic tissue (Fig. 8-7).

F. Treatment

1. The mainstay of treatment for AP is supportive, with the first step being vigorous fluid resuscitation, as fluid sequestration and lack of fluid intake leads to dehydration and shock.

2. Adequate analgesia is also paramount. Morphine is relatively contraindicated in this setting because of its stimulatory effect on the sphincter of Oddi.

3. Ventilatory support is necessary in respiratory failure and ARDS.

4. "Resting" the pancreas by making the patient NPO, and supporting fluid and nutritional requirements with total parenteral nutrition (TPN), is important. Starting TPN early in this highly catabolic state may be beneficial.

5. Studies have shown that enteral feeding beyond the ligament of Treitz causes minimal stimulation of the pancreas. Enteral feeds have the advantage of maintaining the integrity of the intestinal mucosa and decreasing bacterial translocation.

6. Nasogastric decompression of the stomach is only indicated for persistent nausea or vomiting, and intestinal obstruction.

7. Stress ulcer prophylaxis is an important adjunct to therapy.

8. Inhibition of pancreatic secretions using H_2-blockers, somatostatin, octreotide, glucagons, calcitonin, and atropine, although theoretically sound, has had no impact on the course of AP.

9. Similarly, cytokine inhibitors, platelet-activating factor antagonists, and gastrointestinal inhibitory hormones such as peptide YY (PYY) have so far only been effective in experimental models.

10. The current recommendations for the prophylactic use of antibiotics include severe AP, large fluid collections, and sterile pancreatic necrosis of greater than 30% of the gland. Antibiotics with good pancreatic tissue penetration include ciprofloxacin, ofloxacin, and imipenem.

11. ERCP is useful in disimpacting common bile duct stones.
    a. ERCP is the therapeutic modality of choice when the biliary system is dilated, and/or liver function tests are elevated in the setting of AP. Studies have shown that it also decreases the morbidity and mortality of severe biliary AP if performed within 24 to 72 hours.
    b. In addition, ERCP is useful when the etiology of the AP is unclear.

12. Visualizing common bile duct stones, sampling bile for sludge, and inspecting the anatomy of the region can help identify biliary causes for the AP.

13. Occasionally tumors or strictures may be diagnosed.

14. Early cholecystectomy, once the clinical pancreatitis has resolved, is currently recommended for almost all patients after the first attack of biliary pancreatitis. Most surgeons favor cholecystectomy during the same hospitalization because of the 25% to 40% incidence of recurrent attacks if the traditional 6-week "cooling off" period is observed.

G. Complications
  1. Pancreatic pseudocysts
     a. These loculated effusions are rich in amylase, and are enclosed by a nonepithelialized wall composed of fibrous and granulation tissue.
     b. Pseudocysts are more common in alcoholic pancreatitis (15%) than in gallstone pancreatitis (3%).
     c. They are typically appreciated about 4 weeks after the onset of an attack. More than half of all pseudocysts resolve within 4 to 6 weeks.
     d. Pseudocysts greater than 6 cm in diameter are far more likely to require surgical therapy than those less than 6 cm (Fig. 8-8).
  2. Pancreatic necrosis
     a. Pancreatic necrosis is defined as diffuse or focal area(s) of nonviable pancreatic parenchyma, often associated with peripancreatic fat necrosis.

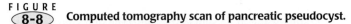

FIGURE 8-8 Computed tomography scan of pancreatic pseudocyst.

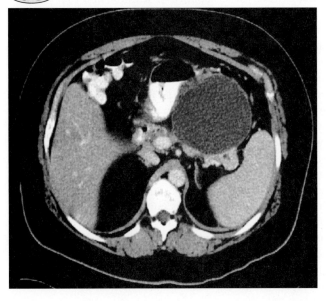

FIGURE
8-9 Computed tomography scan of acute necrotizing pancreatitis.

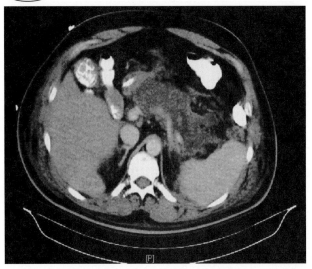

    b. CT is diagnostic in more than 90% of the cases. Focal or diffuse well-circumscribed areas of nonenhanced pancreatic parenchyma larger than 3 cm, or involving more than 30% of the gland, are required for CT diagnosis.

    c. Infected pancreatic necrosis is an indication for surgical debridement. Therefore, the clinical differentiation between sterile and infected pancreatic necrosis is essential.

    d. Because clinical and laboratory findings in these two groups can be identical, the distinction is best made by cultures and Gram stains from percutaneously attained needle aspirates (Fig. 8-9).

3. Pancreatic abscesses

    a. Pancreatic abscesses are defined as a circumscribed intra-abdominal collection of pus in proximity to the pancreas, containing little or no pancreatic necrosis. They can be insidious, are frequently multiple, and are evenly divided among head, body, and tail of the gland.

    b. Abscesses are frequently polymicrobial, containing enteric bacteria as well as *Candida* species.

    c. For both pancreatic abscess and infected necrosis, the treatment consists of adequate drainage. Without it, virtually all patients die. Drainage can be achieved either by image-guided placement of percutaneous drains or a formal surgical debridement.

    d. Aggressive wide debridement **is** necessary.

    e. Most surgeons prefer to leave large caliber sump drains in the pancreatic abscess cavity or cavities with closure of the abdomen.

    f. Irrigation of the pancreatic bed may be performed with saline or antibiotic-containing saline for prolonged periods (3–21 days).

4. Pancreatic fistulas

    a. Both internal and external fistulas may result from inflammation and pancreatic duct disruption.

    b. Fluid may track into the left pleural cavity through the retroperitoneum, causing an effusion.

    c. Other complications include splenic vein thrombosis and false aneurysms, which may lead to bleeding either into the pancreatic duct (hemosuccus pancreaticus) or free rupture leading to hemoperitoneum.

H. Prognosis

1. C-reactive protein and polymorphonuclear-elastase have been used clinically as predictors of disease severity.

2. Several scoring systems have been applied to acute pancreatitis.

TABLE 8-2	Ranson Criteria for Assessing Severity of Pancreatitis
At Admission	
Age	>55 yr
WBC count	>16,000/mm³
Glucose	>200 mg/dL
LDH	>350 IU/L
AST	>250 IU/L
Within 48 hours	
Hematocrit decrease	>10 pt
BUN increase	>5 mg/dL
Calcium	<8 mg/dL
PaO₂	<60 mm Hg
Base deficit	>4 mEq/L
Fluid requirement	>6 L

WBC, white blood count; LDH, lactate dehydrogenase; AST, aspartate aminotransferase; BUN, blood urea nitrogen; PaO_2, arterial oxygen pressure. (Reprinted, with permission, from Mulholland MW, Lillemoe KD, Doherty GM, et al. Acute pancreatitis. In: *Greenfield's Surgery*, 4th ed. Baltimore: Lippincott Williams & Wilkins; 2006:845.)

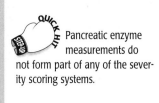

Pancreatic enzyme measurements do not form part of any of the severity scoring systems.

a. Ranson reported the first, and most commonly used, in 1974. This system uses 11 clinical and biochemical measurements available within the first 48 hours of disease onset. These were tabulated on a cohort of patients with alcohol-induced pancreatitis (Table 8-2).

b. Imrie, from Glasgow, has reported a similar scoring system based on patients with mostly gallstone pancreatitis.

c. The Acute Physiology And Chronic Health Evaluation, or APACHE II, score has had much recent support.

   (1) This system is based on the evaluation of clinical data such as blood pressure, pulse, and temperature, biochemical data such as urea and electrolytes, and renal and pulmonary functional parameters.

   (2) Within 24 hours of hospital admission, this system has an approximate 70% sensitivity in the detection of severe acute pancreatitis, with a specificity of 80% to 90%.

III. Chronic Pancreatitis

   A. General principles

   1. Chronic pancreatitis is an inflammatory disease of the pancreas that is marked by the gradual destruction of pancreatic exocrine and endocrine tissues. Fibrous scar replaces the pancreatic parenchyma.

   2. Pancreatic calcifications are seen in one-third of patients with alcoholic chronic pancreatitis.

   3. Significant degrees of weight loss are common, because food tends to worsen the pain. Narcotic addiction is common.

   4. The usual age of onset is in the mid-30s, and men are affected more commonly than women.

   B. Etiology

   1. Alcoholism is the cause of 75% of the cases of chronic pancreatitis in the United States.

   2. Less common causes include cystic fibrosis, pancreas divisum, hyperparathyroidism, and familial pancreatitis.

3. A specific type of chronic pancreatitis is seen in children with severe protein-calorie malnutrition and kwashiorkor. Adequate dietary replenishment is curative, provided parenchymal fibrosis is minimal.

4. Another kind of chronic pancreatitis, possibly related to malnutrition, occurs only in certain tropical areas.

C. Clinical presentation

1. The presenting symptom in up to 95% of patients with chronic pancreatitis is abdominal pain.

2. Malabsorption (steatorrhea) and/or diabetes mellitus are hallmarks of significant pancreatic insufficiency.

D. Laboratory findings. No laboratory test is diagnostic of chronic pancreatitis.

1. CT scanning provides the most reliable overall assessment of the pancreas and peripancreatic area. The most common CT findings in chronic pancreatitis include duct dilatation, calcifications, and cystic lesions (Fig. 8-10).

2. ERCP should be done in most patients with chronic pancreatitis who are being evaluated for operation. The radiologic appearance of the ductal system may show ductal filling defects consistent with stones, areas of stricture alternating with segments of dilatation ("chain of lakes" appearance; Fig. 8-11).

E. Treatment

1. Medical management

a. This includes total abstinence from alcohol, pancreatic enzyme supplements, and optimal nutrition (high-calorie, high-protein diet).

b. Patients are very sensitive to exogenous insulin, which is the only option as oral hypoglycemics are rarely effective.

c. Oral opioids are useful, although dependence is common.

d. Neuroablative procedures such as celiac plexus block have produced inconsistent results.

2. Surgical treatment. The aims of surgery in chronic pancreatitis are to relieve intractable pain, to treat complications, and to preserve as much functioning pancreatic tissue as possible. Three approaches have been used with mixed success:

a. Ductal drainage. When the diameter in the head and body enlarges to 7 to 8 mm or more, an anastomosis between the pancreatic duct and the jejunum, also known as a pancreaticojejunostomy or Puestow procedure, is technically feasible, and has a good chance of producing lasting pain relief (Color Fig. 8-12).

QUICK HIT Symptoms of malabsorption (diarrhea, steatorrhea) do not occur until 90% of the secretory capacity of the pancreas is lost.

FIGURE
8-10 Abdominal computed tomography in a patient with chronic pancreatitis shows dilatation of the main pancreatic duct (*arrows*).

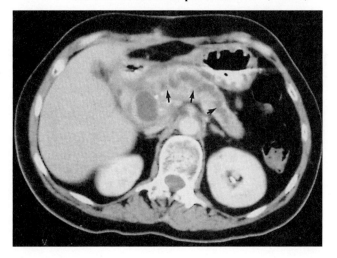

FIGURE
8-11
Endoscopic retrograde cholangiopancreatography (ERCP) illustrates moderate dilation of the main pancreatic duct and ectasia of the secondary ducts associated with moderately advanced chronic pancreatitis. *Arrows* indicate intraductal pancreatic stones.

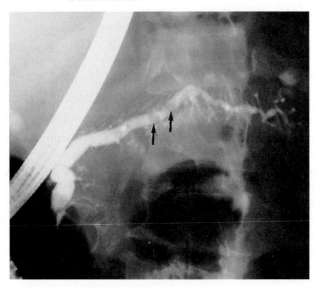

FIGURE
8-12
Lateral pancreaticojejunostomy.

A

B

Jejunum

Jejunal mucosa

Dilated
pancreatic duct

C

b. Resection
   (1) Resection is the treatment of choice when operation is indicated in patients whose ducts are normal or narrow in diameter.
   (2) The type of operation depends on the area of the pancreas affected the most. Therefore, a pancreaticoduodenectomy (Whipple procedure) is performed for disease affecting pancreatic head.
      (a) Beger, who advocates a duodenum sparing resection of the head of pancreas, has described alternatives to the Whipple operation.
      (b) Frey described an operation, which involves coring out the involved pancreatic head without resection, and draining the ductal system into a loop of small bowel.
   (3) Distal pancreatectomy is performed for extensive distal disease.
   (4) Total pancreatectomy is hardly ever performed, because it guarantees diabetes mellitus and pancreatic exocrine insufficiency.
   (5) Pancreatic autotransplant and islet cell transplants have been attempted postpancreatic resection to preserve glandular function, but are only offered at a few centers worldwide.

c. Pancreatic denervation
   (1) Surgical sympathectomy and celiac ganglionectomy have relieved pain effectively in many patients.
   (2) Transthoracic splanchnicectomy and bilateral truncal vagotomy have also been reported to alleviate pain from chronic pancreatitis.

IV. Tumors

A. Types
   1. Exocrine pancreatic neoplasms
      a. These tumors, which are either cystic or solid, are the most common "cystic lesions" in the pancreas and is an inflammatory pseudocyst that are obviously non-neoplastic.
      b. Although many of the cystic lesions are small and benign, they do have malignant potential.
      c. The three common types of cystic pancreatic lesions with their characteristic features are given in Table 8-3.
      d. Remember that the overall postresection survival for malignant cystic lesions is markedly better than for pancreatic ductal adenocarcinoma, which unfortunately is the most common pancreatic neoplasm.

TABLE 8-3 Cystic Pancreatic Neoplasms

	Serous Cystic Neoplasm	Mucinous Cystic Neoplasm	Intraductal Papillary Mucinous Neoplasm
Age	60–70	60–70	60–70
Gender	F > M	F > M	M > F
Location	Anywhere	Body/tail	Head/neck
Communication with pancreatic duct	No	No	Yes
Malignant potential	Low	High	High
"High yield"	Honeycomb septation with central calcification on computed tomography scan	Cyst wall has ovarian type stroma	Mucin at ampulla of Vater

2. Malignant pancreatic neoplasms
   a. Ductal adenocarcinomas account for 90% of all malignant pancreatic cancers, and these will be discussed here. Approximately 65% arise in the pancreatic head and uncinate process, and 15% arise in the body and tail. 20% are diffuse. Uncommon malignant conditions include acinar cell carcinoma, nonepithelial tumors, and lymphomas.
   b. Every year, 30,000 new cases of malignant pancreatic cancers are diagnosed in the United States.
   c. This form of cancer is more common in African-Americans and men, and occurs mostly in the sixth to eighth decades.
   d. Risk factors include hereditary or chronic pancreatitis, smoking, and Peutz–Jeghers syndrome.
   e. Genetic alterations include overexpression of K-ras oncogene and inactivation of p16 and p53.
3. Endocrine tumors
   a. Pancreatic endocrine tumors are rare, with an annual collective incidence of about 5 cases per million population.
   b. Salient features of important pancreatic endocrine cells and their associated tumors are listed in Table 8-4.
B. Clinical presentation
   1. Early symptoms are nonspecific, and include anorexia, nausea, abdominal discomfort, and weight loss. Unlike the liver or the kidney, the pancreas does not have a strong capsule, and consequently the tumor may advance

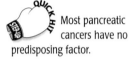

Most pancreatic cancers have no predisposing factor.

TABLE 8-4 Pancreatic Endocrine Neoplasms

Cells	Content	Tumor Syndromes	Clinical Features	Diagnostic Test	% Malignant	Treatment
A	Glucagon	Glucagonoma	Necrolytic migratory erythema, stomatitis, diabetes, weight loss	Elevated glucagon levels (>200 pg/mL) Hyperglycemia	Nearly all	Mostly found in the body and tail and therefore require distal pancreatectomy
B	Insulin	Insulinoma	Hypoglycemic symptoms (catecholamine release), confusion Whipple's triad[a] 10% multiple, 10% associated with MEN-1, 10% malignant	Monitored fast, Insulin-to-glucose ratio >0.4 after fasting. Elevated C-peptide levels	10	Surgical resection Streptozocin, dacarbazine, doxorubicin, and 5-fluorouracil for malignant lesions
D	Somatostatin	Somatostatinoma	Diabetes, gallstones, steatorrhea	Elevated somatostatin levels (>100 pg/mL)	Nearly all	Mostly present in the head Enucleate and debulk liver metastases
D2	Vasoactive intestinal peptide (VIP)	VIPoma (watery diarrhea, hypokalemia, achlorhydria [Verner–Morrison])	High-volume secretory diarrhea, hypokalemia, metabolic acidosis, hypochlorhydria	Elevated VIP levels (>200 pg/mL)	50	Mostly seen in the body and tail Surgical resection
G	Gastrin	Gastrinoma (Zollinger–Ellison syndrome)	Abdominal pain with severe peptic ulcer disease, diarrhea, esophagitis 25% associated with MEN-1 syndrome	Gastrin level >1,000 pg/mL diagnostic; secretin stimulation test increase >200 pg/mL is diagnostic	70	Mostly found in the duodenum and head of the pancreas (gastrinoma triangle) Surgical resection

[a]Whipple's triad: fasting hypoglycemia (< 50 mg/dL), symptoms of hypoglycemia, and symptoms of hypoglycemia relieved by glucose administration.

locally to involve the celiac plexus of nerves, with intractable abdominal and back pain being the first sign.

2. Jaundice is the most common physical sign. Certain physical findings have been historically associated with advanced pancreatic cancer.
   a. Sister Mary Joseph node: periumbilical adenopathy.
   b. Virchow node: left supraclavicular lymphadenopathy.
   c. Blumer shelf: pelvic drop metastases.
   d. Courvoisier sign: a palpable gallbladder in the presence of obstructive jaundice, which indicates noncalculous biliary obstruction (may result from cancer of the pancreatic head).

3. Cancer involving the pancreatic head may cause painless obstructive jaundice with pale stools, dark urine, and pruritus.

4. Unusual presentations may include diabetes or steatorrhea.

C. Laboratory findings
1. Cancer of the pancreatic head may lead to elevation of ductal enzymes, such as alkaline phosphatase and gamma glutamyl transferase, in addition to total bilirubin.
2. Fat malabsorption may result in an abnormally prolonged prothrombin time.
3. Cancer antigen (CA) 19-9 is a tumor marker whose normal upper limit is 37 U/mL. Levels greater than 200 U/mL, when combined with ultrasound, CT, or ERCP, improve the diagnostic accuracy for pancreatic cancer to nearly 100%. Like carcinoembryonic antigen for colon cancer, CA 19-9 can be followed serially as a tool for monitoring response to adjuvant treatment and tumor recurrence.

D. Radiology
1. Transabdominal ultrasound, although useful in detecting gallstones, offers little else.
2. A spiral CT scan with both arterial and portal venous phase is very sensitive in identifying the typical *hypodense lesion* along with invasion into important local structures such as the SMV/portal vein, which would preclude surgical resection (Fig. 8-13).
3. Traditional MRI has not been shown to be superior to CT scan. However, magnetic resonance cholangiopancreatography provides useful information on the biliary and pancreatic ducts, and has the added advantage of being noninvasive, unlike ERCP.
4. ERCP is highly sensitive for detecting pancreatic cancer. However, it is an invasive test and should not be done routinely.

FIGURE 8-13 Computed tomography of the abdomen of a patient with adenocarcinoma of the pancreas. **A.** The obstructed and dilated common bile duct (*light arrow*) and pancreatic duct (*dark arrow*) can be seen. In the adjacent cross-section (**B**), a large mass is present in the head of the pancreas (*arrow*).

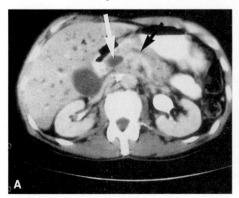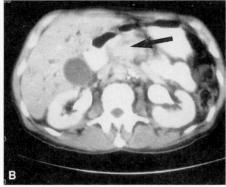

FIGURE
8-14 Endoscopic retrograde cholangiopancreatography in a patient with adenocarcinoma of the pancreas demonstrates a stricture of both the distal common bile duct and the pancreatic duct (*arrow*).

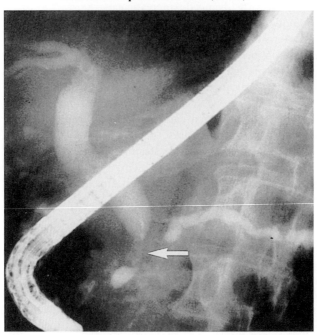

    a. Diagnostic ERCP should be done selectively in patients with presumed pancreatic cancer and obstructive jaundice, without an obvious mass.

    b. Therapeutic ERCP should, of course, be done for palliation of symptomatic obstructive jaundice (Fig. 8-14).

  5. Endoluminal ultrasound and diagnostic laparoscopy are useful tools for staging the tumor in order to establish resectability.

E. Treatment

  1. Resection of pancreatic carcinoma. Only 10% to 20% of all patients diagnosed with adenocarcinoma of the pancreas are candidates for pancreatic resection.

    a. The principles of operative management of pancreatic cancer are quite simple:

      (1) Assess tumor resectability, and determine whether tumor is respectable.

      (2) Do a pancreaticoduodenectomy in case of tumors arising from head, neck, or uncinate process (Color Fig. 8-15).

      (3) Do a distal pancreatectomy, with or without splenectomy, for tumors arising from the body and tail.

    b. The additional consideration in the pancreatic head/neck/uncinate tumors is reestablishment of gastrointestinal continuity after resection.

    c. In cases of advanced malignancy with limited life expectancy, palliative biliary or duodenal bypass can help alleviate symptoms. Preoperative and postoperative chemoradiation have been used with mixed success.

    d. For advanced unresectable pancreatic cancer, the deoxycytidine analogue gemcitabine has shown some benefit in reducing pain, inducing weight gain, and improving performance status. The overall survival benefit has been modest.

QUICK HIT
The 5-year survival for patients undergoing pancreaticoduodenectomy for pancreatic cancer is approximately 20% in the best centers.

QUICK HIT
The most common complication after pancreaticuduodenectomy is pancreatic fistula.

FIGURE
8-15 Pancreaticoduodenectomy. **A.** The tissue to be resected in a standard pancreaticoduodenectomy. **B.** Reconstruction after a standard pancreaticoduodenectomy. **C.** Reconstruction after the pylorus-sparing variation.

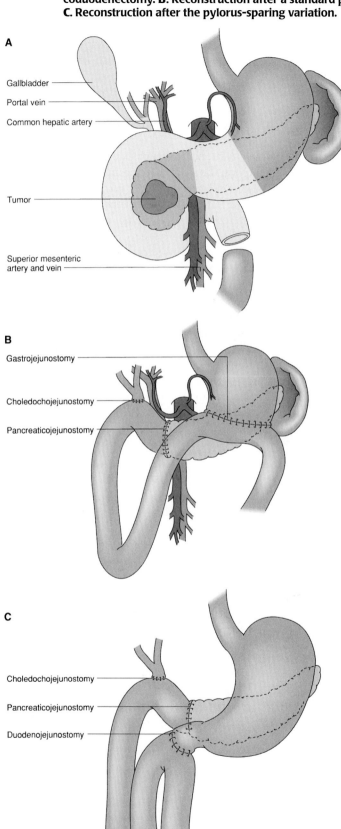

A

Gallbladder

Portal vein

Common hepatic artery

Tumor

Superior mesenteric
artery and vein

B

Gastrojejunostomy

Choledochojejunostomy

Pancreaticojejunostomy

C

Choledochojejunostomy

Pancreaticojejunostomy

Duodenojejunostomy

SPLEEN

I. Anatomy and Physiology

A. Anatomy

1. The spleen develops in the left leaf of the dorsal mesogastrium during the fifth intrauterine week.

2. The odd numbers 1, 3, 5, 7, 9, and 11 summarize certain statistical features of the spleen. It measures $1 \times 3 \times 5$ inches, weighs 7 oz, and lies between the ninth and eleventh ribs

3. In order to be palpable, below the left costal margin, the spleen has to at least double in size.

4. The spleen is enveloped in parietal peritoneum, which extends from it in different directions, creating folds that form the suspensory ligaments of the spleen. Two important folds are the *splenorenal ligament* and the *gastrosplenic ligament*.

   a. The former extends between the anterior surface of the left kidney to the splenic hilum, and invests splenic vessels and the tail of the pancreas.

   b. The latter is a conduit for the short gastric vessels.

5. The splenocolic and splenophrenic ligaments are short and usually avascular. Wandering spleens result from the absence of normal ligamentous attachments.

6. The splenic artery is one of the main branches of the celiac axis, and runs a serpentine course over the pancreas to the splenic hilum. The splenic vein joins the inferior mesenteric vein along its course, until it reaches behind the neck of the pancreas, to join the superior mesenteric artery and forms the portal vein.

7. Accessory spleens are tiny nodules of splenic tissue completely separate from the gland, yet most commonly found in the splenic hilum. Their importance arises in disease processes such as immune thrombocytopenic purpura (ITP), where a total splenectomy is mandatory for cure (Color Figs. 8-16 and 8-17).

FIGURE 8-16 The relations of the spleen to the abdominal and retroperitoneal viscera are seen in a cross-section of the left-facing torso.

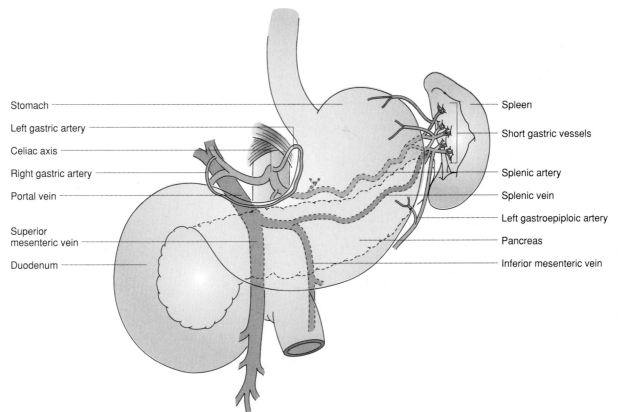

Stomach

Left gastric artery

Celiac axis

Right gastric artery

Portal vein

Superior mesenteric vein

Duodenum

Spleen

Short gastric vessels

Splenic artery

Splenic vein

Left gastroepiploic artery

Pancreas

Inferior mesenteric vein

PANCREAS AND SPLEEN

FIGURE 8-17

The arterial blood flow to the spleen is derived from the splenic artery, the left gastroepiploic artery, and the short gastric arteries (vasa brevia). The venous drainage into this portal vein is also shown.

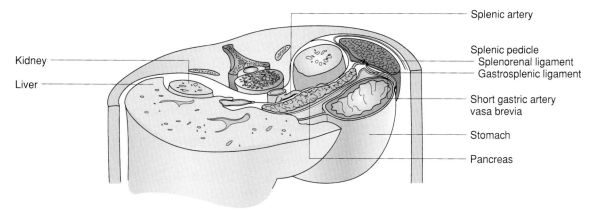

Kidney

Liver

Splenic artery

Splenic pedicle
Splenorenal ligament
Gastrosplenic ligament

Short gastric artery
vasa brevia

Stomach

Pancreas

8. The splenic parenchyma is divided by trabeculae, which are inward extensions of the fibroelastic splenic capsule. The trabeculae carry branches of the splenic vessels in the parenchyma.
   a. The central mass of *red pulp* makes up the bulk of the splenic parenchyma.
   b. The rim of lymphatic tissue around the vessels forms the *white pulp*.
   c. The marginal zone separates white and red pulps (Color Fig. 8-18).
9. The spleen is prone to torsion, and splenopexy is indicated in this instance.
B. Physiology. Functions of the spleen include:
   1. Mechanical filtration of senescent erythrocytes, and circulating antigens/pathogens.
   2. Lymphocyte stimulation and antibody production.
   3. Production of opsonins: tuftsin and properdin.
   4. Reservoir for platelets and granulocytes.
   5. Hematopiesis in fetal life, or later in conditions associated with bone marrow destruction.

FIGURE 8-18

The splenic microanatomy is shown with depictions of both the open and closed circulations.

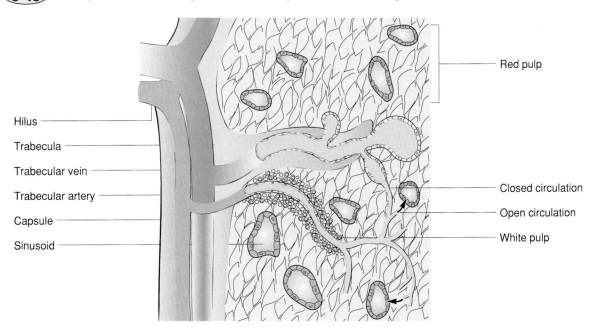

Hilus

Trabecula

Trabecular vein

Trabecular artery

Capsule

Sinusoid

Red pulp

Closed circulation

Open circulation

White pulp

II. Indications for Splenectomy

A. General principles
1. Despite a move towards nonoperative management, blunt trauma remains the most common indication for splenectomy or a splenic salvage procedure in the United States. It is discussed in another section of this book.
2. To better understand the indications for elective surgical removal of the spleen, it helps to categorize them conceptually.

B. Hypersplenism
1. This syndrome is characterized by a decrease in circulating cell count of erythrocytes, platelets, and leukocytes in any combination.
2. The bone marrow shows normal compensatory hematopoietic response.
3. The spleen itself is enlarged as a result of infiltration of stored products of metabolism or neoplastic tissue.
4. Examples include:
   a. Chronic lymphocytic leukemia.
      (1) Most common of all chronic leukemias.
      (2) Patients develop splenomegaly, anemia, and thrombocytopenia.
      (3) Splenectomy is highly successful in relieving these symptoms.
   b. Chronic myelogenous leukemia. Splenectomy is indicated in a select group of patients in advanced stages of chronic myelogenous leukemia, who either have severe transfusion requirements or symptoms due to mass effect.
   c. Other neoplastic conditions in which splenectomy might be indicated, either for relief of pressure-related symptoms or decreased-transfusion requirements are non-Hodgkin lymphoma, myelodysplastic syndrome, and hairy cell leukemia.
   d. Immunologic disorders such as Chediak–Higashi syndrome, and mastocytosis may in rare cases benefit from splenectomy.
   e. Metabolic diseases: Gaucher disease is an autosomal recessive lipid storage disorder. It is the only metabolic disorder where partial splenectomy is the operation of choice.

C. Autoimmune/erythrocyte disorders
1. In these conditions, the abnormality does not lie with the spleen, but results from antibodies against platelets, erythrocytes, or leukocytes. Alternatively, there may be structural changes in the erythrocytes that make them susceptible to destruction by spleen.
2. ITP
   a. This autoimmune disorder is classified as either acute or chronic.
      (1) Acute ITP occurs mostly in children, secondary to a viral illness and is self-limiting.
      (2) Chronic ITP is seen almost exclusively in adults.
   b. Disease results from an antibody production (IgG) against platelet antigen.
      (1) The spleen is the site of antibody production. Most patients with ITP have spleens that are either normal in size, or slightly smaller than normal.
      (2) Assays are now available for detection of antiplatelet IgG antibody.
   c. The platelet count drops to less than 100,000, but patients do not become symptomatic until it drops to considerably less than 50,000.
   d. The bone marrow compensates for systemic platelet destruction by increasing production of megakaryocytes. Therefore, a bone marrow aspiration is a useful test for confirming the diagnosis.
   e. Treatment
      (1) Management is mostly medical, and includes steroids, gammaglobulins, and platelet transfusion.
      (2) Elective splenectomy is indicated in patients who fail medical therapy.
      (3) Splenectomy is also indicated in selected cases of thrombotic thrombocytopenic purpura, and autoimmune hemolytic anemia of the warm antibody type.

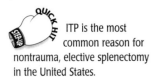

ITP is the most common reason for nontrauma, elective splenectomy in the United States.

3. Autoimmune anemia
   a. A triad of rheumatoid arthritis, neutropenia, and splenomegaly character-izes autoimmune anemia or Felty syndrome.
   b. It affects 1% of patients with chronic rheumatoid arthritis.
   c. The neutropenia is induced by an IgG antibody, and responds effectively to splenectomy.
4. Hereditary spherocytosis
   a. This condition is the most common congenital hemolytic anemia, and has an autosomal dominant transmission.
   b. The defect lies in the cytoskeleton of erythrocytes, and results in decreased plasticity of red blood cells. Erythrocyte proteins *spectrin* and *ankyrin* are primarily affected.
   c. The spleen is the site of destruction of red cells, and splenectomy is indi-cated in all patients. However, in children younger than 6 years of age, the procedure should be avoided because of the risks of overwhelming postsplenectomy sepsis.
5. Hereditary elliptocytosis
   a. This condition is related to hereditary spherocytosis, but is much less severe.
   b. Symptomatic patients respond to splenectomy.

D. Incidental splenectomy
   1. This involves removal of a spleen as part of a major operation on an adja-cent organ (for example, distal pancreatectomy [with splenectomy] or proxi-mal gastric resection for cancer [with splenectomy]).
   2. Removal of the spleen is necessary in these instances, either for complete-ness of resection or technical reasons.

E. Iatrogenic splenectomy. When the spleen is traumatized during surgery in an adjacent area and cannot be salvaged (for example, left adrenalectomy, mobi-lization of splenic flexure of the colon), it is necessary to remove it.

F. Vascular conditions
   1. The splenic artery is the second most common intra-abdominal artery to undergo aneurysmal changes.
      a. Splenic artery aneurysms are twice as common in women.
      b. They are asymptomatic, but may undergo spontaneous rupture especially during pregnancy.
      c. Treatment involves splenectomy.
   2. Splenic vein thrombosis results from a pancreatic or gastric pathology, and is an uncommon cause of upper gastrointestinal bleed curable by splenectomy.

G. Miscellaneous
   1. Staging laparotomies to diagnose Hodgkin lymphoma have decreased con-siderably over the last decade.
   2. Parasitic infection such as *Echinococcus granulosus* can form hydatid cysts in the spleen, and the treatment is a splenectomy.

III. Technique of Splenectomy (Color Fig. 8-19)

A. Open approach
   1. Make midline incision.
   2. Draw off all the blood and clots.
   3. Deliver the spleen in the wound by placing the left hand on its convex sur-face, and cutting the lateral attachments.
   4. Ligate, and divide the short gastric and left gastroepiploic vessels.
   5. Dissect the pancreatic tail free of the splenic artery and vein. Separately ligate and cut those vessels.
   6. Remove spleen. Look for accessory spleens.

B. Laparoscopic splenectomy
   1. This can be performed via either an anterior or a lateral approach.
   2. It is increasingly being used for elective splenectomies, mostly ITP.

FIGURE
8-19 Technique for elective splenectomy. **A.** The inferior pole is reflected laterally by the assistant's fingers, exposing the lower edge of the hilar peritoneal envelope. **B.** The hilar peritoneum is opened, here shown progressing from inferior to superior. **C.** Individual vessels are identified and suture-ligated.

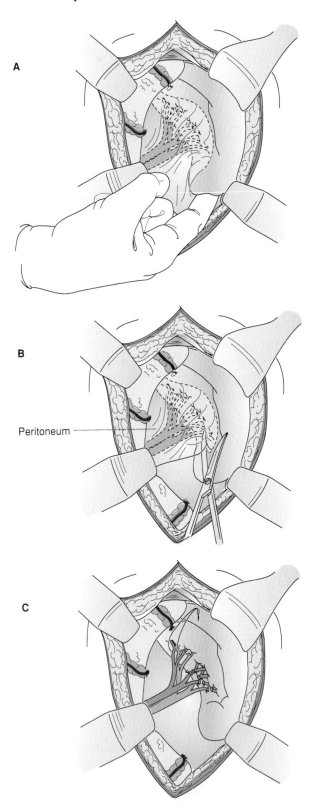

Peritoneum

PANCREAS AND SPLEEN

IV. Changes after Splenectomy

A. Changes in peripheral smear
1. Intraerythrocytic inclusions and cells make an appearance postsplenectomy.
   a. Howell–Jolly bodies (nuclear fragments).
   b. Heinz bodies (hemoglobin deposits).
   c. Pappenheimer bodies (iron deposits).
   d. Target cells.
   e. Spur cells (acanthocytes).
2. Additionally, platelet and leukocyte counts show a transient increase postsplenectomy.

B. Immunologic changes
1. Overwhelming postsplenectomy sepsis (OPSI) is a phenomenon that results from uncontrolled sepsis due to encapsulated microorganisms. The most significant of these bacteria is *Streptococcus pneumoniae*, followed by *Haemophilus influenzae, Neisseria meningitides*, beta-hemolytic *Streptococcus, Staphylococcus aureus, Escherichia coli,* and *Pseudomonas* species.
2. OPSI is more severe in children, and the risks of developing it are the highest in the first 2 years postsplenectomy.
3. To prevent this dreaded complication, patients are vaccinated with pneumococcal, meningococcal, and *Haemophilus* vaccines prior to elective splenectomy. For emergent cases, the vaccine is ideally given 2 weeks postsurgery.

Endocrine Surgery

Bradford Mitchell, MD
Jennifer Knight, MD

THYROID

I. Anatomy and Physiology

A. Anatomy

1. Arterial blood supply

a. The superior thyroid artery originates from the external carotid artery, which is the first branch beyond bifurcation of the common carotid artery.

b. The inferior thyroid artery is a branch of the thyrocervical trunk of the subclavian artery.

2. Venous blood supply

a. The superior and inferior thyroid veins are paired with the superior and inferior thyroid arteries.

b. All venous drainage is to the internal jugular vein.

3. Nerve supply

a. Recurrent laryngeal nerve (RLN).

(1) A branch of the vagus nerve that descends along the internal carotid artery, the RLN is located in close proximity to the inferior thyroid artery branches.

(a) The right RLN loops around the subclavian artery.

(b) The left RLN loops around the aortic arch.

(2) The RLN innervates all intrinsic muscles of the larynx except the cricothyroideus.

(3) The tubercule of Zuckerkandl (pyramidal extension of superior thyroid tissue) and the notch of the cricothyroid membrane are landmarks for RLN insertion.

(4) The nerve may be nonrecurrent (more common on the right, 0.5–0.7%, than on the left, 0.04%), and may be a direct branch from the vagus without an inferior route around the major vessels.

b. External branch of superior laryngeal nerve (EBSLN).

(1) The superior laryngeal nerve is a branch of the vagus nerve, and divides into external and internal branches.

(2) The EBSLN innervates the cricothyroideus muscle and inferior pharyngeal constrictor.

(3) The internal branch provides sensation to the larynx above the vocal cords. Injury results in the inability to phonate in high-pitched sound, yelling, and "voice fatigue." This is described as the voice becoming softer at the end of the day or with prolonged use.

4. Anomalies of thyroid development

a. Lingual thyroid. Thyroid tissue at the base of the tongue may require resection.

b. Thyroglossal duct cyst. This is located in the midline between the base of the tongue and the isthmus, and resection may require removal of the central portion of the hyoid bone.

QUICK HIT The inferior thyroid artery supplies both the superior and the inferior parathyroid glands. Ligation of the main trunk can cause ischemia of the parathyroids.

QUICK HIT The recurrent laryngeal nerve is in close proximity to bifurcation of inferior thyroid artery, and the tubercle of Zuckerkandl.

QUICK HIT Because the thyroidea ima artery is a direct branch of the aorta, it may be relevant in patients with relation to large substernal goiters.

QUICK HIT Venous drainage is important to venous sampling of parathyroid hormone for parathyroid adenoma localization.

QUICK HIT The RLN controls the vocal cords. Unilateral injury results in hoarseness with paralysis of the ipsilateral vocal cord, and carries risk of aspiration. Bilateral injury results in inability to protect the airway, with paralysis of bilateral vocal cords, and may require urgent tracheostomy.

c. Pyramidal lobe. Should be excised during operation to avoid excess tissue as antigenic stimulus in Graves disease, or hindrance to remnant ablation in cancer, or persistent hormone production in hyperthyroidism.

B. Physiology

1. Makes thyroid hormones—triiodothyronine (T3) and thyroxine (T4) from iodine and tyrosine. T3 and T4 are stored in the gland when bound to thyroglobulin.

a. The secretion of T3 and T4 is under the control of thyrotropin-releasing hormone (TRH) secreted by the hypothalamus, which regulates thyroid-stimulating hormone (TSH) from the anterior pituitary.

b. Increased plasma levels of T3 and T4 result in negative feedback on TRH and TSH.

2. Calcitonin is secreted by parafollicular or C-cells, which are involved in medullary thyroid cancer.

II. Hyperthyroidism (Table 9-1)

A. Causes

1. Grave disease (diffuse toxic goiter)

a. Autoimmune disorder with development of antibodies that stimulate thyroid hormone production or secretion.

b. Hyperthyroid symptoms include nervousness, irritability, heat intolerance, involuntary weight loss, palpitations, sweating, and tachycardia secondary to enhanced effect of catecholamines. It is also associated with exophthalmos, edema of the eyelids, pretibial edema, hypertension, arrhythmias, osteoporosis, and amenorrhea.

c. The TSH level is suppressed, and T3 and T4 levels are elevated.

d. Radioactive iodine (RAI) scan and tracer uptake are diagnostic.

2. Hashimoto thyroiditis (hashitoxicosis)

a. 5% of patients with Hashimoto thyroiditis are hyperthyroid.

b. This is generally a transient process, and eventually hypothyroidism ensues.

3. Toxic multinodular goiter

a. This is adenomatous hyperplasia of the thyroid gland.

b. The most common type of multinodular goiter is usually euthyroid.

4. Toxic adenoma. Treatment is radioactive iodine ablation or lobectomy for control of hyperthyroidism.

QUICK HIT The recurrent laryngeal nerves are at risk during surgery at three sites: (i) division of inferior thyroid artery (nerve can be closely applied to artery), (ii) division of ligament of Berry (nerve fibers can traverse ligament), and (iii) the main trunks low in the neck during exploration for ectopic parathyroid glands.

QUICK HIT The lingual thyroid may be the only thyroid tissue present, and resection may result in hypothyroidism. Autotransplantation or hormone replacement should be considered in this circumstance.

QUICK HIT T3 is mainly produced by peripheral conversion of T4 by deiodinase in the liver, muscle, and kidney. T4 is secreted exclusively by the thyroid gland.

TABLE 9-1	Management of Causes of Hyperthyroidism		
	Medical Management	**Radioactive Iodine**	**Surgical Resection**
Graves disease	Treatment of choice Rare but serious side effect is aplastic anemia	Second-line; some advocate this as first-line due to low risk and complications of medical treatment	For patients who fail RAI or who cannot receive RAI, or failure/complication of antithyroid drug or if tracheoesophageal compressive symptoms of goiter
Hashimoto thyroiditis	Transient phenomenon		Reserved for those with symptoms of goiter
Multinodular goiter			First option for symptomatic goiters due to size of the disease, which limits medical therapy
Toxic adenoma		Treatment of choice	If RAI fails

5. Amiodarone-induced thyrotoxicosis
   a. This is very difficult to treat due to cardiac condition and arrhythmias.
   b. Hyperthyroidism is controlled with antithyroid medications or iopanoic acid, and then surgery if amiodarone cannot be discontinued permanently.

B. Medical management
   1. Antithyroid drugs (propylthiouracil [PTU], methimazole, and Tapazole) may be useful.
      a. Functions
         (1) Block organification of iodine, and formation of thyroid hormone.
         (2) Prevent peripheral conversion of T4 to T3 by deiodinase (PTU).
      b. Complications include aplastic anemia and liver function abnormalities.
      c. Failure also occurs with noncompliance.
   2. Beta-blockers control symptoms mediated by catecholamines.

C. RAI
   1. I-131 destroys the thyrocytes with minimal effect to surrounding structures. Its therapeutic effect is not immediate. Sometimes it requires repeat treatment.
   2. Relative contraindications include large gland, Grave ophthalmopathy, concerns for radiation exposure in the pregnant patient or the patient considering pregnancy in the near future, and the risk of hyperparathyroidism.

D. Surgical management
   1. Near-total thyroidectomy
   2. Preoperative preparation for surgery
      a. This most often includes beta-blockers to prevent thyroid storm and control symptoms. It may be necessary to taper these drugs postoperatively.
      b. Lugol solution (iodine solution) orally to decrease vascularity of the thyroid gland and decrease hyperthyroidism. There is an "escape effect." If there is no operation within 10 days, the patient becomes more hyperthyroid.

III. Goiter

A. Iodine deficiency is a major cause of goiter
B. Classification is by function or anatomy (toxic, nontoxic, diffuse, focal, and smooth).
   1. Primary
      a. Intrathoracic location (substernal).
      b. Intrathoracic blood supply.
      c. Venous drainage into the chest.
      d. No connection to the cervical thyroid gland.
   2. Secondary
      a. Direct extension of normally located tissue in the neck.
      b. Normal blood supply.
   3. Intrathoracic or substernal goiters
      a. From 10% to 15% of these goiters are primary.
      b. If located in a posterior position, they are associated with symptoms of compression of esophagus and displacement of trachea. This location is most likely at the thoracic inlet at the level of the sternal notch secondary to bony confinement.
      c. Diagnosis of airway compromise involves a flow loop spirogram on pulmonary function test.
C. Treatment
   1. Near-total thyroidectomy is the mainstay when symptoms arise.
   2. Most can be done through a cervical incision, rarely require median sternotomy.
D. Symptomatic goiters
   1. Most goiters are multinodular and benign, and patients are euthyroid. The presence of cancer within a goiter is less than 1%, and within a multinodular goiter 2% to 4%.

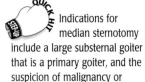

Indications for median sternotomy include a large substernal goiter that is a primary goiter, and the suspicion of malignancy or recurrence.

2. Symptoms of aerodigestive obstruction should be sought.

3. Dysphagia, odynophagia, dyspnea, orthopnea, and changes in these symptoms related to position of head, neck, and arms should be assessed.

    a. Persistent and consistent hoarseness warrants further evaluation to exclude nerve involvement by tumor.

    b. Episodic voice and swallowing changes are common in patients with a large goiter.

4. Studies to evaluate for obstruction of esophagus and trachea are rarely indicated, and do not show evidence of narrowing in most cases. They are of limited value in surgical planning or decision to operate.

IV. Thyroid Nodule

A. This discrete lesion within the thyroid gland is palpably and/or ultrasonographically distinct from the surrounding parenchyma. These nodules are palpable in 5% of the population.

B. In the United States, approximately 50% of individuals older than 50 have thyroid nodules by ultrasonic evaluation (more in women than in men).

C. Less than 5% of nodules prove to be malignant. The risk of malignancy is related to history of radiation, age (extremes of age lead to greater malignancy), number of nodules (solitary more worrisome), and sex (men are more likely to have malignant nodules).

D. Diagnosis

1. Fine-needle aspiration (FNA) biopsy. The most accurate, cost-effective method for evaluating thyroid nodules, this is the procedure of choice.

    a. FNA is safe, minimally invasive, and accurate. The false-negative rate for a benign finding is less than 5%.

    b. FNA should be performed in any nodule greater than 1.5 cm. Some authors now suggest 8 to 10 mm, particularly if it has worrisome ultrasound characteristics. FNA can be done under ultrasound guidance.

    c. Diagnostic categories

        (1) Nondiagnostic or inadequate: repeat FNA. If first attempt not done under ultrasound guidance, do so now (more than two repetitions is of limited benefit).

        (2) Indeterminate: consider repeat FNA or follow with serial ultrasound. If there is an increase in size, consider repeat FNA, or total thyroidectomy or lobectomy.

        (3) Malignant: perform surgical excision.

        (4) Benign: no further diagnostic studies or treatment is necessary.

2. Ultrasound

    a. Accurate at determining size, number, and character (solid versus cystic) of nodules.

    b. Used to diagnose multinodular goiter.

    c. Used to assess malignant features: calcifications, irregular borders, increased blood flow.

3. Radionuclide scanning

    a. Done with radioiodine or technetium-99m pertechnetate.

    b. Rarely useful for evaluation of nodular disease (ultrasound and TSH allow accurate prediction of what scan will show).

4. Measurement of TSH and a history of symptoms (mobility, firmness, solitary nodule, adenopathy, voice changes) are used to exclude toxic adenoma.

5. RAI scans are of limited value.

6. Thyroid function tests are of little value, because most nodules are nonfunctional.

E. Treatment. Indications for surgical removal without use of ultrasound or FNA include:

1. Tracheoesophageal compressive symptoms of a nodule.

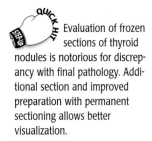
QUICK HIT Evaluation of frozen sections of thyroid nodules is notorious for discrepancy with final pathology. Additional section and improved preparation with permanent sectioning allows better visualization.

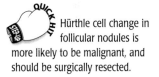
QUICK HIT Hürthle cell change in follicular nodules is more likely to be malignant, and should be surgically resected.

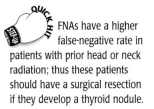
QUICK HIT FNAs have a higher false-negative rate in patients with prior head or neck radiation; thus these patients should have a surgical resection if they develop a thyroid nodule.

ENDOCRINE SURGERY

2. History of significant radiation exposure, or radiation therapy to head and neck, or mediastinum (nodule in this setting has a 30% risk of malignancy).
3. Large nodule (solid or cystic) greater than 4 cm with or without symptoms, which carries high risk of malignancy (FNA may have sampling error due to size).

V. Thyroid Cancer

A. The incidence is 1/10,000 per year, with deaths occurring in 1/200,000 individuals per year (Table 9-2).
B. Well-differentiated cancers (~95%; papillary 80% and follicular 15%).
   1. 10% are associated with a history of radiation exposure (typically papillary variant).
   2. These cancers most common present as asymptomatic thyroid nodules.
   3. Treatment involves surgery. Lobectomy or total thyroidectomy is indicated.
      a. Advantages of lobectomy.
         (1) Eliminates possibility of permanent hypoparathyroidism.
         (2) Decreases the risk of nerve injury.
         (3) Does not require thyroid hormone replacement.
      b. Disadvantages of lobectomy (most physicians would recommend thyroid hormone suppression for prevention of recurrence of benign or malignant nodule in the remaining lobe).
         (1) Thyroglobulin cannot be used as a tumor marker as evidence of recurrence of cancer.
         (2) Whole body RAI scanning cannot be performed to look for recurrent or metastatic disease.
   4. Follow-up involves serial neck examinations and ultrasound, thyroglobulin, and RAI scans if total thyroidectomy was performed in patients at moderate to high risk of recurrence.

> **QUICK HIT**
> Hürthle cell, tall cell, or papillary variants are described, are rare, and carry a poorer prognosis than well-differentiated thyroid cancer.

ENDOCRINE SURGERY

TABLE 9-2 Histologic Types of Thyroid Cancer and Their Treatment

Histologic Type	Characteristics	Lymph Node Metastases	Distant Metastases	Treatment
Papillary	XRT therapy, "psammoma bodies," multicentric	Common	Uncommon	Thyroidectomy and I-131 therapy
Follicular	See invasion of capsule, unifocal, thickly encapsulated	Uncommon	Occasional	Thyroidectomy and I-131 therapy
Hürthle cell	Intermediate differentiation, variants of follicular, multicentric and bilateral	Common	Occasional	Thyroidectomy and I-131 therapy
Anaplastic	Aggressive, older population	Common	Common	Palliative
Medullary thyroid	Arise from C-cells, associated with multiple endocrine neoplasia (MEN) syndromes, contain amyloid RET proto-oncogene	Common	Common	Thyroidectomy and functional neck dissection on the side of the cancer and central node dissection on contralateral side

5. Prognosis makes use of prognostic scoring indices to stratify patients into three risk groups—low-, intermediate-, and high-risk. AMES/AGES and MACIS age is 40 for men and 50 for women (45 for both in tumor-node-metastases system).

    a. AMES: age, metastases, extent, and size.

    b. AGES: age, grade, extent, and size (limitation is subjective interpretation of pathologic grade).

    c. MACIS: metastases, age, completeness of resection, invasion, and size.

C. Medullary thyroid carcinoma (approximately 4%)

    1. Total thyroidectomy with ipsilateral functional neck dissection.

    2. No sex or age predilection. This form of thyroid carcinoma is sporadic in 60% to 70% of cases, and familial in the rest.

        a. Sporadic cases typically have a single focus, with spread to the lymphatics.

        b. Familial cases are typically multifocal and more aggressive.

            (1) These cases carry a worse prognosis. However, even in the face of metastatic disease (miliary liver metastases), patients can live for more than 10 years.

            (2) They can also be associated with multiple endocrine neoplasia (MEN) type II syndrome.

            (3) Spread occurs through the lymphatics and bloodstream.

    3. The tumors secrete calcitonin, so calcitonin is followed as a tumor marker.

    4. Serial ultrasounds are followed to look for recurrence. If there is no evidence of neck disease and consistently rising calcitonin levels, multiple small liver metastases should be considered.

    5. Medullary thyroid carcinoma has a parafollicular C-cell origin, and therefore radioactive iodine and thyroglobulin are not effective in following or treating disease.

    6. Medullary thyroid cancer has a poorer prognosis than well-differentiated thyroid cancer.

D. Lymphoma, anaplastic, and metastatic thyroid carcinoma (1%).

    1. Lymphoma may present like thyroiditis with rapidly enlarging tender gland.

        a. A rare condition, it affects mainly older women (aged 50–70 years).

        b. Open biopsy may be required to distinguish from thyroiditis. FNA shows lymphocytes and thyroid follicles.

        c. If focal, it can be treated with radiation therapy.

        d. If diffuse, it can be treated with chemotherapy.

        e. The prognosis is variable, and depends on the type and extent of disease.

    2. Anaplastic thyroid cancer is one of the most aggressive cancers, and usually presents with advanced disease.

        a. This form of cancer affects the older population (aged 50–70) years, and it has no sex predilection.

        b. It is rapidly growing, with early invasion of adjacent structures.

        c. Metastasis occurs early via lymphatics and bloodstream.

        d. It is usually incurable with a poor prognosis.

            (1) Surgical resection is usually palliative, and for control of respiratory compressive symptoms.

            (2) Radiation therapy may have limited benefit.

VI. Thyroid Positron Emission Tomography for Incidentaloma

A. Thyroid nodules are frequently identified on positron emission tomography (PET) scan when it is performed for patients with other malignancy.

B. Nodules that are found incidentally on PET have a 50% chance of being malignant.

C. Neck ultrasound and FNA may be used to biopsy, but surgical excision is generally advised.

D. As the frequency of PET scans increases, the incidence of malignancy in thyroid nodule incidentalomas may decrease.

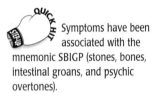

Knowledge of parathyroid gland embryology is essential when searching for an ectopic gland. If the inferior gland is not in the usual location, it is most often found in the fat along the thyrothymic ligament or in the thymus.

Surgical localization of the parathyroid glands can be aided by following the arterial supply from the thyrocervical trunk.

Symptoms have been associated with the mnemonic SBIGP (stones, bones, intestinal groans, and psychic overtones).

PARATHYROID GLANDS AND HYPERPARATHYROIDISM

I. Embryology and Anatomy

A. Embryology
1. The superior gland comes from the fourth brachial cleft.
2. The inferior gland comes from the third brachial cleft, with the thymus derived from the same source.

B. Anatomy
1. Blood supply: the inferior thyroid artery and its branches carry the blood to the glands.
2. Location: both glands are usually located within 1 cm of the insertion of the recurrent laryngeal nerve at the cricothyroid membrane. The superior gland is posterior and superior to the nerve, and the inferior gland is anterior to the nerve and inferior to the insertion (Fig. 9-1).
3. Size and color: normal glands are less than 8 mm in length, 2 to 4 mm in width, and 0.5 to 2 mm in depth. They are described as mustard-colored, and may have a slight purple-to-gray hue when adenomatous or hyperplastic. They are difficult to distinguish from blood-stained fat or small lymph nodes. Normal glands weigh 30 to 50 mg.

II. Hyperparathyroidism and Hypercalcemia

A. Hyperparathyroidism
1. Symptoms are subtle, and are often attributed to aging or other medical condition (Table 9-3). Hypertension, osteoporosis, and heart dysfunction and premature cardiac death not from atherosclerosis have all been associated with hyperparathyroidism.

FIGURE 9-1 Ectopic parathyroid gland locations secondary to aberrant migration found on reoperation for persistent hyperparathyroidism.

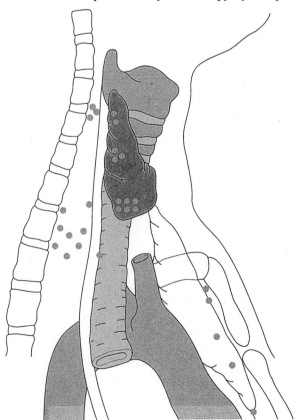

(Reprinted, with permission, from Karp SJ, Morris JPG. *Blueprints Surgery,* 4th ed. Baltimore: Lippincott Williams & Wilkins; 123.

ENDOCRINE SURGERY

TABLE 9-3 Symptoms in Patients with Hyperparathyroidism	
Symptom	Percent
Stones	30
Bone pain	2
Peptic ulcer disease	12
Psychiatric complaints	15
Weakness	70
Constipation	32
Polyuria	28
Pancreatitis	1
Myalgia	54
Arthralgia	54

(Reprinted, with permission, from Wells AB, Doherty GM, Greenfield LG. *Surgery: Scientific Practice and Principles,* 2nd ed. New York: Lippincott-Raven)

2. Diagnosis
   a. Most often, the diagnosis is not suspected. The condition is found when elevated calcium is noted on routine testing.
      (1) Elevated calcium level should not be ignored, and evaluation should begin with parathyroid hormone (PTH) level.
      (2) Low total calcium may be the result of low protein, and serum albumin is first test of choice.
   b. In addition to elevated calcium, elevated PTH is also found.
   c. To exclude familial hypocalciuric hypercalcemia, use normal or elevated 24-hour urine calcium.
3. Secondary and tertiary hyperparathyroidism
   a. Mechanism
      (1) Low serum calcium is secondary to low vitamin D and elevated phosphorus levels.
      (2) With aggressive calcium and vitamin D supplements and phosphate binders, this is less common today.
   b. Treatment
      (1) Calcimimetic (Sensipar) is approved to treat refractory secondary hyperparathyroidism and parathyroid carcinoma. Mimics calcium at the calcium sensing receptor and causes reduction of PTH excretion (and calcium levels in parathyroid carcinoma).
      (2) Surgery is indicated when medications have failed to control the hyperparathyroidism.
         (a) Indications: patients with renal osteodystrophy, bone pain, pruritus, soft tissue calcification, and necrosis, as well as renal transplant candidates.
         (b) Purpose: to avoid tertiary hyperparathyroidism (severe hypercalcemia and hyperparathyroidism occurring following transplant, when calcium and vitamin D mechanisms are restored in patients with hyperplasia from secondary hyperparathyroidism).
      (3) Surgical treatment: subtotal parathyroidectomy or total parathyroidectomy with autotransplantation, and cervical thymectomy to minimize risk of recurrence.
4. Asymptomatic hyperparathyroidism
   a. A careful history shows subtle symptoms in most patients thought to be asymptomatic.

b. Operative management has morbidity of less than 3%. Blood loss is minimal, and the operation can be performed under local or regional anesthesia as an outpatient in most hospitals.

c. Cost of continued medical evaluation to follow patients exceeds surgical costs after several years, and the natural history of untreated disease is poorly delineated.

d. The 1990 National Institutes of Health consensus conference on management of asymptomatic patients was not for *minimally symptomatic* patients. Signs and symptoms must be assessed carefully, and most patients note improvement or resolution of these symptoms after surgical resection.

(1) All truly asymptomatic patients require every 6-month follow-up.

(2) Bone densitometry, 24-hour urine calcium, and creatinine clearance need to be followed.

(3) Patients younger than 50 years of age should be offered surgical correction.

(4) Cost of medical follow-up exceeds cost of surgical therapy in short period.

B. Hypercalcemia
1. Differential diagnosis
a. Hyperparathyroidism
b. Malignancy/multiple myeloma
c. Thiazide diuretics
d. Hyperthyroidism
e. Excess of vitamins A or D
f. Sarcoidosis
g. Miscellaneous conditions: milk-alkali syndrome, familial hypocalciuric hypercalcemia, immobilization, Paget disease, Addisonian crisis
2. Routine (cost-effective) testing
a. Based on frequency of these diagnoses, a reasonable approach would include a careful history and physical examination, chest x-ray, urinalysis with attention to protein and red blood cells, and a PTH level.
b. Based on the results, consider ordering PTHrP, serum protein electrophoresis, 24-hour urine calcium level.
3. Treatment for severe or symptomatic hypercalcemia
a. The mainstay of acute therapy is hydration followed by furosemide after the patient is adequately rehydrated.
b. Bisphosphonates, calcitonin, mithramycin, and steroids each have varied duration of onset and action and degree of efficacies.

III. Thyroid Surgery

A. Localization studies
1. These are all limited by the difficulty in locating ectopic glands and by the expertise and experience of surgeons performing the studies.
2. Recently, many studies have shown potential cost savings with preoperative localization by decreasing time of exploration when limited explorations are performed.
3. The lack of numbers and prospective randomized controls is the main limitation of all studies of parathyroid localization.

B. Considerations for **surgery**
1. Risks
a. Recurrence, persistence, nerve injuries
b. Increased risks in reoperation
(1) Prior thyroid, parathyroid, carotid surgery, or anterior cervical fusion mandates formal vocal cord evaluation and preoperative localization studies to minimize unnecessary exploration.
(2) Nerve monitoring is adjunct with possible benefit of preventing injury.

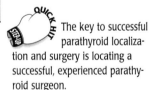

The key to successful parathyroid localization and surgery is locating a successful, experienced parathyroid surgeon.

ENDOCRINE SURGERY

c. Recurrence and persistence of hyperparathyroidism is best avoided by:
  (1) Recognition of familial disease by careful history preoperatively.
  (2) Suspicion of multigland disease or double adenomas based on change in intraoperative PTH assay.

d. Rough handling of parathyroid tissue can lead to implantation of fragments of viable parathyroid tissue. Parathyromatosis (implantation of significant volume of spilled benign tissue) can behave like parathyroid carcinoma.

e. This ability of implantation with subsequent functional hormonal production is exploited in the care of patients with hyperplasia to allow for autotransplantation and cryopreservation, and subsequent implantation to prevent or treat hypoparathyroidism.

> **QUICK HIT** PTH levels at 5 and 10 minutes postexcision are anticipated to fall to 50% of pre-excision or baseline peak levels and/or into the normal range in adenomatous disease.

IV. Parathyroid Carcinoma

A. Fewer than 1% of cases of primary hyperparathyroidism are cancerous.

B. This form of carcinoma is usually associated with a three- to ten-fold elevation of PTH, and higher calcium levels than adenomatous disease (>14 versus 10.5–11.5). There is a palpable nodule in 50% of patients.

C. Treatment is excision, ipsilateral thyroid lobectomy, and ipsilateral lymph node dissection.
  1. Sensipar may significantly lower calcium and control growth.
  2. Reoperation for carcinoma requires use of all the previously mentioned adjuncts and may offer significant duration of control of calcium.

D. Prognosis is poor

ADRENAL GLANDS

I. Embryology and Anatomy

A. Embryology
  1. Adrenal cortex
    a. Derived from mesodermal cells near urogenital ridge.
    b. Occasionally form adrenocortical rests (ectopic location), most commonly in the ovary, testis, or kidney.
  2. Adrenal medulla
    a. Derived from ectodermal cells of neural crest origin, which migrate from the sympathetic ganglion.
    b. Occasionally, ectopic locations include the paraganglia, the organ of Zuckerkandl (just below bifurcation of the aorta), and the mediastinum.

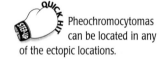

> **QUICK HIT** Pheochromocytomas can be located in any of the ectopic locations.

B. Anatomy
  1. Location. These glands lie on medial aspect of superior pole of each kidney.
    a. The right gland is just posterior to the inferior vena cava, adjacent to the liver and the right diaphragmatic crus.
    b. The left gland is near the aorta, tail of the pancreas, and the spleen.
  2. Arterial supply. Blood is supplied by the phrenic artery, the aorta, and the renal artery.
  3. Venous drainage
    a. A single vein drains into the inferior vena cava on the right and into the renal vein on the left.
    b. The adrenal portal system allows blood from the cortex to drain directly to the medulla.

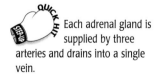

> **QUICK HIT** Each adrenal gland is supplied by three arteries and drains into a single vein.

  4. Histology
    a. Zona glomerulosa: outer zone, which produces aldosterone.
    b. Zona fasciculata: middle zone, which produces cortisol and other glucocorticoids.
    c. Zona reticularis: inner zone, which produces sex hormones.
    d. Medulla: produces catecholamines (epinephrine, norepinephrine, and dopamine).
  5. For details about the adrenal hormones, see Table 9-4.

TABLE 9-4	Adrenal Hormones			
Hormone	**Stimulated By**	**Inhibited By**	**Actions**	**Diagnostic Tests**
Cortisol	Adrenocorticotropic hormone (ACTH) from pituitary	Negative feedback of cortisol on ACTH	Increases gluconeogenesis, lipolysis, and proteolysis; positive chronotropic and inotropic effects on the heart; immunosuppressive and anti-inflammatory effects	Can measure serum free cortisol (diurnal variation) or 24-hour urinary 17- hydroxy-corticosteroids
Aldosterone	Decreased blood volume via angiotensin II, hyperkalemia, hyponatremia, slightly by ACTH and sympathetic nervous system	Hypernatremia, hypokalemia, fluid overload	Stimulates sodium and free water resorption, potassium and hydrogen ion excretion	Serum aldosterone, 24-hour urinary aldosterone
Androgens	ACTH	Negative feedback	Promote development of secondary sexual characteristics	24-hour urine for 17-ketosteroids
Catecholamines	Sympathetic nervous system	Negative feedback	"Fight or flight" response	Serum metanephrines, 24-hour urine for vanillylmandelic acid (VMA), normetanephrines, metanephrines

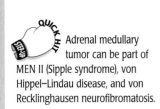

QUICK HIT

Adrenal medullary tumor can be part of MEN II (Sipple syndrome), von Hippel–Lindau disease, and von Recklinghausen neurofibromatosis.

II. Adrenal Medullary Tumor. Pheochromocytoma

A. Epidemiology
1. There are 400 cases per year in the United States.
2. This tumor follows the 10% rule: 10% are bilateral, 10% are familial, 10% are extra-adrenal, 10% are malignant, 10% are multiple, and 10% occur in children.
3. This tumor occurs rarely during pregnancy, but if it is unrecognized, very high infant and maternal mortality results. The condition may be misdiagnosed as preeclampsia.
4. Rarely, ectopic urinary bladder occurrence is associated with flushing and hypertensive episodes incited by contraction of the bladder.

B. Etiology
1. Adrenal tumors (90%).
2. Extra-adrenal tumors (10% are paraganglia, organ of Zuckerkandl, urinary bladder, or mediastinum).

C. Signs and symptoms include palpitations, tachycardia, flushing, headache, and "sense of impending doom."

D. Diagnosis
1. A 24-hour urine catecholamines and venous assay
   a. Limited by episodic nature of secretion and sensitivity of assay.
   b. Vanillylmandelic acid (VMA) and total metanephrines.
   c. Other cautions: monoamine oxidase inhibitor agents, stresses for other reasons and angiographic dyes may give false-positive results. Aldomet may falsely raise plasma levels.
2. Imaging for localization

a. CT scan: 90% to 95% accuracy

b. I-metaiodobenzylguanidine (MIBG) scan: to show absorption by pheochromocytomas and paraganglionomas (sympathetic chain tumors that also secrete catecholamines).

E. Treatment: surgery

1. Preparation for surgery to avoid hypertensive crisis.

a. Alpha blockade with phenoxybenzamine, until symptoms resolve in 10 to 14 days.

b. Intravenous hydration when dehydration is secondary to catecholamine excess.

c. Then add beta-blockers, and continue both until the time of surgery.

d. Calcium-channel blockers alone may be used.

e. May require vasopressor management intraoperatively, as tumor is manipulated and removed.

2. Surgery can be performed with open or laparoscopic technique from anterior posterior or flank approaches.

a. Laparoscopic anterior approach seems to be gaining greatest favor.

b. Minimal handling is necessary, with early ligation of vein and avoidance of capsular rupture.

c. Rupture of pheochromocytomas can cause implantation and recurrence, even with benign pheochromocytoma.

III. Cushing Syndrome and Cushing Disease

A. Hypercortisolism

B. Adrenocorticotropic hormone (ACTH)-secreting pituitary adenoma: Cushing disease

1. Overproduction of ACTH from pituitary leads to bilateral adrenal hyperplasia.

2. Treatment involves resection of pituitary adenoma.

C. Hypercortisolism and/or ACTH excess from other source: Cushing syndrome

1. May have cortisol secreting tumor.

a. Primary adrenal adenoma or hyperplasia.

b. Paraneoplastic syndrome: oat cell lung cancer, bronchial carcinoids, thymomas, and tumors of the pancreas and liver.

2. Iatrogenic from steroid use.

D. Signs and symptoms: hyperglycemia, truncal obesity, hypertension, striae, immunocompromise, muscle wasting

E. Diagnosis

1. A 24-hour urine cortisol and 24-hour urine creatinine.

2. Overnight 1-mg dexamethasone suppression test.

3. If positive, do high-dose dexamethasone suppression test.

a. If ACTH is high, look for pituitary causes; and if very high, this may indicate an ectopic source. Perform CT, magnetic resonance imaging (MRI), or positron emission tomography of the chest, abdomen, or pelvis.

b. If ACTH is low, perform imaging of adrenals.

IV. Hyperaldosteronism: Conn Syndrome

A. Signs and symptoms: hypertension, hypokalemia, polyuria, polydipsia, headache

B. Diagnosis

1. Look for evidence of dehydration.

2. Plasma renin activity: look for plasma aldosterone /plasma renin activity ratio greater than 30, and plasma aldosterone greater than 20, which indicates aldosteronoma (90% sensitive).

3. If CT or MRI does not show a 1 cm or greater tumor, adrenal vein sampling may be used to localize hyperfunctioning adrenal. This involves simultaneous sampling of adrenal veins after ACTH intravenous injection. Cortisol ratios from adrenal vein/plasma ensure adequacy of adrenal vein cannulation. A 4 × aldosterone ratio gives appropriate lateralization.

C. Treatment
1. For nodular adrenal hyperplasia or bilateral masses, use spironolactone.
2. For adenoma, use adrenalectomy.
D. Secondary hyperaldosteronism: due to renal artery stenosis, congestive heart failure, cirrhosis, malignant hypertension.

V. Incidentaloma

A. Diagnosis: discovery of an asymptomatic adrenal lesion on imaging done for another indication.
1. 1% to 10% are found in healthy patients on routine imaging.
2. Most are benign and nonfunctioning tumors.
3. Adrenal masses increase in incidence with age.
4. Patients need thorough physical examination, routine laboratory studies, serum potassium, aldosterone/renin, cortisol, and 24-hour urine for VMA, normetanephrines, and metanephrines. Laboratory studies for assessment purposes should be repeated at 1 year.
B. Treatment
1. If nonfunctional and less than 4 cm, serial imaging every 6 to 12 months × 2.
   a. If mass grows, then surgical resection
   b. If stable after 2 years, then stop following.
2. If nonfunctional and greater than, or equal to 6 cm, adrenalectomy is indicated due to higher chance of malignancy.
3. If functional and of any size, adrenalectomy is required.

VI. Adrenal Cortical Carcinoma

A. There are 0.5 to 2 cases per million per year. 60% have hormone production and may have mixed hormone secretion.
B. Needle biopsies should be avoided.
C. Treated with adrenalectomy, with complete resection is only chance for cure.
1. Tumors may be slow growing, and debulking a tumor may eliminate symptoms of hormone excess but will not alter prognosis.
2. Chemotherapy is of limited benefit.

VII. Adrenal Insufficiency

A. Signs and symptoms: lethargy, abdominal pain, nausea, vomiting, confusion, hypotension, hyponatremia, hyperkalemia, fever.
B. Diagnosis: serum cortisol and ACTH stimulation test. Then 250 μg of ACTH is given, and cortisol is checked at 30 and 60 minutes.
C. Treatment: give 4 mg of dexamethasone to initial treatment, and hydrocortisone replacement every 6 to 8 hours, plus intravenous hydration.

VIII. Multiple Endocrine Neoplasia

A. Tumor characteristics
1. They tend to be multicentric.
2. They may be benign or malignant.
B. Etiology: autosomal dominant
C. MEN I: pancreatic islet cell tumors 10%, parathyroid hyperplasia 80%, pituitary adenomas 20%
1. Tumor suppressor (*MEN-I*): the first mutation is inherited, and requires a second mutation to have evident disease.
2. Careful family history allows detection of MEN I in families.
3. Parathyroid hyperplasia.
   a. Treated with 3 1/2 gland resection, or total parathyroidectomy with autotransplantation.
   b. Many advocate cervical thymectomy to prevent recurrence.
4. Pancreatic islet cell tumors.
   a. Tumors may be isolated, multicentric, or diffuse hyperplasia.
   b. Somatostatin receptor scintigraphy may be helpful to locate tumor.

ENDOCRINE SURGERY

All symptoms of adrenal insufficiency are also common symptoms after abdominal surgery, and may confuse management of a surgical patient after adrenalectomy.

Adrenalectomy may result in adrenal insufficiency, even if a nonfunctional adenoma was resected, because contralateral adrenal suppression may occur.

c. Gastrinoma is the most frequent functional tumor.
   (1) Diagnosis is indicated by gastrin levels greater than 200 pg/mL.
   (2) The tumor may be in the pancreas or in the submucosa of the duodenal wall.
   (3) The gastrinoma triangle is bounded by the junction of the cystic and common bile duct, the junction of the second and third portions of the duodenum, and the junction of the neck and body of the pancreas.
   (4) Treatment with histamine$_2$-receptor antagonists or proton-pump inhibitors is usually successful. Surgical enucleation may be necessary.
d. Insulinoma is the next most frequent tumor.
   (1) The tumor is small, solitary, and benign.
   (2) Diagnosis involves fasting hypoglycemia and inappropriately elevated insulin.
   (3) The tumor can be localized with CT and angiography, and preoperative and intraoperative ultrasound can be used.
   (4) Enucleation of the tumor is usually successful.
e. Other pancreatic endocrine tumors are rare.
5. Pituitary adenoma
   a. Prolactin-secreting tumors are most common, but Cushing disease and acromegaly may occur.
   b. Signs and symptoms.
      (1) Compression of the optic chiasm.
      (2) Prolactin excess: amenorrhea, galactorrhea in females or hypogonadism in males.
D. MEN IIA medullary thyroid carcinoma, pheochromocytoma, parathyroid hyperplasia
   1. Etiology: oncogene RET proto-oncogene on chromosome 10
   2. Medullary thyroid carcinoma
      a. This condition occurs in 90% patients with MEN II.
      b. Early total resection of the thyroid gland by age 2 to 5 years is curative therapy for genetically affected.
      c. This carcinoma is virtually always bilateral and multicentric.
      d. Patients may develop C-cell hyperplasia, a diffuse proliferation of parafollicular C-cells, and elevated stimulated or basal calcitonin without frank invasive carcinoma first.
   3. Pheochromocytoma (40%): 80% of these are bilateral, and occur in the second or third decade of life
   4. Parathyroid hyperplasia (60%)
E. MEN IIB pheochromocytoma, medullary thyroid carcinoma, mucosal neuromas, and a distinctive marfanoid habitus. Medullary thyroid carcinoma usually occurs at an earlier age, and is more aggressive.

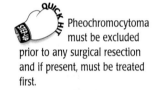

Compression of the optic chiasm causes bitemporal hemianopsia or loss of peripheral vision.

Pheochromocytoma must be excluded prior to any surgical resection and if present, must be treated first.

PANCREAS

I. Gastrinomas (Zollinger–Ellison syndrome): See Discussion in MEN I
A. Sporadic tumors are more likely solitary and benign.
B. Caution is used in interpreting levels in patients taking acid-blocking medications or prior gastric surgery.
C. Gastrinomas are sporadic in 75% and familial in 25% of patients (MEN I).

II. Insulinomas: See Discussion in MEN I
A. Sporadic tumors are more likely solitary and benign.
B. Sulfonylurea and C-peptide levels are used to exclude surreptitious hypoglycemia.

III. VIPomas (Verner–Morrison Syndrome)
A. Symptoms are watery diarrhea, hypokalemia, achlorhydria, and flushing.
B. Cell origin is nonbeta.

IV. **Somatostatinomas**
   A. Symptoms are steatorrhea and hyperglycemia.
   B. Cell origin is delta.

V. **Glucagonoma**
   A. Symptoms are dermatitis (necrolytic migratory erythema) and hyperglycemia.
   B. Cell origin is delta.

VI. **Nonfunctioning Islet Cell Tumors**
   A. Tumors are of islet cell origin but without functional hormone secretion.
   B. They are often found at later stage due to lack of secretion.
   C. Behavior and treatment are similar to pancreatic adenocarcinoma.
   D. Consider octreotide therapy to slow growth.

VII. **Localization of Islet Cell Tumors**
   A. CT and MRI may be used.
   B. Nuclear medicine octreotide scanning with possible use of gamma detector intraoperatively may help finding occult tumors or metastases.

CARCINOID TUMORS

I. **Characteristics**
   A. Arise from enterochromaffin cells in the crypts of Lieberkühn. Tumors are composed of multipotential cells with the ability to secrete a variety of hormones, most commonly serotonin and substance P.
   B. Most common locations are in the gastrointestinal tract; particularly the appendix (46%), small bowel (28%), and rectum (16%).
      1. Foregut (respiratory tract, thymus) carcinoids secrete low levels of serotonin.
      2. Midgut (jejunum, ileum, and right colon, stomach and proximal duodenum) carcinoids.
         a. These tumors secrete high levels of serotonin.
         b. Small bowel carcinoid is multicentric in 20% to 30% of cases.
      3. Hindgut (distal colon and rectum) carcinoids rarely secrete serotonin—usually other hormones such as somatostatin or peptide YY.
   C. The majority of tumors (75%) are less than 1 cm and are slow growing.
   D. The tumors occur in the fifth decade of life.
   E. Invasion into serosa produces an intense desmoplastic reaction in causing fibrosis, intestinal kinking, and obstruction.
   F. Tumors have a variable malignant potential, and are likely to metastasize, especially ileal carcinoid greater than 1 cm.

II. **Signs and Symptoms**
   A. 80% of tumors are asymptomatic, and found incidentally at the time of surgery.
   B. Most common symptoms are abdominal pain, partial or complete small bowel obstruction from intussusception or from a desmoplastic reaction, diarrhea, and weight loss.
   C. Carcinoid syndrome is characterized by episodic attacks of cutaneous flushing, bronchospasm, diarrhea, and vasomotor collapse. This condition occurs only in 10% of patients, most commonly with massive hepatic replacement by metastatic disease.

III. **Diagnosis**
   A. Laboratory tests
      1. Elevated urinary levels of 5-hydroxyindoleacetic acid in 24-hour urine
      2. Serum chromogranin A: elevated in 80% of carcinoid tumors

    B. Localization
       1. Barium radiographic studies may show filling defects in the small bowel.
       2. Somatostatin receptor scintigraphy 111-in-labeled pentetreotide detects somatostatin receptors.
       3. CT or ultrasound may be useful in evaluating metastatic disease.

IV. Treatment

    A. Dependent on tumor size, site, and presence of metastatic disease
       1. Tumors less than 1 cm without evidence of metastatic disease: segmental intestinal resection
       2. Tumors larger than 1 cm, multiple tumors, or lymph node involvement: wide excision of bowel and mesentery
       3. Tumors in terminal ileum: right hemicolectomy
       4. Small duodenal tumors: local excision
       5. Large duodenal tumors: pancreaticoduodenectomy
       6. Extensive disease: surgical debulking can provide symptomatic relief
    B. Anesthetic considerations: carcinoid crisis
       1. Symptoms: hypotension, bronchospasm, flushing, tachycardia, and arrhythmias
       2. Treatment: octreotide, antihistamine, and hydrocortisone
    C. Medical treatment
       1. Symptomatic treatment
       2. Octreotide: may relieve diarrhea and flushing

Breast

Jessica Partin, MD
Marissa Howard-McNatt, MD
Hannah Hazard, MD

ANATOMY AND DEVELOPMENT

I. Anatomy

A. Boundaries: sternum, axilla, pectoralis major, serratus anterior
B. Breast tissue: epithelial parenchyma elements (10–15%) and stroma
   1. Composition: 15 to 20 lobes of glandular tissue, supported by connective tissue framework with adipose tissue in between.
   2. Cooper ligaments: bands of fibrous tissue extending from fascia to dermis that support the breast. Breast size varies depending on the amount of adipose tissue.
   3. Lobes: divided into lobules made up of branched tubuloalveolar glands. Lobes end in 2- to 4-mm lactiferous ducts, which dilate to sinuses beneath the areola and open into a nipple orifice.
   4. Radially arranged smooth muscle fiber with rich sensory innervation below nipple/areola: causes nipple erection.
   5. Sebaceous glands, apocrine sweat glands, no hair follicles.
   6. Tubercles of Morgagni: nodular elevations formed by Montgomery gland openings at periphery of areola which secrete milk.
C. Blood supply
   1. Internal mammary artery (IMA) and lateral thoracic arteries.
      a. IMA artery perforators: supply the medial and central breast.
      b. Lateral thoracic: supply the upper outer quadrant.
   2. Venous drainage follows arterial supply.
D. Lymphatics
   1. Skin and nipple (areolar complex): drain initially to superficial subareolar plexus, and then to a deeper plexus.
   2. Sites of drainage: 97% to the axilla and 3% to the internal mammary nodes. All quadrants can drain into the internal mammary nodes.
E. Axilla: borders include the axillary vein (superior), latissimus dorsi (lateral), serratus anterior (medial), pectoralis major (anterior), and subscapularis (posterior)
   1. Nerves: long thoracic nerve (serratus), thoracodorsal bundle (latissimus), and intercostobrachial nerves (sensory upper middle arm)
   2. Node levels
      a. Level I: inferior and lateral to pectoralis minor
      b. Level II: behind pectoralis minor
      c. Level III: medial to pectoralis minor against chest wall

II. Development

A. Role of hormones
   1. Estrogen promotes ductal dilation in primordial breast bud. Androgen causes destruction.
   2. Growth hormone in puberty causes ductal elongation and branching. Estrogen and progesterone are needed as well. During puberty, growth of both

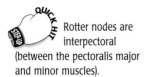

Rotter nodes are interpectoral (between the pectoralis major and minor muscles).

glandular and stromal elements occurs. Cyclical increases in menstrual cycle influence breast macroscopic and microscopic structure.

B. Premenstrual period: patient may feel fullness, nodularity, and sensitivity

C. Pregnancy
1. Breast enlargement, dilation of superficial veins, and terminal epithelium differentiation leads to development of secretory cells. Lobular-alveolar differentiation produces three types of lobules.
2. Oxytocin causes myoepithelial proliferation and differentiation.
3. Lactation/involution.
   a. Prolactin, growth hormone, and insulin, which lead to milk production initially colostrums (rich in growth factors).
   b. Secretion regulated by oxytocin; release by neuronal reflex.
   c. Secretory activity decreases gradually after weaning, with gland, duct, and stromal atrophy.

D. Menopause
1. Breast tissue: predominantly fat and stroma.
2. Breast regression and predominance of type I lobules.

BREAST WORKUP

I. History and Physical Examination

A. History
1. Presenting complaint
   a. Most common presenting complaint is breast mass.
   b. Other presenting complaints: pain, change in size or shape of breast, nipple discharge, or skin changes.
   c. Radiographic abnormalities may include calcifications or architectural distortion on mammogram, mass on ultrasound or MRI finding.
2. Baseline menstrual status and breast cancer risk factors (see Breast Cancer discussion)
   a. Current menopausal status.
   b. Risk factor assessment: menstrual history, use of oral contraceptives and hormone replacement therapy, number and age of pregnancies, family history of breast and/or ovarian cancer and age of diagnosis.

B. Physical Examination
1. Inspection
   a. Comparison of bilateral chest.
   b. Check nipple-areola complex for symmetry, retraction, and skin changes
   c. Inspect the skin for erythema, ulceration, dimpling, or eczematous changes.
   d. Inspect the breasts in varying arm positions – relaxed, above head, and on hips with pectoralis muscles contracted.
2. Palpation
   a. Palpate for cervical and supraclavicular lymphadenopathy.
   b. Palpate breast for masses/lumps/ridges.
   c. Palpate axilla for lymphadenopathy
   d. Examine abdomen for hepatomegaly.
   e. Examine extremities for peripheral edema or bone pain.

II. Radiologic Tests

A. Screening mammography
1. Two views of the breast: craniocaudal and mediolateral oblique
2. Research validation
   a. Randomized trials have shown a 20% to 30% reduction in mortality with screening mammograms in women older than 50 years of age.

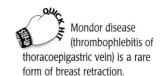

Mondor disease (thrombophlebitis of thoracoepigastric vein) is a rare form of breast retraction.

TABLE 10-1	Breast Imaging Reporting and Data System (BI-RADS) Classification	
Category	Assessment	Recommendations
1	Negative	Routine screening
2	Benign finding	Routine screening
3	Probably benign finding	Short-interval follow-up (repeat in 6 months)
4	Suspicious abnormality	Definite probability of malignancy; consider biopsy
5	Highly suggestive of malignancy	High probability of cancer; appropriate action should be taken

(Reproduced, with permission, from Michael W. Mulholland, et al. *Greenfield's Surgery: Principles and Practice.* Philadelphia: Lippincott Williams & Wilkins; 2006.)

  b. Meta-analysis has suggested a 29% reduction in mortality in 40- to 49-year-old women.
 3. Reduction in mortality: a result of detection of nonpalpable abnormalities (i.e., microcalcifications, nodules <1 cm).
 4. Sensitive but not specific. Only 20% to 30% of abnormalities found are malignant. For the Breast Imaging and Reporting and Data System (BI-RADS) classification, see Table 10-1.
  a. BI-RADS 3: Less than 2% risk of malignancy.
  b. BI-RADS 4: 2% to 50% risk of malignancy.
B. Ultrasound
 1. Performed on all patients with a palpable mass.
 2. Differentiates cystic from solid mass.
 3. Benign lesions:
  a. Simple cysts
  b. Solid masses that are oval or round with circumscribed margins.
 4. Malignant lesions are solid with irregular shape, speculated margins, posterior acoustic shadowing and are often taller than wide.
C. Magnetic resonance imaging (MRI)
 1. Evolving technology for the breast–now with specific coils for imaging acquisition.
 2. Useful for screening women with known breast cancer genetic abnormalities (BRCA) or women with a strong family history of breast cancer without a known BRCA mutation
  a. American Cancer Society recommends screening MRI for women with approximately 20–25% lifetime risk of breast cancer regardless of BRCA status.
 3. Useful in women with lobular carcinoma as this is less readily seen on mammogram.
 4. Maybe useful in women with dense breast tissue as seen on mammogram.
 5. Aids in detecting capsular leaks in patients with implants.

III. Patients at High Risk for Breast Cancer
A. Definition
 1. BRCA-positive status or with a strong family history of breast or ovarian cancer.
 2. Personal history of: atypical ductal hyperplasia (ADH), atypical lobular hyperplasia (ALH), or lobular carcinoma in situ (LCIS).
B. Increased monitoring
 1. Augment screening mammogram with liberal use of ultrasound.
 2. Addition of screening bilateral breast MRI alternating every 6 months with screening mammography.

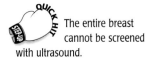
The entire breast cannot be screened with ultrasound.

BREAST

C. Strategies to reduce the risk of breast cancer
1. Tamoxifen, a selective estrogen receptor modulator (SERM).
   a. National Surgical Adjuvant Breast and Bowel Project (NSABP) – P1 showed that women taking Tamoxifen had a 49% reduction in risk of invasive breast cancer and a 50% reduction in risk of noninvasive breast cancer in estrogen receptor (ER)- positive tumors.
   b. Tamoxifen reduced the risk of breast cancer in women with personal history of LCIS and atypical hyperplasia (AH) by 65% and 85%, respectively.
2. Raloxifene, a newer SERM, may reduce the risk of breast cancer in ER-positive postmenopausal patients.
   a. NSABP P-2 (STAR trial) showed raloxifene is as effective as Tamoxifen in reducing the risk of invasive breast cancer with a lower side effect profile.
   b. Raloxifene does not reduce the risk of noninvasive breast cancers.
3. Oophrectomy
   a. Removal of both ovaries can reduce the risk of breast cancer by approximately 50% in high risk women.
4. Prophylactic mastectomy
   a. Should be performed only after complete risk assessment and thorough discussion with the patient.
   b. Should remove the entire breast using the same boundaries as therapeutic mastectomy, including resection of the nipple-areolar complex.
   c. Skin-sparing mastectomy may be used to facilitate immediate reconstruction.

> **QUICK HIT**
> Prophylactic mastectomy reduces the risk of breast cancer by only approximately 90% (not 100%).

BREAST COMPLAINTS AND DISORDERS

I. Breast Pain
A. Common condition that is rarely a sign of carcinoma.
B. Pain may originate from breast or be referred from other structures (ribs, vertebrae, teeth). There are two categories: cyclical and noncyclical.
1. Cyclical: waxes and wanes with menstrual cycle, often bilateral, frequently in upper outer quadrants into axilla; most severe immediately prior to menses.
2. Noncyclical: occurs in postmenopausal women, or no relation to menstrual cycle in premenopausal women.
C. Hormonally related: more common in premenopausal women, and often precipitated by a hormonal change.
D. Workup: history, physical examination (fibrocystic changes), mammogram in women age 35 and older.
E. Majority of patients have no breast disease and require only reassurance.
F. About 5% of patients have disabling breast pain. Further treatment includes danazol, bromocriptine, and tamoxifen. Surgery should be avoided.
G. Mondor disease
1. Tender, subcutaneous cord in lateral breast, with or without skin retraction.
   a. The condition can be secondary to trauma, surgery, or irradiation.
   b. Thrombophlebitis of the lateral thoracic or superior thoracoepigastric vein) is an uncommon cause.
2. Anti-inflammatory agents may be necessary.
3. Because the condition is occasionally seen with nonpalpable breast cancer, a mammogram is indicated if the patient older than 35.

> **QUICK HIT**
> Always illicit patient's primary concern–the fear of cancer (predominant complaint) or need for pain relief.

II. Nipple Discharge
A. Common complaint, especially in premenopausal women. The cause is benign in 95% of cases.

1. Patients with nipple discharge that occurs with compression of the breast and is nonbloody need only reassurance.
2. Except for galactorrhea (nonpuerperal discharge of milky fluid bilateral), nipple discharge is usually not indicative of primary breast disease.

B. Etiology (bloody nipple discharge)
  1. Commonly due to intraductal papilloma (60%), and mostly in subareolar ducts.
  2. Peripheral papillomas are usually multiple, and less often present with discharge.
  3. Of the women who undergo duct excision, 15% to 20% have duct hyperplasia and 5% to 20% have DCIS.
  4. Single papillomas without atypia carry a three-fold risk factor, and a four-fold risk factor when there is atypical hyperplasia in the papilloma.
  5. Other causes: DCIS or invasive breast cancer.

C. Clinical evaluation (spontaneous bloody nipple discharge without breast compression)
  1. History. Determine that symptoms are not side effects of medication (oral contraceptive pills, phenothiazines, tricyclic antidepressants, metoclopramide, reserpine).
  2. Physical examination. Evaluate for endocrine disorder, pituitary adenoma, and chest trauma.
  3. Measure prolactin level.
  4. Order mammography and ultrasound (any palpable mass).
  5. Cytology is not very useful.

D. Management
  1. Attempt to localize the source (physical examination, ductoscopy). Galactography is controversial.
  2. Perform duct excision with lacrimal duct probe via a circumareolar incision. Visualize the duct, and excise to a depth of 2 cm.

III. Breast Masses

A. Masses may be cystic or solid
B. Cysts: a common cause of breast masses
  1. Peak in women in their 40s and in perimenopause. Uncommon in post-menopausal women who are not taking hormone replacement therapy.
  2. Well-demarcated, mobile, firm, and may fluctuate with menstrual cycle.
  3. Evaluate with needle aspiration or ultrasound.
    a. If fluid is nonbloody on aspiration, discard. Only send bloody fluid for cytology.
    b. If fluid is bloody on aspiration, the mass does not resolve, or the cyst recurs multiple times, then biopsy is necessary (for malignant lesion in cyst wall).
    c. If the ultrasound shows cyst is simple and/or if cyst is asymptomatic, it can be left alone.

C. Solid masses
  1. May be fibrocystic changes, fibroadenoma, AH, and carcinoma
  2. History and physical examination
  3. Diagnostic imaging
    a. Diagnostic mammogram (versus screening mammogram) should be obtained before biopsy of palpable mass. This involves placing a marker on an area of palpable concern and includes magnification/compression views of lesion.
    b. Ultrasound is performed on all palpable masses. This can determine cyst from solid lesion and can show characteristics typical of malignancy.

D. Biopsy of palpable breast mass
  1. Fine-needle aspiration biopsy (FNA)
    a. Sensitivity: 65%–98%, with a higher chance of false-negative results with tumors that are small and fibrotic.
    b. Advantages: simple, quick, available in office, low cost.

      c. Disadvantages: need cytopathologist, poor sample size, and if malignant, can not distinguish between invasive and noninvasive disease.

   2. Core needle biopsy

      a. Core of tissue obtained as opposed to individual cells.

      b. Preferred method to diagnose breast mass prior to surgery.

      c. Advantages: more detailed evaluation of the tissue including receptor status, and invasive vs. noninvasive disease.

      d. Disadvantages: more labor intensive, increased risk of bleeding.

   3. Excisional biopsy

      a. Complete removal of the mass

      b. May be performed if patient cannot tolerate core needle biopsy or pathology from core biopsy is indeterminate or discordant with imaging findings.

      c. Outpatient procedure

      d. Specimen should be oriented

  E. Nonpalpable radiographic abnormality

   1. Lesions can be sampled by core needle biopsy either via ultrasound guidance if seen on ultrasound or via stereotaxis if only seen on mammogram.

   2. For suspicious calcifications or architectural distortion seen on imaging which cannot be biopsied by noninvasive techniques, needle guided excisional biopsy may be performed.

IV. Benign Breast Disease

  A. Fibrocystic changes

   1. This ambiguous term includes most types of benign breast disease.

   2. Autopsy studies show that more than 50% of women have microscopic changes consistent with fibrocystic breast disease.

   3. Fibrocystic change is not premalignant.

   4. This condition is found in women in their 30s and 40s.

   5. These changes are usually diffuse and ill-defined.

   6. They occur cyclically with menses and are painful and prominent beforehand. They disappear after menopause.

  B. Fibroadenomas

   1. These well-defined, palpable, rubbery, mobile masses occur as multiple lesions in 10% to 15% of patients.

   2. They usually present between 20 and 50 years of age.

   3. They involute after menopause, and they may increase in women taking estrogen alone.

   4. On ultrasound, they appear round or oval, well-circumscribed, solid, and homogeneous, with low-level internal echoes and intermediate acoustic attenuation.

  C. Cysts (see Breast Masses)

  D. Intraductal papilloma (see Nipple Discharge)

  E. Lipoma: benign encapsulated adipose tissue

  F. Pseudoangiomatous hyperplasia

   1. Benign stromal proliferation that simulates a vascular lesion.

   2. It is necessary to rule out angiosarcoma by obtaining a larger tissue sample.

  G. Mammary duct ectasia

   1. Occurs in perimenopausal and postmenopausal women.

   2. Characterized by dilatation of subareolar ducts. Periductal inflammation leads to fibrosis and duct dilatation.

V. Proliferative Lesions

  A. Atypical lobular hyperplasia (ALH)

   1. Composed of cells similar to those found in LCIS, but less than half the acini are filled or distorted.

   2. Associated with a five times relative risk of developing breast cancer.

  B. Atypical ductal hyperplasia (ADH)

   1. Marked proliferation and atypia of the epithelium.

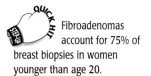

Fibroadenomas account for 75% of breast biopsies in women younger than age 20.

BREAST

2. Found in 3% of benign breast biopsies.
3. Associated with a 13% development of breast cancer (4 × risk).
4. Diagnosed by the same criteria as DCIS, but does not have all the characteristics necessary to diagnose intraductal cancer.

C. Lobular carcinoma in situ (LCIS)
1. An incidental finding or core or excisional biopsy or marker.
2. Patients have an 8 to 10 times risk, or about a 1% per year risk of developing invasive carcinoma in the same or opposite breast.
3. Treatment may be observation, hormonal (tamoxifen), or bilateral mastectomies depending on patient preference.

VI. Paget Disease
A. Eczematoid lesion of the nipple and areolar complex caused by large malignant cells
1. A nonpalpable mass is usually due to DCIS.
2. A palpable mass usually indicates invasive ductal carcinoma.

B. Diagnosis
1. Tissue is obtained by scrape cytology, epidermal shave biopsy, punch biopsy, wedge incision biopsy, or nipple excision.
2. Retroareolar spot compression views should be added to the standard bilateral mammogram.

C. Management
1. Patients with disease extending beyond the central portion of the breast by physical examination or imaging studies should undergo mastectomy.
2. Patients choosing breast conservation (lumpectomy with excision of nipple–areolar complex) should combine surgery and radiation.
3. Sentinel lymph node biopsy may be performed if invasive breast cancer is present.

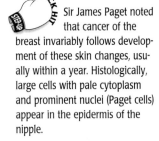

QUICK HIT

Sir James Paget noted that cancer of the breast invariably follows development of these skin changes, usually within a year. Histologically, large cells with pale cytoplasm and prominent nuclei (Paget cells) appear in the epidermis of the nipple.

BREAST CANCER

I. Epidemiology
A. Incidence
1. Estimated number of new invasive breast cancer (2008) is 182,400 females and 2000 males.
2. Potentially 1 in 8 American women affected.
3. Estimated number of deaths (2008) 42,000 and mortality is decreasing.

B. Risk factors
1. Age: most common risk factor
   a. The risk is 2.5% for women aged 35 to 55 years.
   b. The risk is higher in younger African-American women, but becomes higher in Caucasian women after age 40.
2. Family history. Between 20% and 30% of women with breast cancer have a positive family history.
3. Prior personal history of breast cancer
4. Hereditary factors
   a. Of women with breast cancer, 5% to 10% have an inherited mutation in a breast cancer susceptibility gene.
      (1) Most involve BRCA1 or BRCA2 autosomal dominant mutations.
      (2) Having either gene gives a 37% to 85% risk of breast cancer, high risk of contralateral breast cancer, and elevated risk of ovarian cancer (greater with BRCA1) during life.
      (3) BRCA2 increases risk of male breast cancer, prostate cancer, and pancreatic cancer. Both maternally and paternally inherited.
   b. Chance of mutation varies with ethnicity (higher in Ashkenazi Jews).

c. Genetic testing is available for patients with suggestive family history, and a counseling session should always precede testing.

d. Infrequent breast cancer syndromes: Li-Fraumeni syndrome, Cowden syndrome, the Lynch syndromes.

5. Hormonal factors
   a. Lifetime exposure to estrogens linked to breast cancer risk
   b. Early age at menarche, late age at first pregnancy, postmenopausal obesity
   c. Relative risk ranges from 1.5 to 2.0 for hormonal factors
   d. Long duration of lactation reduces risk in premenopausal women
   e. Small increase in risk with combination postmenopausal hormone replacement, but not contraceptive use

6. Environmental factors and diet
   a. Exposure to ionizing radiation (accidental or medical) increases risk, which is greater for childhood and adolescent exposures.
   b. Most commonly encountered group is patients with Hodgkin lymphoma, who received treatment with mediastinal irradiation.

7. Diet and weight gain
   a. Diet has not been shown to have a relationship with breast cancer.
   b. There may be a link between weight gain as an adult and the development of breast cancer.

8. LCIS
9. ADH

II. Breast Cancer

A. Noninvasive breast cancer:
1. Ductal carcinoma in situ (DCIS)
   a. Pathology
      (1) Proliferation of malignant epithelial cells is confined by the basement membrane of the duct-lobular system.
      (2) Classification: comedo, cribriform, micropapillary, papillary, solid
         (a) Up to 30–60% of mass may be mixed.
         (b) Newer systems use grading of DCIS–high, intermediate and low grade.
      (3) Cannot spread to lymphatics because the disease is confined to the duct.
2. Clinical presentation
   a. Nipple discharge, Paget's disease of the nipple, mass
3. Mammographic presentation (most common)
   a. Pleomorphic microcalcifications.
   b. Frequency of diagnosis of DCIS is increasing because of mammography.
      (1) DCIS represents 30-50% of malignancies seen on biopsy of suspicious mammogram abnormalities.
      (2) DCIS may also be an incidental finding when invasive cancer is present.
4. Surgical management
   a. Lumpectomy and radiation : most common treatment
      (1) NSABP–B17 (randomized trial studying lumpectomy with and without radiation therapy).
         (a) Overall survival rates of lumpectomy both with and without radiation compared favorably with those of mastectomy.
         (b) There was a clear reduction in local recurrence when lumpectomy was combined with radiation, but this did not affect overall survival.
   b. Mastectomy
      (1) Curative in about 98% of patients.
      (2) Up to 26% of patients may have invasive cancer not identified preoperatively. Invasive cancer is usually found in larger, high-grade DCIS lesions.

TABLE 10-2	The Van Nuys Prognostic Index for Ductal Carcinoma *in Situ*		
Score	**1**	**2**	**3**
Size	<15 mm	16–40 mm	>40 mm
Margin	>10 mm	1–9 mm	<1 mm
Pathology	Low grade, no necrosis	Non-high grade, plus necrosis	High grade, plus or minus necrosis

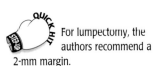

For lumpectomy, the authors recommend a 2-mm margin.

        (3) Mastectomy is usually reserved for diffuse DCIS throughout the breast or because of patient preference.

        (4) In performing mastectomy for DCIS, sentinel lymph node biopsy is used in the event incidental invasive cancer is identified on final pathology.

    c. Excision alone

        (1) Silverstein and associates developed the Van Nuys prognostic index (Table 10-2) dependent on certain risk factors: size, surgical margins, nuclear grade, and comedo necrosis.

          (a) Patients with a score of 3–4 can be treated with lumpectomy alone.

          (b) Scores of 5–7 require the addition of radiation therapy.

        (2) Excision alone may be offered to some patients with small, favorable tumors with wide negative surgical margins.

    d. Adjuvant therapy for DCIS

        (1) Tamoxifen, as determined by NSABP–B24, was found to reduce the risk of ipsilateral breast cancer recurrence by 38% and contralateral disease by 52%.

          (a) It is recommended for patients with ER-positive tumors.

        (2) Systemic chemotherapy is not needed for DCIS alone.

        (3) Radiation therapy is recommended in most patients undergoing breast conservation with the exception being some patients with small, favorable tumors.

  B. Invasive Cancer

    1. Types

      a. Ductal: the most common type (approximately 80%).

      b. Lobular: second most common type.

        (1) Can be difficult to detect on mammography.

        (2) Consider bilateral breast MRI.

      c. Mammary: tumor with ductal and lobular features.

      d. Medullary: less likely to have axillary node involvement

      e. Others: (incidence in parenthesis)

        (1) Mucoid or colloid (2.4%)

        (2) Tubular (1.2%)

        (3) Adenoid cystic (0.4%)

        (4) Cribiform (0.3%)

        (5) Carcinosarcoma (0.1%)

        (6) Papillary

    2. Pathology

      a. Infiltration of cells across the basement membrane and into surrounding stroma.

      b. Final pathology should contain tumor types, histologic grade, and hormonal receptor status.

      c. Estrogen receptors (ER) and progesterone receptors (PR) are members of a nuclear hormone receptor family that act as transcription factors when bound by their ligands.

(1) ER-positive tumors account for approximately 70% of breast cancers

(2) Greatest numbers receptor positive tumors are seen in well-differentiated tumors and in tumors in older postmenopausal women.

   d. Her-2/neu protein is a member of the tyrosine kinase receptor family. Her-2/neu gene is amplified in almost 1/3 of breast cancer patients.

(1) This is associated with a shortened disease-free survival and a decreased overall survival.

3. Diagnosis

   a. History (see above)

   b. Physical examination (see above)

   c. Imaging

(1) All patients need bilateral mammogram.

(2) Ultrasound for all palpable masses.

(3) Consider adding bilateral breast MRI in certain circumstances.

   d. Biopsy

(1) All patients with palpable lesions can undergo core or vacuum-assisted needle biopsy without image guidance.

(2) All patients with nonpalpable mammographic abnormalities need stereotactic core biopsy.

(3) All patients with nonpalpable ultrasound abnormalities should undergo ultrasound guided core biopsy.

   e. Surgical management

(1) Lumpectomy (also known as partial mastectomy)

     (a) Most commonly recommended for stages I/II disease, depending on patient preference

     (b) Surgeon must achieve negative surgical margins

     (c) If the tissue removed does not have negative margins, additional operations to remove more tissue may be necessary

     (d) Specimen should be oriented

     (e) May use neoadjuvant chemotherapy for larger tumors, or low breast to rumor ratio to shrink the tumor in order to perform lumpectomy

     (f) Contraindications to lumpectomy (Table 10-3)

TABLE 10-3	Contraindications to Breast-Conserving Therapy in Invasive Carcinoma
Absolute contraindications	• Two or more primary tumors in separate quadrants • Persistent positive margins after reasonable surgical efforts • Pregnancy (with use of radiation therapy) • History of previous radiation therapy that would result in excessive radiation dose to the breast region • Diffuse microcalcifications that appear malignant
Relative contraindications	• Active systemic lupus erythematosus or history of scleroderma • Extensive, gross, multifocal disease • Large tumor in a small breast, resulting in unacceptable cosmesis • Very large or pendulous breasts (if adequate and reproducible homogeneity of radiation dose is not possible)
Contraindications to sentinel lymph node biopsy	• Clinically suspicious axillary lymphadenopathy • Inflammatory carcinoma or other locally advanced breast cancer • Patient is pregnant or lactating • Prior axillary surgery

(Reproduced, with permission, from *Greenfield's Surgery: Principles and Practice.* Philadelphia: Lippincott Williams & Wilkins; 2006.)

(2) Mastectomy (with or without immediate reconstruction)
  (a) Borders: superiorly to inferior border of clavicle, medial to the lateral sternal border, laterally to the latissimus dorsi muscle, and inferiorly to the superior border of the rectus sheath
  (b) Performed for patients with large tumors, all patients with inflammatory breast cancer, and for patient preference
  (c) Skin-sparing mastectomy (removal of nipple-areolar complex only) is used in patients who desire immediate reconstruction
(3) Reconstruction
  (a) Implant reconstruction: initial placement of a tissue expander under the pectoralis muscle followed by removal and placement of a permanent implant
  (b) Autologous reconstruction: transverse rectus abdominis myocutaneous (TRAM) flap
    i. More natural look and feel
    ii. Significant increase in operative time, hospital stay and recovery period
(4) Lumpectomy vs. mastectomy (NSABP–B06)
  (a) Enrolled 1,257 patients who either had total mastectomy, lumpectomy alone, or lumpectomy with radiation therapy.
  (b) Incidence of local recurrence was approximately 10% for those with mastectomy, 9% with lumpectomy alone, and 3% for those with lumpectomy with radiation.
  (c) There is no difference in disease-free survival.
f. Axillary Staging: required for invasive cancer
  (1) Sentinel lymph node biopsy (SLNB)
    (a) Lymphatics of the brest drain into the axilla and the first nodes in the lymphatic basin are the sentinel lymph nodes (SLN).
    (b) SLN can be identified in two ways
      i. Radionucleotide (technetium-labeled sulfur colloid).
        (i) Radioactivity is measured by a hand-helded gamma probe and nodes are removed in the OR.
      ii. Isosulfan blue dye (peritumoral or subareolar injection).
        (i) Blue lymph nodes are removed in the OR.
      iii. SLN are blue, radioactive or both
      iv. Be wary of firm, enlarged lymph nodes in the axilla that are neither blue nor radioactive as they may be completely replaced by tumor and therefore unable to uptake tracers.
    (c) SLNB can be performed with lumpectomy or mastectomy.
    (d) If SLN is negative for tumor, no further axillary surgery is necessary.
    (e) If SLN is positive for tumor, the recommendation is an axillary lymph node dissection.
    (f) SLNB is not recommended for patients with clinically involved axillary nodes and in inflammatory cancer and contraindicated in pregnancy.
  (2) Axillary lymph node dissection (ALND)
    (a) Definition: removal of level 1 & 2 axillary nodes.
    (b) Morbidity associated with ALND include lymphedema (10–15%), decreased range of motion at the shoulder, numbness axilla and/or arm.
4. Staging (Tables 10-4 and 10-5)
5. Systemic therapy
  a. Chemotherapy
    (1) Should be considered for all patients with receptor negative disease.
    (2) Should be considered for all patients with positive nodal involvement.

TABLE 10-4 Tumor-Node-Metastasis Classification in Breast Cancer

Primary Tumor

Tx	Primary tumor cannot be assessed
T0	No evidence of primary tumor
Tis	Carcinoma *in situ,* ductal or lobular or Paget disease of the nipple without tumor
T1	Tumor 2 cm or less
T2	Tumor more than 2 cm and less than 5 cm
T3	Tumor greater than 5 cm
T4	Tumor of any size directly extending into chest wall (not including pectoralis muscle), skin edema or ulceration, satellite skin lesions, or inflammatory carcinoma

Regional Lymph Nodes (Pathologic)

Nx	Lymph nodes cannot be assessed
N0	No histologic evidence for regional node metastases
N1	Metastases in 1 to 3 axillary nodes or internal mammary nodes with microscopic disease detected by biopsy
N2	Metastases in 4 to 9 axillary nodes or clinically apparent disease in internal mammary nodes
N3	Metastases in: 1. 10 or more axillary nodes 2. Disease in infraclavicular or supraclavicular nodes 3. Internal mammary nodes with 1 or more positive axillary nodes 4. More than 3 axillary nodes with internal mammary metastases

Distant Metastases

Mx	Distant metastases cannot be assessed
M0	No distant metastases
M1	Distant metastases

TABLE 10-5 Stages of Breast Cancer Using the Tumor-Node-Metastasis Classification

Stage 0	Tis	N0	M0
Stage I	T1	N0	M0
Stage IIA	T0	N1	M0
	T1	N1	M0
	T2	N0	M0
Stage IIB	T2	N1	M0
	T3	N0	M0
Stage IIIA	T0	N2	M0
	T1	N2	M0
	T2	N2	M0
	T3	N1	M0
	T3	N2	M0
Stage IIIB	T4	N0	M0
	T4	N1	M0
	T4	N2	M0
Stage IIIC	Any T	N3	MM0
Stage IV	Any T	Any N	M1

(Reproduced, with permission, from *Greenfield's Surgery: Principles and Practice.* Philadelphia: Lippincott Williams & Wilkins; 2006.)

(3) Should be considered for all patients with tumors greater than 1cm.

(4) Most common regimen includes Adriamycin and cyclophosphamide.

    (a) Side effects of Adriamycin include cardiotoxicity, bone marrow suppression, fatique and hair loss.

(5) A taxane may be added for tumors with poor prognosis or increased lymph node involvement.

    (a) Side effects of taxanes include neuropathy and arthralgias.

b. Hormonal therapy: for ER-positive and PR-positive cancers

(1) SERMs (Tamoxifen)

    (a) Only hormonal agent for premenopausal women.

    (b) When used for 5 years, it is associated with a significant reduction in the risk of recurrence, and the risk of dying from breast cancer in the affected and contralateral breast.

    (c) Side effects include hot flashes, small increase risk of deep vein thrombosis (including pulmonary embolus), and small increase risk of uterine cancer.

    (d) Can be used in premenopausal and postmenopausal women.

(2) Aromatase inhibitors (AI) (i.e. Arimidex, Femara, Aromasin)

    (a) Inhibit the synthesis of estrogens from androgens.

    (b) Only used in postmenopausal patients.

    (c) The Arimidex or Tamoxifen Alone or in Combination (ATAC) trial showed advantages to Arimidex over Tamoxifen for postmenopausal women with early stage, hormone receptor positive disease.

    (d) AIs have fewer rare but serious side effects in comparison to Tamoxifen but the AIs are associated with more bone loss and fractures.

    (e) ATAC trial showed that Arimidex is better than Tamoxifen in:

       i. Preventing or delaying recurrence

       ii. Lowering the risk of contralateral breast cancer.

c. Antibody therapy (Traztusamab)

(1) Trastuzumab (Herceptin) is a murine monoclonal antibody that can be used to treat Her-2/neu positive cancers.

(2) Clinical studies have confirmed trastuzumab, in combination with Adriomycin or taxanes, improves survival in patients with Her-2/neu overexpression in metastatic disease.

(3) Used only in patients with Her-2/neu overexpression.

6. Radiation therapy

a. High energy beams of radiation are focused on the affected breast.

b. In whole breast radiation, patients receive radiation treatment as an outpatient in daily sessions over 5-7 weeks. Delivery is delayed until after chemotherapy if chemotherapy is required.

c. In partial breast radiation, patients receive focused radiation to the lumpectomy cavity and 1cm of surrounding tissue twice daily for 5 days.

(1) This is a newer form of radiation delivery and long-term trials are still necessary for validation.

d. Radiation after mastectomy:

(1) Tumor is greater than 5cm.

(2) Positive margins of resection.

(3) Four or more lymph nodes with metastatic disease.

e. Radiation after lumpectomy:

(1) Broadly speaking, radiation is necessary after lumpectomy to affect adequate local control.

f. Radiation is felt to be a contraindication or a relative contraindication in the following:

(1) Prior radiation to the affected are of the body.

(2) Patient with connective tissue disorders like lupus or vasculitis.

(3) Pregnancy.

(4) Unable to commit to the rigorous schedule required to complete treatment.

SPECIAL PROBLEMS

I. Breast Cancer in the Elderly

A. Approximately half of breast cancers in the United States are diagnosed in women 65 years old and over.

B. Either mastectomy or breast conservation therapy may be offered, depending on physiologic (not chronologic) age. Some studies suggest lower failure rates with lumpectomy in older women than in those younger than 65 years.

C. Radiation therapy is fairly well tolerated, but limited mobility may make daily visits difficult. If the tumor is less than 2 cm, radiation therapy may offer only marginal benefit. Wide excision combined with hormonal therapy may be offered.

D. Tamoxifen alone as an alternative to surgical treatment has been studied, and although local recurrence was better controlled in women treated surgically, there was no survival benefit to surgical therapy.

E. Endocrine therapy is a viable alternative for the elderly patient with a limited life span, or significant comorbid conditions that may preclude surgery.

II. Breast Cancer in Pregnancy

A. This is a relatively uncommon occurrence, and only 7% to 14% of breast cancer patients of child-bearing age are pregnant at diagnosis. Approximately 2.2 breast cancers per 10,000 pregnancies are seen.

B. Clinical presentation is the same as in patients who are not pregnant, with a palpable mass being the most common presenting symptom.

C. Mammography is indicated, and ultrasound should be performed for all palpable masses.

D. Diagnosis is commonly delayed. Pregnant women may safely undergo core needle biopsy or biopsy under local anesthesia.

E. If the patient wishes to continue the pregnancy, treatment options are limited.

1. Lumpectomy may be performed with delayed radiation, depending on the trimester.

2. Radiation therapy is contraindicated at all times, because the fetus cannot be shielded from internal scatter.

3. Mastectomy is recommended if cancer is diagnosed in the early trimester.

4. Staging is performed by axillary dissection, because the effects of radiocolloids and blue dyes in sentinel lymph node biopsy are unknown.

5. Termination of pregnancy has not been shown to confer survival advantage.

6. Chemotherapy may be offered after the first trimester (risk of fetal malformation during first trimester is 20%, and declines to 2% in the second and third trimesters).

7. Tamoxifen is contraindicated in pregnancy.

III. Male Breast Cancer

A. Uncommon disease, where the mean age at presentation is 10 years more than in women

B. Risk factors

1. Klinefelter syndrome, BRCA2 mutations, family history, hepatic disorders, radiation exposure.

2. There is no clear association with gynecomastia, except in Klinefelter syndrome.

C. Typical presentation is a mass under the nipple–areolar complex with ulceration or retraction of the nipple. Approximately 80% are hormone-receptor positive.

TABLE 10-6 Recommendations for Adjuvant Therapy in Breast Cancer	
Node Negative, Low Risk	
Tumor <1 cm Special histologic types 1–2 cm, grade 1, estrogen receptor (ER) positive	No treatment, or endocrine therapy is tumor is ER positive
Node Negative, High Risk	
ER positive ER negative	Endocrine therapy or chemotherapy + endocrine therapy Chemotherapy
Node Positive	
ER positive Premenopausal Postmenopausal ER negative	 Chemotherapy + endocrine therapy Chemotherapy + endocrine therapy or endocrine therapy alone Chemotherapy

(Reproduced, with permission, from *Greenfield's Surgery: Principles and Practice.* Philadelphia: Lippincott Williams & Wilkins; 2006.)

D. Management
  1. Mastectomy is the most common treatment; may have to excise some of the pectoralis muscle.
  2. If the mass is small, can offer lumpectomy and radiation.
E. Sentinel lymph node biopsy is used to stage the patient, unless palpable FNA-positive axillary lymphadenopathy is present (mandating axillary dissection).
F. Compared to women of the same stage, survival is similar in men. Axillary nodal status is the major predictor of outcome as it is in women.
G. Largest advantage of systemic adjuvant therapy is seen with hormonal therapy (Table 10-6).
  1. Tamoxifen improved 5-year survival to 55% (compared to 28% with no systemic therapy) but may be less well tolerated in men.
  2. Orchiectomy is a second-line hormonal therapy in metastatic disease, resulting in an 80% response rate in receptor-positive male breast cancer.

IV. Occult Primary Tumor Presenting with Nodal Metastases
A. Breast cancer is the most common type of metastatic adenocarcinoma presenting in the axillary lymph nodes.
B. Fewer than 1% of cases in most large series of patients.
C. MRI may be able to detect primary tumor when an ultrasound and a mammogram are negative.
D. If breast cancer is presumed, treatment is mastectomy, as in other patients with similar stage.

V. Locally Recurrent Breast Cancer
A. After breast conservation therapy
  1. Causal factors: inappropriate patient selection, poor surgical or radiotherapy technique, or tumor biology
  2. Frequency
    a. Uncommon in the first 2 postoperative years.
    b. Develops at a constant rate, usually adjacent to site of primary tumor, during years 2 to 6.
    c. Develops in other quadrants after year 6, and may be new primary tumors (supported by 1% annual risk, which is equal to risk for developing a new contralateral tumor).
  3. Most tumors recur in the breast parenchyma (5–10% occur in the skin). Evaluation for metastatic disease is mandatory prior to local therapy, which is mastectomy in the absence of metastases.

BREAST

4. Treatment for ipsilateral recurrence is mastectomy as the breast can only be radiated once.

5. 5-year survival ranges from 60% to 79%.

B. After mastectomy

1. Frequency

a. Different time frame than after breast conservation.

b. About 75% of local recurrences occur in first 3 postoperative years; half of these have distant metastases at the time of recurrence.

2. Best predictor of chest wall recurrence is the number of axillary nodes with metastases.

3. Evaluation for distant metastases is mandatory.

a. Check computed tomography scans of brain, chest, abdomen, and pelvis. Order bone scans.

b. Locally excise recurrences if possible.

c. Radiation therapy is indicated to include chest wall. This field includes supraclavicular space (second most frequent site of recurrence).

CHAPTER 11

Skin and Soft Tissue

Bruce Freeman, MD, PhD
Mathew Loos, MD

ANATOMY

See Color Figure 11-1.

I. Epidermis
   A. Layers
      1. Stratum corneum: outermost layer consisting of mostly dead keratinocytes, typically 20 to 30 cells thick, and making up approximately 75% of the thickness of the skin.
      2. Stratum lucidum: few flattened rows of dead keratinocytes.
      3. Stratum granulosum: 3 to 5 layers of cells with increased levels of keratin.
      4. Stratum spinosum: several rows of mature keratinocytes.
      5. Stratum basale: single row of continuously dividing cells that produce keratin. This layer is attached to the dermis via a basement membrane that acts to selectively filter substances passing up from the dermis.
   B. Cell types
      1. Melanocytes
         a. Produce melanin, which protects the skin from the harmful effects of ultraviolet (UV) light.
         b. Act to pigment the skin so that those individuals with more melanin have darker skin, and those with less have lighter skin.
      2. Merkel cells: mechanoreceptors that provide information of light touch sensation
      3. Langerhans cells: act to protect the body by attacking and engulfing foreign material
   C. Appendages
      1. Hair follicles: regulate body temperature and contain sebaceous glands that produce sebum to aid in lubricating the skin and hair
      2. Sudoriferous glands: produce sweat to aid in temperature regulation and fight infection
      3. Nails: are hard keratin produced at the tips of the fingers and toes

II. Dermis
   A. Thickness: 2 to 4 mm
   B. Consists of two layers
      1. Papillary dermis: thin and loosely woven fibers that conform to the stratum basale, and aid in anchoring the epidermis and protecting the appendages.
      2. Reticular dermis: dense, irregularly arranged fibers that contribute to the strength of the skin.
   C. Highly vascular and provides the more superficial layers of skin with nutrient supply
   D. Contains lymphatics

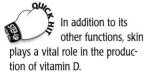

In addition to its other functions, skin plays a vital role in the production of vitamin D.

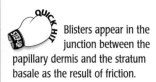

Blisters appear in the junction between the papillary dermis and the stratum basale as the result of friction.

FIGURE 11-1 **Anatomy of the skin.**

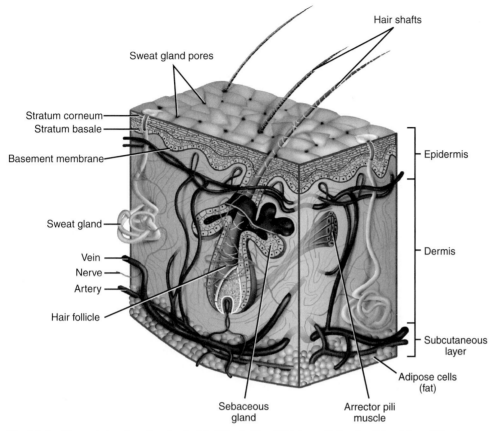

Hair shafts

Sweat gland pores

Stratum corneum
Stratum basale
Basement membrane

Epidermis

Sweat gland

Vein
Nerve
Artery

Hair follicle

Dermis

Subcutaneous
layer

Adipose cells
(fat)

Sebaceous
gland

Arrector pili
muscle

(Reprinted, with permission, from Eroschenko VP. *DiFiore's Atlas of Histology with Functional Correlations.* 10th ed. Baltimore: Lippincott Williams & Wilkins; 2005:184.)

E. Cell types
1. Fibroblasts: produce collagen and elastin for strength and flexibility
2. Macrophages and white blood cells: for fighting infection
3. Mast cells: for secretion of numerous mediators such as histamine, tumor necrosis factor-alpha (TNF-α), and interleukin-1 (IL-1)
4. Sensory receptors: for touch, pressure, vibration, and temperature

III. Subcutaneous Tissues
A. Adipose tissue
B. Fascia
C. Deep lymphatics

WOUNDS AND SCARS

I. Wounds
A. Phases of wound healing
1. Inflammation
a. Vascular response
(1) Injured vessels allow leakage and edema formation.
(2) Vasoconstriction then reduces further blood loss.
(3) Platelets arrive, and adhere to the exposed endothelial lining (collagen). They release growth factors and chemotactic agents, such as vascular endothelial growth factor, prostaglandin E2, platelet-dervied growth factor, TGF-α, thrombin, and thromboxane A2.

> **QUICK HIT**
> Wounds are classified by the depth of the injury. Superficial wounds involve the epidermis only, partial-thickness wounds involve the epidermis and dermis, and full-thickness wounds are through the dermis and into the subcutaneous tissues or deeper.

SKIN AND SOFT TISSUE

TABLE 11-1	Inflammatory Cytokines	
Cytokine	**Cellular Source**	**Action**
Proinflammatory		
TNF-α	Macrophages	PMN margination and cytotoxicity, collagen synthesis
IL-1	Macrophages, keratinocytes	Chemotaxis and collagen synthesis
IL-2	T-lymphocytes	Fibroblast metabolism and infiltration
IL-6	Macrophages, PMNs, fibroblasts	Fibroblast proliferation, protein synthesis
IL-8	Macrophages, fibroblasts	Chemotaxis
IFN-γ	Macrophages, T-lymphocytes	Activation of macrophages and PMNs, increase collagenase action
Anti-Inflammatory		
IL-4	T-lymphocytes, basophils, mast cells	Inhibits TNF, IL-1, IL-6, fibroblast proliferation
IL-10	T-lymphocytes, macrophages, keratinocytes	Inhibits TNF, IL-1, IL-6, inhibits macrophage and PMN activation

QUICK HIT

Five signs of inflammation: tumor (swelling), rubor (redness), calor (heat), dolor (pain), and function laesa (loss of function).

(4) Vasodilatation then resumes and contributes to the pain, swelling, and redness seen in most acute wounds.

b. Cellular response (Table 11-1)

(1) Reduced blood flow through the area of injury forces the traveling white blood cells (WBCs) to be pushed against the sidewalls of the vessel (margination). These WBCs then migrate through the vessel walls and move toward the zone of injury during the first 24 hours.

(a) The WBCs are guided by changes in pH, chemotaxins produced by dead or dying cells, and bacterial toxins.

(b) This begins the process of clearing the wound of foreign material.

(2) Monocytes arrive next (2–3 days) and become macrophages in the interstitium.

(a) These contribute to wound cleaning not only by direct phagocytosis but also as the source of over 30 growth factors as well as cytokines.

(b) Mast cells also contribute to the wound clearance at this point.

2. Proliferation

Proliferative cytokines and inflammatory mediators are defined and described in Table 11-2.

a. Typically begins within about 48 hours of injury

b. Has four major elements

(1) Angiogenesis: endothelial cells adjacent to the zone of injury bud, and grow into the wound

(a) Led by ischemia and chemical mediators

(b) Form new capillary beds, thus providing nutrition and avenues for removal of waste products

(c) Lymphatics also regenerate, and aid in lessening the edema within the wound

(2) Granulation: temporary connective tissue that fills the wound

(a) Fibroblasts are important elements in the formation of the extracellular matrix.

(b) Fibroblasts are drawn into the wound by ischemia.

TABLE 11-2	Proliferative Cytokines	
Cytokine	**Source**	**Function**
PDGF	Platelets, macrophages, endothelial cells, keratinocytes	Chemotaxis, angiogenesis, wound contraction, remodeling
TGF-β	Platelets, macrophages, endothelial cells, keratinocytes, fibroblasts, T-lymphocytes	Chemotaxis, angiogenesis Inhibits keratinocytes and MMPs Induces TGF-β
EGF	Platelets, macrophages,	Mitogenic
TGF-a	Macrophages, T-lymphocytes, keratinocytes	Mitogenic
FGF	Macrophages, endothelial cells, keratinocytes, mast cells, T-lymphocytes, fibroblasts	Chemotaxis, angiogenesis, wound contraction, matrix deposition
KGF	Fibroblasts	Keratinocyte migration, proliferation, differentiation
IGF-1	Macrophages, fibroblasts	Like growth hormone, stimulates collagen, fibroblasts, keratinocytes
VEGF	Keratinocytes	Increases vasopermeability, mitogenic

(3) Contraction: fibroblasts are transformed into myofibroblasts and are capable of action similar to smooth muscle. Myofibroblasts are actin rich and stretch the dermis to attempt to cover the wound.

(4) Epithelialization: keratinocytes from the wound margins and appendages multiply and migrate across the wound.

    (a) Keratinocytes further debride the wound and require an oxygen-rich environment.

    (b) Thus, if the wound is full of debris or has poor blood supply, reepithelialization is hindered.

3. Maturation

  a. Collagen within granulation tissue is further remodeled through a process of creation and destruction via collagenases.

    (1) This process can take up to 2 years to complete, but is primarily complete by 6 to 12 months.

    (2) The collagenases convert immature collagen (type III) to mature collagen (type I).

  b. The collagen realigns itself through an interaction of forces both internal and external.

    (1) Internal alignment comes when the collagen attempt to match the collagen found at the wound edges.

    (2) External alignment is based on the forces applied to the wound.

B. Wound closure

  1. Primary intention

    a. Clean wounds in which the edges are approximated either by suture, staples, or other adhesives.

    b. This limits the inflammatory and proliferative phases. In fact, epithelialization begins in as early as 24 hours.

  2. Secondary intention

    a. The wounds are not approximated.

    b. This requires all phases of healing, and is therefore longer and requires more energy.

    c. This allows for contaminated wounds to be removed by the body or mechanical means, and thus reduces the risk of infection.

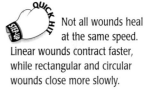 Not all wounds heal at the same speed. Linear wounds contract faster, while rectangular and circular wounds close more slowly.

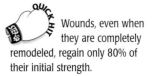 Wounds, even when they are completely remodeled, regain only 80% of their initial strength.

3. Tertiary intention: also known as a delayed primary closure
   a. The wound is left open initially for a certain period of time while the wound is cleaned and observed.
   b. The wound edges are then approximated in usual fashion with stitches or adhesive.

C. Factors that affect wound healing
   1. Cause of wound: sharply incised wounds heal faster than blunt traumatic wounds.
   2. Time since injury: delay in presentation and cleaning can prolong the inflammatory phase, and thus delay wound healing.
   3. Location: wounds that occur in areas with reduced vascular supply heal more slowly.
   4. Size: wounds heal from the periphery, thus the larger the area affected the longer it will take for the wound to progress through the phases of healing.
   5. Temperature: decreased temperature inhibits wound healing.
   6. Hydration: dry wounds progress through the phases of healing more slowly than those in a moist environment.
   7. Foreign bodies: prolong the inflammatory phase and delay wound healing.
   8. Necrotic tissue: impairs wound healing by providing a medium for microbes to exist.
   9. Irradiation: causes endothelial cell damage and hypoxia.
      a. Inhibits angiogenesis.
      b. Impairs keratinocytes and fibroblasts in their G2-phase and S-phase of replication.
   10. Diabetes: impaired microcirculation and red cell function, resulting in poor blood flow to the wound.
       a. Decreased leukocyte and lymphocyte function.
       b. Increased collagen degradation and poor collagen reformation.
   11. Infection: prolongs inflammation and slows healing overall.
       a. For a wound to be considered infected, the quantitative amount of bacteria is greater than 10^5 microbes per gram of tissue.
       b. Amounts less than this imply colonization, and may still impair wound healing through their competition for oxygen within the wound.
   12. Age: as people age, their macrophage and fibroblast functions are reduced. Cellular turnover is decreased, and microvasculature is reduced.
   13. Nutrition: adequate nutrition is vital to the healing process, as all of the phases of wound healing require energy to complete.
       a. Vitamins A and C are especially important.
       b. Zinc deficiency inhibits collagen formation and delays wound healing.
   14. Smoking: nicotine acts to constrict the microvasculature, thereby reducing the blood flow within a wound.
       a. Nicotine causes platelet aggregation and clot, thus impairing blood flow to the wound.
       b. Carbon monoxide binds to the red blood cells, and thus limits the amount of oxygen available to the wound bed.
   15. Medications that impair wound healing:
       a. Glucocorticosteriods
       b. Doxorubicin
       c. Tamoxifen
       d. High-dose nonsteroidal anti-inflammatory drugs
   16. Oxygen content: polymorphonuclear neutrophils require PaO_2 levels greater than 50 mm Hg to produce superoxide derivatives.
       a. Typically, oxygen levels at the center of a wound are significantly lower than those in the surrounding tissue. In areas of hypoxia, collagen synthesis is driven by glycolysis, but oxygen is essential for formation of the triple-helix and cross-linking.
       b. The role of hyperbaric oxygen in wound healing is to increase the oxygen levels in the bed of the wound and thus stimulate growth.

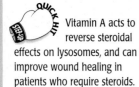

QUICK HIT

Vitamin A acts to reverse steroidal effects on lysosomes, and can improve wound healing in patients who require steroids.

SKIN AND SOFT TISSUE

D. Wound management
  1. Description of the wound
    a. Depth
      (1) Superficial (stage I)
      (2) Violating the dermis (stage II)
      (3) Violating the subcutaneous tissue (stage III)
      (4) Violating to the deep structures of muscle or bone (stage IV)
    b. Dimension
    c. Location
    d. Presence of infection
      (1) Purulence
      (2) Erythema
      (3) Crepitus
      (4) Induration
  2. Debridement
    a. Benefits
      (1) Reduce bacterial load of a wound
      (2) Increase effectiveness of antibacterials applied to the wound
      (3) Improve action of leukocytes: provide an aerobic environment for the opsonization and phagocytosis of bacteria
      (4) Shorten the inflammatory phase of wound healing
      (5) Decrease the energy required for wound healing
      (6) Decrease the physical barrier to wound healing
    b. Indications for debridement
      (1) Necrotic tissue
      (2) Foreign material
      (3) Debris
      (4) Blisters
      (5) Callus
    c. Contraindications for debridement
      (1) Granulation tissue
      (2) Viable tissue
      (3) Stable heel ulcers
      (4) Healthy deep tissues (e.g., muscle, tendon, ligament, nerve, capsule of joint)
    d. Types of debridement
      (1) Sharp: removal of tissue with scalpel, or scissors
        (a) This is commonly performed at the bedside or in the operating room.
        (b) This is the fastest means of debridement, but is associated with pain and other complications such as bleeding.
      (2) Autolytic: removal of tissue by providing an environment for the body's own defenses to work
        (a) Application of a moisture retentive dressing to allow for the body's own collagenases and inflammatory cells to soften and debride the wound
        (b) Principles of topical therapy
          (i) Remove necrotic tissue
          (ii) Identify and eliminate infection
          (iii) Obliterate dead space
          (iv) Absorb excess exudates
          (v) Maintain moist environment
          (vi) Thermal insulation
          (vii) Protection from trauma
        (c) Labor intensive, and requires more time to clean the wound
        (d) Lower rate of infection than with traditional gauze dressings
      (3) Enzymatic: application of enzymes exogenously

(a) Three major categories of enzymatic debriders:
  (i) Fibrinolytics
  (ii) Proteolytics
  (iii) Collagenases: this appears to be the quickest and most effective at debriding a wound
(b) Time consuming
(c) Labor intensive and costly
(4) Mechanical
(a) Wet-to-dry dressings
  (i) Inexpensive and easy
  (ii) Good for removing debris within the wound
  (iii) May traumatize the wound and remove viable tissues
  (iv) Do not maintain a moist environment
(b) Whirlpool
  (i) Nonspecific
  (ii) Good for removing debris within the wound
(c) Scrubbing
  (i) Nonspecific
  (ii) Cytotoxic: hydrogen peroxide and Betadine are especially toxic to tissues, and should be avoided in open wounds
  (iii) Painful and traumatic to tissues

II. Scars
A. Keloid
  1. Uncommon, occur mainly in dark-skinned patients
  2. Extend beyond the boundary of the original scar and invades the surrounding normal tissue
  3. Genetic predisposition
  4. Characterized by an overabundance of collagen. Collagen formation outpaces the actions of collagenases.
  5. Treatment
    a. Steroid injection
    b. Re-excision followed by radiation
    c. No single therapy with good results
B. Hypertrophic scars
  1. Overabundance of collagen
  2. Contained within the borders of the original scar
  3. Treatment
    a. Re-excision, especially for wounds allowed to close by secondary intention
    b. Application of silicone sheets
    c. Pressure garments
    d. Steroid injections

NEOPLASMS OF THE SKIN

I. Melanoma
A. Risk factors
  1. Fair skin
  2. UV light exposure
  3. History of precursor lesions
    a. Dysplastic nevi
    b. Xeroderma pigmentosa
    c. Congenital nevi
  4. History of blistering or peeling sunburns
  5. Immunosuppression

6. Family history
   a. Some cases (5–10%) of melanoma are familial. Individuals who have one first-degree relative with melanoma have a 70 times increased risk of the disease.
   b. Earlier age of onset
   c. Chromosomes 1p and 9p
7. CDKN2A/p16/MC1R mutation

B. Diagnosis
   1. The ABCD rule:
      Asymmetry
      Border irregularity
      Color (nonuniform, varying shades of brown, black, blue, red, and/or yellow)
      Diameter (greater than 6 mm [the diameter of a pencil eraser], or different from the rest)
   2. Early detection is the key. Monitor precursor lesions for any change in size, shape, color, or persistent itching.
   3. Education of the patient to monitor lesions and report any changing moles can play a vital role in early detection.

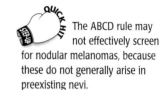
QUICK HIT
The ABCD rule may not effectively screen for nodular melanomas, because these do not generally arise in preexisting nevi.

C. Types of melanoma (based on histologic and clinical characteristics)
   1. Superficial spreading melanoma
      a. This type accounts for 70% of cases.
      b. The lesions typically arise from a preexisting nevus.
      c. This type often displays the classic melanoma features of ABCD.
   2. Lentigo maligna melanoma (Hutchinson freckle)
      a. This type accounts for 10% to 15% of cases.
      b. Lesions are usually on sun-exposed areas of the skin, especially the face.
      c. Usually seen in the elderly, the disease typically starts as a brown lesion that grows and becomes mottled with black.
      d. The substantial diameter of these lesions makes excision difficult.
   3. Acral lentiginous melanoma
      a. This type accounts for 2% to 8% of cases.
      b. It is the most common melanoma in people of color.
      c. It affects the palms of the hand, the soles of the feet, the fingers, toes (including under the nails).
      d. Delay in detection is common, because the affected areas are not routinely examined.
   4. Nodular melanoma
      a. This type accounts for 15% to 30% of cases.
      b. The age of onset is lower than that of the superficial spreading variant.
      c. Typically, the most aggressive form of melanoma, it does not often display the classic appearance of the disease.
      d. The majority arise *de novo* in seemingly unaffected skin.
   5. Other: mucocutaneous and amelanotic melanomas can occur.

D. Staging
   1. Thickness
      a. Clark defined melanoma based on the level of invasion through the layers of the skin. (This is now used to define T1 lesions only.)
         (1) Clark I: *in situ*
         (2) Clark II: papillary dermis
         (3) Clark III: papillary/reticular dermis junction
         (4) Clark IV: reticular dermis
         (5) Clark V: subcutaneous involvement
      b. Currently, the Breslow method of classification is most used.
         (1) This defines melanoma by its thickness in millimeters.
         (2) Breslow thickness is linearly correlated with overall survival.
   2. Lymph node status: involvement of regional lymph nodes is a poor prognostic indicator.

SKIN AND SOFT TISSUE

a. A greater number of involved nodes (especially more than 4), and macroscopic involvement of the nodes, adversely influences long-term survival.

b. The 5-year survival rate for persons with involved lymph nodes is 25% to 70%.

3. Staging using the tumor (thickness), nodal status, metastasis (TNM) system (Table 11-3)

TABLE 11-3 AJCC 2002 Revised Melanoma Staging

Stage	Histologic Features/TNM Classification	Overall Survival		
		1-Year (%)	5-Year (%)	10-Year (%)
0	Intraepithelial/*in situ* melanoma (TisN0M0)		100	100
IA	≤1 mm without ulceration and Clark Level II/III (T1aN0M0)		95	88
IB	≤1 mm with ulceration or level IV/V (T1bN0M0)		91	83
	1.01–2 mm without ulceration (T2aN0M0)		89	79
IIA	1.01–2 mm with ulceration (T2bN0M0)		77	64
	2.01–4 mm without ulceration (T3aN0M0)		79	64
IIB	2.01–4 mm with ulceration (T3bN0M0)		63	51
	>4 mm without ulceration (T4aN0M0)		67	54
IIC	>4 mm with ulceration (T4bN0M0)		45	32
IIIA	Single regional nodal micrometastasis, nonulcerated primary (T1-4aN1aM0)		69	63
	2 or 3 microscopic regional nodes, nonulcerated primary (T1-4aN2aM0)		63	57
IIIB	Single regional nodal micrometastasis, ulcerated primary (T1-4bN1aM0)		53	38
	2 or 3 microscopic regional nodes, ulcerated primary (T1-4bN2aM0)		50	36
	Single regional nodal macrometastasis, nonulcerated primary (T1-4aN1bM0)		59	48
	2 or 3 macroscopic regional nodes, nonulcerated primary (T1-4aN2bM0)		46	39
	In-transit met(s)/satellite lesion(s) *without* metastatic lymph nodes (T1-4a/bN2cM0)		30–50	
IIIC	Single microscopic regional node, ulcerated primary (T1-4bN1bM0)		29	24
	2 or 3 macroscopic regional nodes, ulcerated primary (T1-4bN2bM0)		24	15
	4 or more metastatic nodes, matted nodes/gross extracapsular extension, or in-transit met(s)/satellite(s) *and* metastatic nodes (anyTN3M0)		27	18
IV	Distant skin, subcutaneous, or nodal mets with normal LDH (any TanyNM1a)	59	19	16
	Lung mets with normal LDH (anyTanyNM1b)	57	7	3
	All other visceral mets with normal LDH or any distant mets with increased LDH (anyTanyNM1c)	41	9	6

Below thickness is defined as the thickness of the lesion using an ocular micrometer to measure the total vertical height of the melanoma from the granular layer to the area of deepest penetration. The Clark level refers to levels of invasion according to depth of penetration of the dermis.

(Adapted with permission from Balch et al. Final Version of the American Joint Committee on Cancer Staging System for Cutaneous Melanoma. *J Clin Oncol.* 2001;19:3635–3548. Lippincott Williams & Wilkins.)

(Copyright © 2002 The Cleveland Clinic Foundation.)

4. Other prognostic factors
   a. In stages I to III, ulcerated primary lesions portend a worse prognosis.
   b. Mitotic rate greater than $1.0/mm^2$ and the presence of regression also adversely affect outcome.
   c. Both have been shown to be independent prognostic factors.
E. Treatment
   1. Biopsy: full-thickness biopsy down to subcutaneous fat is required for accurate determination of the Breslow depth.
      a. Margins are only required to be 1 to 2 mm.
      b. Taking wider margins is not recommended, because this may inhibit the ability to perform accurate mapping for sentinel lymph node dissection.
   2. Re-excision is required if the biopsy reveals melanoma. The thickness of the lesion determines if there is a need for sentinel lymph node biopsy at this same surgery.
      a. The re-excision should have margins of 0.5 cm to 2.0 cm, depending on the thickness of the original biopsy, as per the World Health Organization recommendations (Table 11-4).
      b. Studies have shown that there may be higher local recurrence with narrower margins. However, there is no survival advantage with wider margins (e.g., 4 cm versus 2 cm).
   3. Metastatic evaluation
      a. Determines staging, prognosis, survival benefit of surgical and adjuvant immunotherapy or chemotherapy, and in conjunction with sentinel lymph node biopsy, prevents unnecessary extensive surgical procedures.
         (1) If the lesion is less than 1mm in depth, current recommendations are to perform no routine testing, but to follow the patient with recurrent check-ups.
         (2) For lesions 1mm or more, no routine tests, but may obtain chest x-ray, lactate dehydrogenase, or sentinel lymph node biopsy.
         (3) For lesions greater than 4 cm, consider computed tomography (CT) evaluation. Sentinel lymph node biopsy is not recommended.
      b. Common sites of metastasis: melanoma can metastasize anywhere, and is one of the few tumors that can cross the placenta and lodge in the fetus.
         (1) Liver, skin, gastrointestinal tract.
         (2) Lung.
            (a) Observation is indicated to see if further metastasis occurs.
            (b) If no further metastasis present, then pulmonary metastectomy may be considered.
         (3) Adrenals: resection if isolated metastases.
         (4) Bone: radiation for palliation.
         (5) Brain/central nervous system: some success with resection or "gamma knife."
      c. If regional nodes are involved (palpable) at presentation with the primary lesion.

TABLE 11-4	Melanoma Thickness and Required Clinical Excision Margin
Melanoma Thickness	**Clinical Excision Margin**
In situ	0.5–1.0 cm
1.0 mm	1.0 cm
1.1–2.0 mm	1.0–2.0 cm
2.1 mm or greater	2.0 cm

(1) Fine-needle aspiration of the node confirms diagnosis of stage III disease.

(2) CT of the chest/abdomen/pelvis and magnetic resonance imaging of the brain rules out distant disease.

(3) The 5-year survival for patients with palpable nodes at presentation is 40% to 50%.

4. Sentinel lymph node biopsy
    a. Two methods for isolating the sentinel lymph node:
        (1) Lymphazurin: blue dye injected at the site of the original lesion is seen during surgical exploration of the lymph node bed.
        (2) Radiolabeled colloid: this too is injected into the skin near the original lesion, and is detected in the lymph node bed by gamma detector probe.
            (a) Take the node with the highest count.
            (b) Also take all nodes that have counts at least 10% of the "hottest" node removed.
    b. These methods have improved the accuracy of finding the sentinel lymph node to over 95%.
    c. If the sentinel lymph node is positive for disease, then the patient must undergo a radical lymphadenectomy.
        (1) The 5-year survival after lymphadenectomy is 25% to 70%.
        (2) Biopsy/removal of the sentinel lymph node has high morbidity, with increased risk of lymphedema, especially in the groin.
    d. Follow-up
        (1) Education of the patient and family for self examination of the skin.
        (2) Clinic visits every 3 to 6 months for the first 3 years following a resection to perform skin survey. By this time, 75% of people who are going to have a recurrence, have one.
    e. Recurrences (local and/or nodal)
        (1) Incidence of 0.2% to 13%
        (2) Long-term survival is less than 20% in those with a recurrence.
        (3) Re-excision is the treatment of choice.

5. Adjuvant therapy: chemotherapy (numerous agents have been tested without demonstration of significant survival advantage)
    a. Interferon-alpha has offered some increased survival, and is generally indicated for patients with stage III disease, and for those with primary tumors greater than 4 mm deep.
    b. Limb perfusion with either melphalan or TNF is useful for limb conservation when there are multiple subcutaneous (in-transit metastases) or skin lesions.
        (1) No improvement in overall survival
        (2) No utility as an adjuvant treatment after surgical resection
    c. IL-2 also has shown some survival advantage, and is usually combined with dacarbazine-containing chemotherapy regimens.

II. Basal Cell Carcinoma
A. Most common form of skin cancer
B. Locally invasive and rarely metastasizes
    1. Main problem is local recurrence, due to difficult locations for wide resections such as nose, ear, and periorbital areas.
    2. Those that do metastasize were generally either neglected by patient or have recurred multiple times, and have a median survival rate of less than 1 year.
C. Types
    1. Nodular
        a. Pearly nodules with central depression
        b. Pruritic
        c. May bleed if irritated (telangiectasias)

QUICK HIT

If the sentinel lymph node is negative, the patient is 96% likely to have the rest of that nodal basin be negative.

SKIN AND SOFT TISSUE

2. Pigmented: dark and often confused with melanoma

3. Morpheaform, sclerosing, or fibrosing: scar-like, flat, aggressive local invasion

4. Squamous metaplasia with keratinization: aggressive and may develop lymphatic spread

5. Ulcerative: raised rolled edges with central ulcer ("rodent")

D. Treatment

    1. Surgical excision with pathologically free margins

       a. Margins are typically only 3 to 4 mm.

       b. Moh surgery has lowest recurrence rate.

    2. Cryotherapy

    3. Radiation therapy

    4. Electrodesiccation

III. Squamous Cell Carcinoma

A. Derived from the keratinocyte, and can deeply invade surrounding structures

B. Appears as a pink, nonhealing sore with ulceration

C. Metastasizes to regional lymph nodes, especially in immunocompromised patients and in those with Marjolin ulcer

    1. Marjolin ulcer is a squamous cell carcinoma that arises in areas of chronic inflammation, such as old burn scars, hydradenitis, pilonidal cysts, draining osteomyelitis, and skin lesions associated with lupus.

    2. Regional nodal metastases account for 80% to 90% of metastatic squamous cell cancer, whereas metastases to the brain, lung, liver, and bone account for 10% to 20%.

    3. Squamous cell cancers of the mucocutaneous areas, such as the perineum and vulva, as well as those involving the ear or scalp, have highest rates of distant metastatic involvement. Patients with distant metastases have a 10-year survival of 10%.

D. Precursor lesions: actinic keratoses, Bowen disease, and erythroplasia of Queyrat

E. Treatment

    1. Surgical excision with pathologically free margins. Margins are typically only 3 to 4 mm for low-risk lesions, and 6 mm for high-risk lesions.

    2. Cryotherapy

    3. Radiation therapy

    4. Electrodesiccation

    5. Topical 5-fluorouracil

IV. Merkel Cell Carcinoma

A. Aggressive, locally invasive, and high rate of metastasis

B. 5-year survival varies from 88% for stage I disease to 0% for distant metastasis

C. Order chest x-ray to rule out pulmonary primary tumor, because tumor pathology resembles small cell carcinoma of the lung

D. Appears as a red or purple papulonodule, or indurated plaque

E. Has characteristic positive immunocytochemical staining for CK-20. The small round blue cell tumor appears neuroendocrine

F. Treatment

    1. Wide local excision with 1 to 2 cm margins

    2. Sentinel lymph node biopsy

    3. Radiation to the primary site and nodal bed, if the latter is involved

    4. Use of adjuvant chemotherapy controversial if node-positive disease, with a regimen similar to that used for small cell cancer of the lung

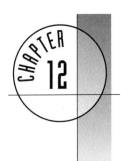

Vascular Surgery

Kumar Pillai, MD, Alexandre D'Audiffret, MD
Kamran Karimi, MD, Giridhar Vedula, MD
Laura Buchanan, MD, Pamela Zimmerman, MD

Every cell in the human body is critically dependent on oxygen in order to function and maintain homeostasis. Oxygen combined with hemoglobin is carried by the blood and delivered to tissues and cells throughout the body. Waste products of cellular metabolism are then carried to organs that can efficiently excrete them. This vital process is dependent on the heart and the vascular system, the pump and the tubes.

The vascular tree is comprised of the arterial, venous, capillary, and lymphatic systems. The arteries carry oxygenated blood from the heart to the tissue. Gas exchange with oxygen delivery and carbon dioxide uptake takes place at the capillary level, and the blood is then carried back to heart via the venous system. The only exception to this rule is the pulmonary vasculature.

The arterial tree is a high-pressure/low-volume system designed to provide the mechanical and kinetic energy needed to transport blood to peripheral tissues in the body. At any given time, less than one-third of the circulating blood volume is contained within the arterial system. The walls of the arteries are thicker and more adept to elastic recoil during cardiac systole and diastole, hence the pulsatile flow pattern. The only one-way valve in this design is at the origin of the system (i.e., the aortic valve).

The venous side is a low-pressure/high-capacitance multibranched conduit. Veins have a tremendous capacity to accommodate increased or backed-up blood volume. Their walls are thinner and flow is nonpulsatile. The venous system depends on unidirectional valves, and action of peripheral skeletal muscles for continued return of blood back to the heart.

In addition to the body's own natural wear and tear, genetic, environmental, dietary, and iatrogenic factors pose a constant threat to the integrity of the vascular tree. Arterial vascular disease can manifest in the form of narrowing (stenosis, occlusive disease), which impedes blood flow; or enlargement (aneurysm), which risks rupture. Venous disease can take the shape of undue clotting (deep venous thrombosis), valvular incompetency (reflux insufficiency), or localized acute infections (thrombophlebitis).

ANEURYSMAL VASCULAR DISEASE

I. **General Principles.** Important Definitions Include:
   A. Aneurysm (derived from the Greek word "aneurysma"): a permanent localized enlargement that is 1.5 times or greater than its expected diameter
   B. Arterial ectasia: a localized enlargement less than 1.5 times of normal diameter
   C. Arteriomegaly: generalized arterial enlargement in contiguous vessels, less than 1.5 times normal, and a well-recognized risk factor for progression to aneurysmal proportions
   D. True aneurysm: enlargement composed of all three layers (tunics) of the vessel wall
   E. False aneurysm: also known as pseudoaneurysms, they lack at least one, and sometimes all three, layers of the vessel wall. Blood is contained by perivascular connective tissue and if present, the tunica adventitia.
   F. Aortic dissection: passage of blood from the arterial lumen into the arterial wall, thereby creating a false lumen. The false lumen may reestablish flow back into the main arterial lumen and become a double-barrel system.

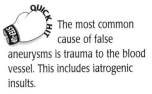

The most common cause of false aneurysms is trauma to the blood vessel. This includes iatrogenic insults.

G. Dissecting aneurysm: aortic dissection with aneurysmal dilatation of the false lumen. These can be prone to rupture.

H. Mycotic aneurysm: refers to any aneurysms that result from direct infectious process resulting in destruction of the supportive tissue in the arterial wall. These compose a small (<5%) proportion of all aneurysms. Bacteria and fungi are the most commonly implicated organisms.

I. Syphilitic aneurysm: although extremely rare in this day and age, this is characteristic of tertiary syphilis, and occurs secondary to inflammatory disease of the ascending thoracic aorta

J. Infrarenal aneurysm: aneurysm with a normal-caliber aorta between the renal arteries and the aneurysm

K. Juxtarenal aneurysm: involve the renal arteries, or are within 1 cm of them

II. Abdominal Aortic Aneurysms

A. Anatomy. The abdominal aorta is a direct continuation of the thoracic aorta as it passes through the aortic hiatus in the diaphragm. It lies in the retroperitoneum, and slightly to the left of midline. It bifurcates into the right and left common iliac arteries at L4.
1. The major branches include the celiac axis, superior mesenteric artery, renal artery, and the inferior mesenteric artery.
2. Other named vessels of clinical interest are the inferior phrenic, gonadal, and lumbar arteries.

B. Epidemiology
1. Abdominal aortic aneurysms (AAAs) affect about 1% to 3% of the general population. Aging of the population and increasing use of routine radiographic studies has resulted in an increase in the prevalence of AAAs.
2. AAAs are the thirteenth leading cause of death in all age groups.
   a. They are the third leading cause of sudden death in males older than 70 years of age.
   b. Ruptured AAAs account for 15,000 deaths per year in the United States.

C. Risk factors for AAAs
1. Age: natural tissue degeneration, and atherosclerosis, increase with age and predispose to the formation of aneurysms. Most patients are 65 years of age and older.
2. Sex: males are at least four times more likely to develop AAAs than women.
3. Smoking: this is by far the single most important environmental risk factor. The prevalence of AAAs in smokers is four times that of nonsmokers.
4. Infections: salmonellosis and tuberculosis have been implicated in the formation of certain aneurysms.
5. Connective tissue disorders: individuals with Marfan syndrome and Ehlers–Danlos type IV have an increased risk of aneurysms.

D. Risk factors for rupture of AAAs—which patients need elective surgery?
1. Size: single most important factor. According to the Laplace law, the tension on the wall of a fluid-containing structure is a product of the radius and pressure ($T = P \times r$). Increasing size not only results in increasing wall tension but also implies weakening of the aortic wall (Fig. 12-1). Generally aneurysms 5 cm or greater should be repaired.

QUICK HIT In males older than 50 years of age, the normal abdominal aortic caliber is between 15 and 24 mm.

QUICK HIT The retroperitoneum can sometimes confine a rupture and prevent fatal exsanguination, which can give surgeons time to repair the aneurysm expeditiously. Such presentations can present with referred flank and groin pain, and can easily be mistaken for renal or ureteral colic.

QUICK HIT In the United States, nearly 100,000 AAAs are diagnosed each year.

QUICK HIT Comparison of the relative risks for different diseases in chronic smokers show that the risk of developing AAAs is threefold more than the risk of developing coronary artery disease, and nearly fivefold more than the risk for cerebrovascular disease.

FIGURE
12-1 Laplace's law. The tension exerted on the wall is determined by the radius and pressure generated by the fluid in the vessel.

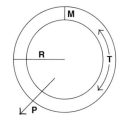

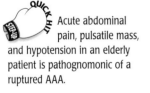
VASCULAR SURGERY

2. Hypertension: the second variable in the Laplace equation, hypertension (uncontrolled) can result in rapid enlargement of the aneurysm, and a higher risk of rupture for any given size of aneurysm.
3. Smoking: especially if there is associated chronic obstructive pulmonary disease (COPD), smoking is an independent risk factor for rapid enlargement and eventual rupture of AAAs.
4. Sex: although AAAs are more common in males, size for size, females are at three times the risk of rupture. The recent increasing popularity of smoking among females is drawing the statistics closer between males and females.
5. Family history: there is a clear association here, as 25% of patients who present with AAA rupture have a first-degree relative with a history of a ruptured AAA.

E. Clinical features and diagnosis
1. Most AAAs are asymptomatic and are discovered incidentally.
2. Symptoms can be due to mass effect and irritation of regional sensory nerves (i.e., back and/or abdominal pain) or due to showering of clots distally (thromboembolism).
3. Abdominal sonography is a good screening and surveillance tool. In experienced hands, the accuracy can reach margins of 3 mm.
4. Computed tomography (CT) scans with intravenous contrast and high resolution serve as confirmatory evidence, and also help with surgical planning and approach.

F. Management
1. The decision to electively repair AAAs is based on size and associated risk factors. The surgeon needs to weigh risk of rupture versus risks and complications of surgery. In the absence of significant risk factors for rupture, aneurysms smaller than 5 cm can be followed by surveillance sonography or CT scans.
2. Aneurysms that are tender to palpation and those that are rapidly enlarging (greater than 5 mm/6 months) should be repaired electively.
3. In patients who warrant surgical treatment, there are three different techniques: the open transperitoneal, open retroperitoneal, and endovascular aneurysm repair (EVAR). Circulation of pressurized blood through the aneurysm sac is responsible for expansion and eventual rupture of all aneurysms.
   a. Choice of procedure is determined by several factors, most importantly the anatomy of the aneurysm. When trying to decide on the most suitable approach, key factors to keep in mind are patient's previous history, including surgical history, unusual anatomic features on the CT scan, and comorbid conditions. One such memory tool is outlined in Table 12-1.
   b. The basic principle of all three techniques is to channel blood from the normal-caliber aorta proximally to the normal-caliber aorta or iliacs distally, thereby excluding the aneurysm from the circulation. This is achieved by placing nonexpansible yet durable synthetic tubes (grafts) in the aorta at the two ends of the aneurysm. In the open approach the graft is sutured to the aorta using a nonabsorbable suture. In EVAR the graft is attached to the aorta by metallic hooks.

G. Ruptured AAAs
1. Most feared complication of AAA
2. Carries an overall mortality rate of more than 80%
3. Presents with acute abdominal pain, back pain, and hypotension
4. Immediate operative intervention is the only treatment that can offer hope for survival.

H. Inflammatory AAAs
1. Inflammatory AAAs represent about 5% of all infrarenal AAAs.
2. There is usually a dense fibroinflammatory tissue that may be adherent to fourth portion of the duodenum, inferior vena cava, and left renal vein.
3. These aneurysms can also have associated ureteral involvement with renal outflow obstruction.

TABLE 12-1 The ABCDEFG of Approaches to AAA Repair

Feature	Open Transperitoneal	Open Retroperitoneal	Endovascular
A Aortic anatomy	Suitable for infrarenal and juxtarenal	Suitable for infrarenal and juxtarenal	Suitable for infrarenal only
B Bifurcation (iliac arteries)	Suitable for aneurysms that involve either of the iliac arteries	Unsuitable in cases of associated right iliac aneurysm	Suitable for aneurysms that involve either of the iliac arteries
C Cava (inferior vena cava)	Suitable for left-sided cava	Unsuitable for left-sided cava	Suitable for left-sided cava
D Diseased abdomen	Multiple previous surgeries, intestinal ostomies a relative contraindication	Suitable in cases of abdominal scarring	Preferred in patients with multiple previous abdominal procedures
E Extra procedures	Preferred approach in patients requiring visceral vessel surgery	Unsuitable in cases where visceral vessel surgery is anticipated, especially right renal artery	Can be combined with additional vessel procedures
F Fat	Morbid obesity makes exposure difficult, although not a strict contraindication	Access to aorta relatively easier through this approach	Preferred approach in morbidly obese patients
G Genitourinary	Preferred in cases of horseshoe kidney where renal artery reimplantation may be needed	Horseshoe kidney is a contraindication to this approach	Suitable if the dominant arterial supply is arising from nonaneurysmal aorta

4. Patients can present with pain, weight loss, and elevated erythrocyte sedimentation rate.
5. CT scan is diagnostic and shows four layers: aortic lumen, luminal clot (thrombus), thickened aortic wall, and adjacent inflammatory tissue.
6. Inflammatory aneurysms are less prone to rupture.
7. These are a technical challenge, and most surgeons prefer either EVAR or the open retroperitoneal approach.

III. Thoracoabdominal Aortic Aneurysms (TAAAs)
A. Anatomy. TAAAs refer to fixed aortic dilatation, starting anywhere from descending thoracic aorta from the left subclavian, to the aortic bifurcation. The aneurysmal segments of the aorta may involve intercostal arteries, celiac axis, superior and inferior mesenterics, renals, and gonadal vessels. There are four types of TAAAs.
B. Etiology. The majority of these aneurysms are due to degenerative changes secondary to abnormal collagen and elastin metabolism. Previous chronic aortic dissections are the second most common cause. Connective tissue disorders, trauma, and vasculitis (especially Takayasu aortitis) make up a small percentage.
C. Clinical features. Most TAAAs, like most AAAs, are discovered incidentally. When symptomatic, TAAAs can present with pain or signs of distal embolization. Mass effect symptoms include dyspnea and dysphagia from compression of the aerodigestive tract or ascites, visceromegaly, and lower extremity swelling from caval compression.
D. Management. Surgical repair, as with AAAs, comprises replacement of diseased aortic segment by an artificial graft. The approach requires gaining exposure in

the thoracic as well as the abdominal cavities. The complex anatomy of TAAAs makes their repair a surgical challenge.

1. Indications for repair include the presence of symptoms that are attributable to the aneurysm. In the absence of symptoms, size greater than 6 cm, or increase in size of more than 0.5 cm per 6-month interval, are accepted criteria for elective repair.
2. To the operating team, perfusion of the spinal cord and abdominal viscera during the aortic clamping is of paramount importance. This is best achieved by a specialized team approach.
3. Like AAAs, TAAAs are also amenable to EVAR.

IV. Femoral and Popliteal Aneurysms

A. Epidemiology and etiology
   1. Almost 90% of the peripheral aneurysms are found in the femoral and popliteal arteries.
   2. Popliteal aneurysms alone make up about 70% of the peripheral aneurysms. The majority are secondary to degenerative atherosclerotic disease, and are predominantly an affliction of men.
B. Clinical features. These aneurysms, although not life threatening, can certainly be limb threatening in a number of ways. Accumulation of thrombus, distal propagation, and limb-threatening ischemia can often be the presenting catastrophic features. Other symptoms include pain secondary to nerve compression or edema, and venous thrombosis secondary to venous outflow obstruction.
C. Diagnosis
   1. Due to its deep location, the popliteal artery is barely palpable in normal individuals. Prominent pulsation in the popliteal fossa is an indication that the patient may be harboring a popliteal aneurysm. Finding an aneurysm in these vessels should prompt a thorough evaluation, as 50% are bilateral, and 30% have an aortic aneurysm associated with them.
   2. If suspected by physical examination, duplex ultrasonography can be used to confirm the anatomic configuration as well as the flow dynamics of the aneurysmal segment.
D. Management. Indications for intervention include thromboembolic complications and size. It is generally agreed that femoral aneurysms of greater than 2.5 cm, and popliteal aneurysms of greater than 2.0 cm, should be repaired. Here, unlike AAAs, replacement with artificial graft is generally unnecessary, and usage of autogenous vein is feasible. Endovascular treatment with placement of covered stents that can exclude the aneurysm from the circulation is also a popular approach.

V. Splenic Artery Aneurysms

A. Splenic artery aneurysms (SAAs) are the most common of the visceral artery aneurysms. After the aorta and iliacs they are the third most common intraabdominal aneurysms.
B. Unlike most aneurysms, SAAs are predominantly a disease of the female sex. Moreover, there is a close association with parity. More than 90% females with SAAs have been pregnant at least once.
C. Like most aneurysms, SAAs are asymptomatic.
D. Indications for treatment are symptoms, documented enlargement, pregnancy or anticipated pregnancy, and diameter of greater than 2.5 cm. SAAs discovered during pregnancy should be repaired, because pregnancy greatly increases the risk of rupture.
E. All potential surgical candidates should receive preoperative immunizations, similar to splenectomy patients. However, aneurysm repair with splenic preservation is the ideal treatment.
F. The main complication of SAAs is rupture.

VI. Renal Artery Aneurysms

A. Aneurysms of the renal artery are the second most common visceral aneurysm. Even so, they occur in about 0.09% of the general population. They are more commonly seen in the female multiparous population.

B. They, like other aneurysms, are discovered as incidental lesions. Most are associated with hypertension.

C. Indications for surgery are difficult-to-control hypertension and size of greater than 2 cm. In the majority of cases, excellent response with blood pressure control is seen.

VII. Mycotic Aneurysms

A. Mycotic aneurysms result from localized infection, which may be a consequence of periaortic infectious process, or due to aortic intimal seeding from blood-borne pathogens. The most common infectious bacteria are *Staphylococcus aureus* and *Salmonella typhi*, and the most common fungal agents are *Candida albicans* and *Aspergillus fumigatus*. Bacterial infections are more common than fungal infections. The usual sites are the femoral arteries and the aorta.

B. Clinical presentation can be nonspecific, but with recurrent bacteremia or fungemia. Fevers, chills, and tenderness not attributable to size alone should prompt the physician to include an infected aneurysm in the differential diagnosis.

C. Management is resection and repair of the aneurysm, thorough debridement of infected tissue, and life-long antibiotic treatment.

VIII. Pseudoaneurysms

A. Pseudoaneurysms (PSAs) are contained arterial disruptions. The main types are traumatic and postsurgical.
   1. Traumatic PSAs are usually iatrogenic, and are a result of arterial punctures for various procedures. Because the femoral artery is the most common site for such procedures, iatrogenic PSAs are predominantly found in this area.
   2. Postsurgical PSAs are due to contained suture line disruptions between the arterial wall and graft material.

B. The diagnosis can be made readily by duplex sonography.

C. Traumatic PSAs greater than 2.5 cm are treated by injection of thrombin, a procoagulant, in the cavity of the PSAs under sonographic guidance. Those that do not respond to this approach require open surgery to repair the localized disruption in the vessel wall.
   1. Asymptomatic, traumatic PSAs less than 2.5 cm do not require treatment.
   2. Postsurgical PSAs most often require revision of the surgical site suture line.

CEREBROVASCULAR OCCLUSIVE DISEASE

I. Anatomy

A. Divisions of the aorta
   1. Ascending aorta courses anteriorly from the left ventricle
   2. Branches of the ascending aorta
      a. Brachiocephalic trunk (innominate artery): aorta courses from a right anterior to left posterior position in the upper mediastinum. The first and most anterior branch is the innominate artery. At the right clavicular head it splits into the right common carotid and the right subclavian artery.
      b. Left common carotid artery: arises 1 cm from the innominate, and courses posteriorly into the left base of the neck.
      c. Left subclavian artery: located posterior, and at the distal end of the aortic arch.

B. Divisions of the common carotid artery
   1. External carotid artery: The common carotid bifurcates at the angle of the mandible to form the internal and external carotid. The external carotid

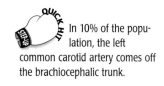
In 10% of the population, the left common carotid artery comes off the brachiocephalic trunk.

Because of the anterior position of the innominate artery, it is accessible for reconstruction by a median sternotomy approach.

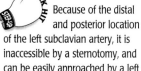
Because of the distal and posterior location of the left subclavian artery, it is inaccessible by a sternotomy, and can be easily approached by a left high anterior or anterolateral thoracotomy.

VASCULAR SURGERY

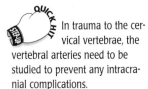
The supraclinoid portion of the carotid, intracranially, gives rise to the ophthalmic, posterior communicating and the anterior choroidal arteries. Ophthalmic artery occlusion is often the initial indicator of carotid occlusive disease (amaurosis fugax).

In trauma to the cervical vertebrae, the vertebral arteries need to be studied to prevent any intracranial complications.

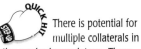
There is potential for multiple collaterals in the cerebral vasculature. These collaterals become the source of blood supply, when arterial occlusive disease develops in one of the four major arteries supplying the brain.

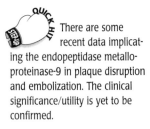
There are some recent data implicating the endopeptidase metalloproteinase-9 in plaque disruption and embolization. The clinical significance/utility is yet to be confirmed.

The carotid bifurcation is most commonly affected due to increased turbulent flow in this area.

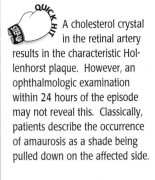
A cholesterol crystal in the retinal artery results in the characteristic Hollenhorst plaque. However, an ophthalmologic examination within 24 hours of the episode may not reveal this. Classically, patients describe the occurrence of amaurosis as a shade being pulled down on the affected side.

splits to form the ascending pharyngeal artery, superior thyroidal artery, lingual artery, occipital artery, posterior auricular artery, and superficial temporal arteries.
2. Internal carotid artery: Main divisions of the internal carotid artery are the intrapetrosal, intracavernous, and supraclinoid arteries.
C. Divisions of the subclavian artery
1. Vertebral artery: This artery arises from the first portion of the subclavian, and enters the foramina transversum at the level of the sixth cervical vertebra. It gains intracerebral access through the foramen magnum.

II. Epidemiology

A. Each year 500,000 individuals suffer from stroke. The Framingham study (1975) noted that 62% of all stroke victims exhibit decreased socialization, 71% are dependent on other means of mobility, and 16% are institution bound.
B. Stroke is the third most common cause of death in the United States. About 200,000 individuals die as a result of stroke annually.
C. Public health costs for disabilities related to stroke exceed $16 trillion a year.

III. Etiology and Pathophysiology

A. Atherosclerotic/embolic strokes
1. Most common cause of cerebrovascular occlusive disease.
2. Risk factors include advanced age, hypertension, diabetes, hyperlipidemia, positive family history, tobacco use, hypercoagulable state, and elevated homocysteine levels.
3. Occlusion is thought to occur secondary to focal vessel wall injury in areas of turbulent blood flow. Brownian movement of blood results in particulate deposition, and atherosclerotic plaque. An endothelium-lined fibrous cap usually covers this plaque. Disruption of the cap causes platelet deposition. Platelet aggregates or plaque material may embolize, resulting in stroke.

IV. Clinical Features

A. Transient ischemic attack (TIA): sudden onset of focal neurologic deficit that resolves in 24 hours. Manifestations include hemispheric deficit (e.g., sensory or motor), transient monocular blindness (amaurosis fugax), and drop attacks/falls (from vertebrobasilar TIA).
B. Hemispheric stroke: An embolic event in the cerebral circulation typically occurs in the watershed area of the brain, and is manifested as contralateral sensory or motor loss, a prominent visual field defect, and aphasia or partial inattention. Strokes of the posterior circulation may cause ataxia, vertigo, diplopia, syncope, and nystagmus.
C. Carotid bruits: These are usually detected on routine physical examination, and are reported in 5% of the population older than 60 years of age.
1. There is a poor correlation between the presence of carotid bruit and stenosis.
2. Less than 23% of patients with a carotid bruit actually have disease greater than 50% stenosis.

V. Management

A. Medical management
1. Lifestyle modification (e.g., weight loss, smoking cessation)
2. Control of hypertension and diabetes
3. Aspirin (acetylsalicylic acid, ASA) to prevent platelet aggregation. Data support the use of ASA for symptomatic disease, with a 22% risk reduction in recurrent TIA when compared to controls. ASA also improves mortality from coronary artery disease.

4. Clopidogrel (antiplatelet agent). This also has been shown to have a relative risk reduction in the incidence of TIA, myocardial infarction (MI), and death.

5. Lipid-lowering agents. The 3-hydroxy-3-methylglutaryl coenzyme A (HMG CoA) reductase inhibitors may be of benefit. However, the data are still inconclusive.

6. Anticoagulation. This treatment is only recommended in patients with embolic stroke from atrial fibrillation.

B. Surgical management
  1. Surgical options
     a. Carotid endarterectomy: exposure of the carotid artery is achieved by an incision over the medial border of the sternocleidomastoid muscle. Following adequate exposure, the common, internal, and external carotid vessels are clamped. It is important to minimize the degree of manipulation in order to prevent embolization of plaque. An arteriotomy is performed. The plaque is gently dissected off the inner vessel wall. The arteriotomy is closed using a vein or synthetic patch. Studies have shown that restenosis rates and thrombosis rates are lower with the use of a patch.
        (1) Indications for carotid endarterectomy. The risk of stroke is substantially increased, irrespective of the degree of stenosis, after a TIA or stroke (10–40%). This clearly indicates the need for an intervention in this scenario. In asymptomatic patients, there is a clear risk reduction in stroke if the degree of luminal stenosis is 80% or greater. Additionally, grafting may be of benefit in carotid repair of patients with high-grade stenosis or bilateral disease prior to coronary artery bypass.
        (2) Contraindications for carotid endarterectomy. The main contraindications to repair include an acute profound stroke, a stroke in evolution, or complete occlusion of the internal carotid.
     b. Carotid angioplasty and stenting: this minimally invasive technique allows access to the carotids using catheters via a femoral arterial puncture. It is still considered investigational.
     c. Aortic root reconstruction: performed in cases of brachiocephalic occlusion via median sternotomy approach.
     d. Vertebral artery reconstruction: performed for vertebral occlusion. The vertebral artery is usually ligated, and the distal portion is transposed to the ipsilateral carotid.
  2. Endovascular therapy. The Food and Drug Administration has approved the use of endovascular therapy for carotid stenosis in very specific instances. For example, it may be used in high-risk patients such as those with recent MI, poor ejection fraction, severe COPD, carotid restenosis, prior neck dissection, radiation to neck, or contralateral recurrent nerve injury.
  3. Postoperative/intervention complications. These include perioperative plaque embolization with stroke, injury to the recurrent laryngeal nerve (causes hoarseness), injury to the hypoglossal nerve (causes the tongue to deviate to the side of the injury), and injury to the superior laryngeal nerve (causes voice to fatigue easily). Nonneurologic complications can also occur postoperatively. Bleeding can result in neck swelling/hematoma, requiring re-exploration.

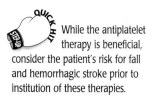
While the antiplatelet therapy is beneficial, consider the patient's risk for fall and hemorrhagic stroke prior to institution of these therapies.

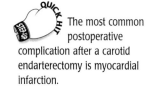
The most common postoperative complication after a carotid endarterectomy is myocardial infarction.

AORTOILIAC OCCLUSIVE DISEASE

I. General Principles
  A. This disease is restricted to the distal aorta, and the bilateral common and external iliac arteries.
  B. Disease of the aorta and the iliac arteries is referred to as "inflow" disease, and disease distal to the groin is referred to as "outflow" disease.
  C. Inflow disease affects the major muscle groups of the pelvis and lower extremities, and can result in disabling symptoms.

II. Anatomy

A. The abdominal aorta enters the diaphragmatic hiatus at the level of the twelfth thoracic vertebra, and bifurcates at the level of the fourth lumbar vertebra.

B. At the level of the bifurcation (approximately the level of the umbilicus) form the right and left common iliac arteries. The common iliacs curve posteriorly into the sacral hollow, and divide into the internal iliac and the external iliac.

C. The internal iliac supplies the pelvic viscera. The external iliac courses anteriorly along the psoas muscle under the inguinal ligament, forming the common femoral artery.

III. Pathophysiology

A. As noted earlier, the disruption in normal laminar flow at the level of the bifurcation results in the formation and organization of plaque. Further plaque deposition results in the augmentation of collaterals around the occlusive segments.

B. These collaterals are not always sufficient to provide flow to the pelvic viscera or lower extremities. When unable to meet the metabolic demands of the lower extremities or pelvis, impotence, buttock claudication, and severe disabling lower extremity pain occurs.

IV. Clinical Features

A. Risk factors. Multiple risk factors have been identified in this disease process. These include smoking, hypertension, hyperlipidemia, diabetes mellitus type 2, male sex, older age (age 50–60), and genetic disposition.

B. Claudication. This denotes an extremely disabling condition with characteristic exercise-induced, cramping pain, when oxygen supply does not meet demand in active muscles. Rest relieves pain.

C. Erectile dysfunction. In men, reduced internal iliac perfusion can lead to erectile dysfunction.

D. Classification
1. Type I disease: confined to the distal aorta and bilateral iliacs (10%). This often presents in young females with claudication of the buttocks and hips.
2. Type II disease: more extensive (80%) and involves the aorta, the iliacs, and often the common femoral artery. Type II disease is the most common.
3. Type III: involves the femoropopliteal and tibial segments (10%). Patients with type III disease usually present with critical limb ischemia.

V. Diagnosis

A. Physical Examination
1. Presence of gangrene
2. Tissue atrophy, especially in the calf
3. Dermal changes such as *livedo reticularis* suggest proximal occlusive disease with showering of distal microemboli
4. Presence/absence of pulses in the groin and along the lower extremity
5. Presence of bruits in the abdomen and groin

B. Noninvasive vascular testing
1. Segmental pressure measurements: ankle-brachial index (ABI) in a patient with claudication ranges from 0.5 to 0.9, whereas patients with rest pain and tissue loss have ABI less than 0.5.
   a. In some scenarios, the ABI at rest may be normal, but with exercise the ABI may decrease.
   b. A drop of 15% in the ABI after exercise is considered significant.
   c. Also realize that patients with medial calcinosis (e.g., diabetes mellitus type 2, renal disease) may have falsely elevated ABI.
2. Duplex scanning. Although this can be used to identify occlusion, utility is limited by such factors as the patient's body habitus and operator expertise.

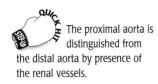
The proximal aorta is distinguished from the distal aorta by presence of the renal vessels.

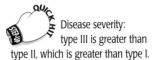
The symptom constellation consisting of lower extremity claudication, gluteal atrophy, impotence, and diminished femoral pulses results in "Leriche syndrome."

Disease severity: type III is greater than type II, which is greater than type I.

C. Arteriography. This technique involves the use of radio-opaque dye to delineate the vascular anatomy/abnormalities of the lower extremity. The patient requires a palpable pulse (either in the femoral artery or an upper extremity artery) to cannulate the vessel for the angiogram.

VI. Management

A. Medical management

1. Smoking cessation: the most important modifiable risk factor that has been shown innumerable times to improve claudicatory symptoms.

2. Vigorous exercise program: must be emphasized in patients who are able to exercise. It is thought that exercise increases the anaerobic tolerance in ischemic muscle tissue.

3. Aspirin (ASA): although no specific data support the use of ASA in aorto-occlusive disease, its use must be recommended, considering the benefit in the treatment of occlusive disease in other vascular territories.

4. Pentoxifylline: the mechanism in its benefit is still unclear; however, trials have shown a small decrease of claudication symptoms with its use.

5. Hypertension, diabetes, and hyperlipidemia control: this approach may not reverse the disease but certainly may prevent its progression.

B. Surgical management

1. Endovascular techniques

a. Percutaneous access followed by balloon angioplasty with a stent has shown some promise for short segment, nonocclusive disease in the iliacs.

b. Complications include perforation, dissection, thrombosis, and distal embolism.

2. Aortoiliac endarterectomy: usually reserved for focal type I disease in the distal aorta. This operation can provide excellent results provided there is no aneurysmal dilation of the distal aorta. The procedure involves an arteriotomy, with careful dissection to remove the plaque from the aortic wall.

3. Arterial reconstruction with anatomically placed prosthesis: involves the use of a Dacron or polytetrafluoroethylene (PTFE) graft from the proximal aorta to the iliacs or femorals. The orientation of the graft is similar to the anatomy of the vasculature.

4. Arterial reconstruction with extra-anatomically placed prosthesis

a. In patients with a hostile abdomen or in poor-risk patients, inflow can be derived from the axillary artery.

b. A PTFE graft is used connecting the axillary artery to the femoral artery. A second piece of graft is used connecting the two femoral arteries. This provides blood flow to the extremities using the axillary artery as inflow. The patency rates are lower than aortobifemoral prosthesis.

FEMOROPOPLITEAL AND TIBIAL OCCLUSIVE DISEASE

I. General Principles

A. This extremely debilitating condition leads to claudication, rest pain, and critical ischemia, resulting in gangrene.

B. There is an increased risk of cardiovascular mortality.

C. Limb loss rates can be as high as 1% to 5% as a result of infrainguinal disease.

II. Anatomy

A. Outflow disease is defined as being distal to the inguinal ligament.

B. Hunter canal (adductor canal): as the superficial femoral artery courses toward the knee, it passes via the adductor canal. This is the most common site of occlusion below the inguinal ligament.

C. It is important to identify the collaterization in the lower extremity via the profunda femoris, and the geniculate branches at the level of the knee.

III. Diagnosis

A. History. Identify patient symptomatology. Patients often present with exercise-induced lower extremity pain, nonhealing ulcer, and muscle wasting. 80% have a history of smoking.

B. Physical examination. Begins with a pulse examination. Identify trophic changes, muscle wasting, thinning of the skin and nails, and loss of hair. Ischemic ulcerations begin as small dry ulcers of the toes or heel, and progress to frank gangrene.

C. Noninvasive testing. Check ABI, segmental pressures, and pulse volume recordings. Magnetic resonance angiography and CT angiography are being increasingly used to identify disease and plan intervention.

D. Diabetes and renal failure make patients more susceptible to arterial insufficiency.

E. In blue toe syndrome, atheroembolic disease moves from an aortoiliac or femoropopliteal source to the distal microvasculature, resulting in digital ischemia.

IV. Management

A. Risk factor modification: cornerstone for management of lower extremity occlusive disease.
   1. Smoking cessation
   2. Dietary modification
   3. Structured exercise program

B. Medical management: use of HMG CoA reductase inhibitors, aspirin, and pentoxifylline

C. Surgical management
   1. Percutaneous angioplasty. With the advent of flexible stents and unique catheters, this option is being considered more frequently as a first-line treatment.
      a. It is can be performed under local anesthesia, with complications primarily related to the contrast agents (such as renal failure and reaction to the agent) and access site.
      b. Other complications include bleeding, pseudoaneurysm, and distal plaque embolism.
      c. Technical success achieved in 88% to 93% of patients, with patency rates up to 60% at 1 year.
   2. Other operative techniques
      a. Autologous vein bypass. The ipsilateral or contralateral saphenous vein is harvested for bypass around the occluded segments. The vein is reversed to allow flow through the venous valves.
      b. In-situ vein bypass. The saphenous vein is identified in its native location. The venous valves are disrupted using a valvulotome, and the bypass is carried out around the occluded segments.
      c. Prosthetic bypass. Cryopreserved vein, Dacron, or PTFE grafts may be utilized to bypass the occlusion. This modality is used primarily for above-the-knee reconstructions when there is well-preserved tibial/peroneal artery blood flow distally.

UPPER EXTREMITY OCCLUSIVE DISEASE

I. General Principles

A. This debilitating condition is associated with severe pain, and patients often are disabled from occupations and are unable to perform daily activities.

B. Lesions that are more proximal are more amenable to surgical correction, and the lesions that are more distal require aggressive medical management.

II. Diagnosis

A. History of pain, exercise-induced fatigue, occupational exposure (such as in cases of thoracic outlet syndrome or vibration syndromes), and medical

---

QUICK HIT Patients with lesions amenable to percutaneous interventions benefit from angiography at the hands of an experienced vascular surgeon. This ensures the identification of appropriate distal targets, and therapeutic interventions such as angioplasty can be performed with stenting, if possible.

QUICK HIT Use of preoperative hydration, N-acetyl cysteine (Mucomyst), sodium bicarbonate hydration, and hypo-osmolar/iso-osmolar contrast agents has markedly decreased the incidence of acute renal failure in this population.

QUICK HIT Identify the possibility of compartment syndrome, and the need for fasciotomy in patients after revascularization for reperfusion injury.

VASCULAR SURGERY

conditions (e.g., arteritis, fibromuscular dysplasia, azotemic arteritis in end-stage renal disease, postradiation arteritis).

B. Raynaud phenomenon. This phenomenon is described as episodic color change in the digits secondary to hypothermia and emotional stimuli. It is thought to occur due to vasospasm (causes pallor), followed by cyanosis (as tissue oxygenation is completed), and finally hyperemia from reperfusion.

C. Examination of the extremity should include palpation of the pulse along the length of the extremity. An Allen test should be performed to evaluate the adequacy of blood flow to the hand.

D. Noninvasive testing, including plethysmography, and transcutaneous Doppler and duplex scanning should be performed to assess for occlusion in the upper extremity.

E. Thoracic outlet syndrome can be a very debilitating condition leading to ischemia and arm pain. This results from compression of nerve, artery, or vein at the space between the first thoracic rib and clavicle, between the pectoralis minor and the coracoid process, or the head of the humerus while the patient externally rotates the arm.

III. Management

A. Lifestyle modification includes smoking cessation, avoidance of cold, and avoidance of occupational exposure (vibratory injury in patients with digital ischemia).

B. Short segments of occlusion in the upper extremity may require bypass grafting or angioplasty, with or without stent, to increase blood flow to the arm.

C. Treatment for thoracic outlet syndrome may involve a first rib resection and anterior scalenectomy to relieve pressure.

D. In cases of occlusions in the palmar arch, which are not amenable to surgical therapy, nifedipine may be helpful.

E. Arteritis may be treated with steroids.

> **QUICK HIT**
> Thromboangiitis obliterans (Buerger disease): this unique disease affects the venoarterial plexus, causing digital/distal ischemia that results in pain and gangrene. It is strongly associated with smoking of an addictive nature. Treatment is supportive, and includes smoking cessation.

SPLANCHNIC OCCLUSIVE DISEASE

A. Occlusive disease of the splanchnic circulation is fairly uncommon.

B. Most patients remain asymptomatic, with occlusion of two of three of the following arteries: the celiac, superior mesenteric, and inferior mesenteric arteries, which have a rich collateral network among the three vessels. These arteries supply the gastrointestinal tract. Symptoms begin when the third becomes occluded.

C. Within this large scope of disease, three specific entities will be discussed.
   1. Chronic splanchnic ischemia.
      a. This syndrome occurs as a result of arteriosclerosis at the origins of the major vascular supply of the intestine.
      b. Symptoms often involve postprandial pain (intestinal angina) with associated profound weight loss. Patients often develop food fear due to pain.
      c. Workup is often undertaken when there is a strong index of suspicion, and involves arterial duplex and possible magnetic resonance angiography or CT angiography.
      d. The treatment is revascularization with vein graft or angioplasty with stent.
   2. Acute splanchnic ischemia.
      a. This occurs primarily due to embolus from a cardiac source, or due to thrombosis of a partially occluded native vessel.
      b. Patients often present with acute onset of pain that is clearly out of proportion to the clinical examination. This warrants urgent attention before the ischemia results in frank necrosis and perforation of the bowel.

QUICK HIT Fibromuscular dysplasia often affects young women, and is related to increased estrogen production. It is amenable, with excellent results, to angioplasty and stenting.

c. Treatment begins with active resuscitation followed by the administration of heparin, and possibly catheter-directed thrombolysis with thrombolytics such as tissue plasminogen activator. Alternatively, a surgical embolectomy may be performed.

3. Renovascular occlusive disease.
   a. This is the most common form of surgically correctable hypertension.
   b. Renal artery occlusion causes decreased blood flow to the kidneys with resultant activation of the renin–angiotensin axis. This activation causes hypertension. Occlusion may either result from arteriosclerosis or fibromuscular dysplasia.
   c. Treatment involves angioplasty with stenting or aortorenal bypass.

VENOUS DISEASE: ACUTE VENOUS THROMBOEMBOLIC DISEASE

I. Acute Lower Extremity Deep Vein Thrombosis: Proximal Vessels

QUICK HIT DVT prophylaxis should be considered for all hospitalized patients. Pneumatic compression boots and early ambulation are the best prophylaxis in surgery patients.

A. Epidemiology
   1. Incidence of deep vein thrombosis (DVT): about 250,000 patients per year, with 200,000 patients also with pulmonary embolism (PE).
   2. Risk factors: age, malignancy, immobilization, surgery and trauma, oral contraceptives, hormone replacement, pregnancy, neurologic disease (spinal cord injury), cardiac disease, obesity, genetic hypercoagulable state.

B. Pathogenesis and clinical features
   1. Most thromboses affect the iliac, femoral, or popliteal lower limb veins. The deep venous system includes the common femoral, femoral (or superficial femoral), deep femoral, popliteal, and tibial veins.
   2. After thrombus formation, an acute and chronic inflammatory response leads to thrombus amplification, organization, and recanalization, often with vein wall and valve damage.

QUICK HIT Virchow triad describes factors predisposing to DVT formation: endothelial damage, stasis, and hypercoagulable state.

   3. Vein wall response is highly dependent on endothelial selectins P- and E-selectin.
   4. Presenting symptoms may include unilateral leg pain and swelling, positive Homans sign (pain on passive dorsiflexion of foot—a nonspecific physical finding), or PE.

C. Diagnosis
   1. 50% of patients with acute DVT may be asymptomatic.
   2. Duplex ultrasound imaging has become the test of choice, with greater than 95% sensitivity and specificity.

QUICK HIT Duplex ultrasound is the best way to diagnose DVT. Circulating D-dimer measurement can rule out DVT, but if positive, is nonspecific.

   3. Differential diagnosis of lower extremity pain and swelling includes muscle strain or contusion, cellulitis, Baker cyst, iliac vein obstruction due to retroperitoneal tumor or mass, and systemic causes of swelling and edema (such as congestive heart failure or venous insufficiency).

D. Management
   1. Treatment for acute DVT is anticoagulation. Initial therapy is often with intravenous unfractionated heparin (UFH), or subcutaneous low-molecular-weight heparin (LMWH), such as enoxaparin.
      a. Intravenous UFH has a narrow therapeutic window and unpredictable dose response. Heparin is administered continuously, requiring inpatient treatment. It is useful for patients with renal failure. The therapeutic response is monitored by following partial thromboplastin time. Patients who do not respond should have antifactor Xa levels measured.
      b. LMWH is more predictable, and has greater bioavailability. Administration is daily or twice a day. LMWH should be avoided in patients with renal failure. No routine blood monitoring is required.
   2. Vena caval interruption via filter placement should be considered when anticoagulation is contraindicated, PE recurs on anticoagulation, or a complication develops from use of anticoagulation.

a. Filters may be retrievable.

b. Contraindications to anticoagulation include evidence of ongoing bleeding, trauma resulting in solid organ injury, intracranial hemorrhage, or spinal hematoma, and complication of anticoagulation such as bleeding.

c. Anticoagulation should be resumed or initiated, when possible, as a filter alone is not effective treatment of DVT.

3. Systemic or catheter directed thrombolysis, and surgical extraction or thrombectomy should be used only in patients with massive iliofemoral DVT at risk of limb gangrene secondary to venous occlusion.

4. Patients who present with idiopathic or recurrent DVT should be evaluated for hypercoagulable state.

5. Ambulation with DVT does not increase the risk of PE, and does decrease the incidence and severity of chronic venous disease after DVT. Ambulation and sequential compression therapy are encouraged in the management of DVT.

6. Long-term treatment

a. Between 15% and 50% of patients often develop symptomatic extension or recurrent events.

b. Long-term treatment involves anticoagulation usually with vitamin K antagonist (warfarin).

(1) Patient with a first episode of DVT with underlying reversible risk factor should receive 3 months of treatment.

(2) Patients with a first episode of idiopathic DVT should receive treatment for 6 to 12 months, and should be considered for indefinite anticoagulant therapy.

(3) Patients with DVT and malignancy should receive 3 to 6 months of LMWH, and indefinite anticoagulation therapy.

(4) Patients with a first episode of DVT and antiphospholipid antibodies, or two or more thrombophilic conditions, should receive 12 months of therapy and be considered for indefinite treatment.

(5) Patients with a first episode of DVT and a documented thrombophilic condition should receive 6 to 12 months of treatment, and be considered for indefinite therapy.

(6) Patients with two or more documented episodes of DVT should receive indefinite treatment.

> **QUICK HIT** A patient with recurrent PE, despite anticoagulation, should have a vena caval filter placed.

II. Upper Extremity Deep Venous Thrombosis

A. Thrombotic obstruction of the subclavian, axillary, or brachial vein

1. Usually associated with central venous catheters or other instrumentation

2. Compression in the thoracic outlet, also known as Paget Schroetter syndrome or "effort thrombosis"

B. Signs and symptoms are edema, dilated collateral circulation, and pain

C. Diagnosis is clinical with venous duplex

D. Management is controversial

1. Generally removal of foreign body is sufficient.

2. Treatment may be similar to lower extremity DVT. However, the level of evidence for this course is lower than for lower extremity DVT.

3. No reliable evidence is available on superior vena cava interruption.

4. Thrombolysis with 3 to 6 months of anticoagulation is indicated for effort thrombosis with possible rib resection.

III. Distal Lower Extremity Deep Venous Thrombosis

A. Between 10% and 15% of patients will propagate to the proximal venous system and require treatment

B. DVT of the calf is treated expectantly

VASCULAR SURGERY

IV. Pulmonary Embolism

A. DVT and pulmonary embolism (PE) are different manifestations of a similar disease process and their treatment is therefore similar.

B. The majority of patients with proximal DVT also have symptomatic or asymptomatic PE, and vice versa.

C. Patients treated for PE are four times more likely to die of recurrent venous thromboembolic disease in the next year when compared with patients treated for DVT (1.5% versus 0.4%).

POSTPHLEBITIC SYNDROME AND CHRONIC VENOUS INSUFFICIENCY

I. Incidence

A. Postphlebitic syndrome (PTS) develops in 20% to 50% of patients after documented DVT. In the absence of DVT, this constellation of symptoms is referred to as chronic venous insufficiency (CVI).

B. CVD affects 50 million Americans, with 500,000 of them developing venous ulcers.

II. Pathology. Development of CVD may be related to venous obstruction, valvular insufficiency, or calf muscle pump malfunction.

III. Clinical Features: Symptoms

A. Chronic postural dependent swelling, pain, local discomfort, and venous ulceration at the ankle.

B. Superficial venous insufficiency that may appear as spider vein, telangiectasias, or varicosities.

C. Pain, hyperpigmentation, stasis dermatitis, or venous ulcers (CVD).

D. Venous ulcers that tend to form just above the medial malleolus.

E. Venous claudication: pain associated with walking from increased swelling and prominence of the superficial venous system usually observed in the setting of both venous obstruction and venous incompetence.

IV. Diagnosis

A. Venous duplex ultrasonography allows imaging of veins as well as analysis of blood flow.

B. Plethysmography uses an air-filled cylinder fitted over the extremity to analyze changes in the extremity with position change and exercise.

C. Venography has no significant role in diagnosis of acute or chronic disease, but may be used to complement noninvasive testing when considering intervention in the deep venous system or in research protocols.

V. Management

A. Elastic compression stockings should be used for 2 years following DVT and for symptom improvement in the setting of PTS or CVD.

B. Conservative medical therapy includes using compressive stockings (30 to 40 mm Hg at the ankle), avoiding prolonged periods of standing, elevating legs intermittently through the day, elevating the foot of the bed at night, and exercising.

C. Sclerotherapy is needle injection of a caustic solution directly into superficial veins, and is used to treat isolated varicosities, telangiectasias, and varicosities remaining after saphenous stripping.

D. Vein stripping/ablation, as well as endovascular laser or radiofrequency ablation, act by disrupting the great saphenous vein, usually at the saphenofemoral junction, with removal of the vein to the level of the knee or below. This is indicated for treatment of saphenous vein insufficiency.

E. Perforator vein ligation can be performed for treatment of isolated perforator vein incompetence.

SUPERFICIAL THROMBOPHLEBITIS

I. Incidence
A. This condition may occur spontaneously, or be associated with intravenous lines, trauma, varicose veins, pregnancy, and the postpartum period.
B. Number of cases is 125,000 per year.
C. Migratory superficial thrombophlebitis may suggest abdominal cancer (Trousseau syndrome).
D. PE is rare.

II. Patients present with localized pain, erythema, and induration.
A. No generalized swelling occurs unless DVT develops.
B. Over time a firm cord forms.
C. Fever and shaking chills may result from septic/suppurative thrombophlebitis with recannulation.

III. Differential Diagnosis. Localization over superficial vein differentiated from cellulitis, ascending lymphangitis, erythema nodosum, erythema induration, and panniculitis.

IV. Management
A. Treatment may involve nonsteroidal anti-inflammatory drugs, local heat, elevation, and support with compressive stocking or elastic wrap.
B. Most cases resolve within 7 to 10 days.
C. Recurrence may be treated with surgical excision usually 6 months after acute inflammation.
D. Septic thrombophlebitis requires intravenous antibiotics, and if the patient becomes septic, surgical excision may be necessary.

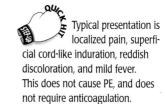

Typical presentation is localized pain, superficial cord-like induration, reddish discoloration, and mild fever. This does not cause PE, and does not require anticoagulation.

VASCULAR NONINVASIVE DIAGNOSTIC STUDIES

I. General Principles
A. Noninvasive testing is a secondary modality, after clinical examination, to help identify vascular disease.
B. The specific indications and the utility in specific scenarios will be described.

II. Arterial Studies
A. Cerebrovascular testing
   1. Oculoplethysmography
      a. This test measures the flow of blood in the ophthalmic artery (indicator of flow in the internal carotid artery), and compares it to the flow of blood in the ipsilateral ear (indicator of flow in the external carotid artery). Rarely performed.
   2. Carotid duplex. The degree of velocity of blood flow in the carotids (duplex scanning) and the arteries luminal diameter is viewed (B-mode analysis).
B. Lower extremity testing
   1. ABI
      a. This test is done by measuring the blood pressure in the ankle and in the arm while the patient is at rest. The measurements may be repeated after 5 minutes of exercise to evaluate for decrease in flow with activity.
      b. The ratio of the ankle pressure to the brachial pressure is a sensitive indicator of degree of peripheral occlusive disease. Normally the ratio should be 1. Mild arterial disease has an ABI of 0.7 to 0.9. Patients with ABIs of 0.5 to 0.7 may have intermittent claudication, and those with ABIs less than 0.5 may have rest pain and/or severe limb-threatening ischemia.

2. Segmental pressures
   a. Blood pressure cuffs are placed around the ankle, upper calf, and thigh.
   b. Decreased pressure in relation to the proximal cuff or to the contralateral pressure at the same level is an indicator of occlusion proximal to measuring site. Pressure considered significant is 20 to 30 mm Hg.
3. Pulse volume recordings.
   a. Doppler waveforms are obtained at the thigh, upper calf, ankle, foot, and toe levels after a pneumatic cuff is inflated to 60 mm Hg. A transducer connected to the cuff records the flow patterns/waveforms at the artery.
   b. Disease is indicated by irregularity within the flow or flattening of the wave.
C. Mesenteric arterial evaluation. Utilizes ultrasound technology to examine aneurysmal disease of the abdominal aorta. Flow velocities in the mesenteric vessels are compared with flow velocity in abdominal aorta and define degrees of stenosis in the vessels.

III. Venous Studies
A. Venous duplex. Ultrasound technology is utilized to examine venous patency, obstruction, and reflux. These data are used to diagnose venous thrombosis and treat venous reflux.
B. Vein mapping. This examines the course and location of the vein prior to planning an operation (e.g., saphenous vein mapping prior to coronary bypass, or jugular vein identification prior to central line placement).

IV. Computed Tomography and Magnetic Resonance Angiography. The utility of these modalities is still under review. They offer the benefit of examining the anatomy of the vasculature and its relation to other surrounding structures. The drawback of these techniques is primarily related to the use of contrast.

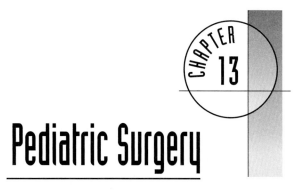
Pediatric Surgery

Kevin Day, MD
Richard Vaughan, MD
Tarun Kumar, MD

HEAD AND NECK

I. Congenital Torticollis
  A. Congenital shortening of the sternocleidomastoid muscle
  B. Clinical features
    1. Incompletely understood, but thought to arise from one of two causes:
      a. Fixed position in utero leads to shortening and tightening of one sternocleidomastoid.
        (1) Higher incidence in breech infants.
        (2) Associated with craniofacial abnormalities, such as asymmetric ears and eyes, flattening of the frontal bone, and/or flattening of the mandible.
      b. Birth trauma leads to a tear and bleeding of the muscle, with resultant scar formation and contracture.
    2. Distinguished from acquired type, which is due to a variety of causes:
      a. Atlantoaxial subluxation.
      b. Brain-stem tumors.
      c. Infectious causes.
        (1) Tonsillitis.
        (2) Retropharyngeal abscess.
        (3) Cervical adenitis.
    3. Spasmodic with gastroesophageal reflux: Sandifer syndrome.
  C. Diagnosis
    1. Purely clinical diagnosis
    2. History
      a. Fetal positioning
        (1) Breech versus vertex
        (2) Was the infant "stuck" in utero: did it seem to move much?
      b. Onset of symptoms
        (1) Congenital type presents immediately, or within weeks of delivery
        (2) Acquired type presents later
      c. Preferred head positioning of the infant
      d. Difficulty with breast-feeding
    3. Physical examination
      a. Head is tilted toward the involved side, with the chin slightly rotated away from the involved muscle.
      b. Test range of motion of the infant's neck.
    4. No imaging required
  D. Treatment
    1. Conservative treatment with physical therapy, stretching of the neck muscles, and range-of-motion exercises is the mainstay of treatment.
    2. If condition fails to resolve by 1 year of age despite aggressive physical therapy, surgical division of the involved sternocleidomastoid may be required.

II. Cystic Hygroma

A. General principles

1. This is a benign multiloculated lymphatic malformation.
2. The majority (65%) present at birth, the remainder present within the first 2 years of life.
3. Most (95%) occur in the neck or axilla, but they may occur anywhere in the body.

B. Clinical features

1. Lymphatics begin to develop from mesenchymal clefts in the sixth gestational week. When lymphatics fail to fuse with the venous system, a disorganized collection of blind-ending lymphatics forms, causing a hygroma.
2. Typically asymptomatic, but complications may occur:
   a. Airway obstruction is possible if the hygroma is large enough, and it may be life threatening.
   b. Infection may occur in 16% of hygromas and presents with redness, fever, and pain.
   c. Hemorrhage into the hygroma occurs in 15% of cases, and presents with rapidly enlarging, painful mass with evidence for blood loss.

C. Diagnosis

1. History
   a. Onset
   b. Enlarging or stable
   c. Fever
   d. Difficulty breathing
2. Physical examination
   a. Look for signs of airway obstruction: tracheal deviation, stridor, and impingement of the neck by the mass.
   b. Palpate to assess size and extent of the mass.
   c. Look for associated congenital abnormalities, because hygromas are associated with chromosomal abnormalities.
3. Diagnosis is typically clinical, with a mass noted in the neck or axilla.
   a. Diagnosis of retroperitoneal or pelvic hygromas may require computed tomography (CT) or magnetic resonance imaging (MRI) scanning.
   b. MRI is essential prior to surgical resection, to rule out adjacent neurovascular structures.

D. Treatment

1. Medical treatment with injection of sclerosing agents has been successful in treating large cystic hygromas, but is less successful in treating smaller lesions.
   a. Bleomycin should be avoided due to toxicity and the resultant scarring, making later surgical resection difficult.
   b. Pure ethanol may be used.
   c. Picibanil (OK-432), a derivative of penicillin and streptococcus pyogenes, is a trial drug that has shown success in shrinking large, unilocular lesions.
   d. Recurrent disease may respond poorly to repeat sclerosis.
2. **Surgical resection** is the mainstay of treatment.
   a. Treatment is generally for cosmetic purposes, and can proceed at the time of diagnosis, unless adjacent neurovascular structures would make risk of morbidity high for a small infant.
   b. If the mass is asymptomatic, surgery may be delayed until 2 years of age, to allow for neurovascular structures to increase in size for better visualization in surgery.
   c. Emergent resection should proceed if there is any airway impingement.
   d. Complications include chylous fistula, chylothorax, hemorrhage, and damage to surrounding neurovascular structures.

III. Brachial Cleft Remnants

A. General principles

1. A congenital anomaly of the neck due to persistence of the fetal branchial clefts. The cause is unknown, but the remnants result from incomplete obliteration of the clefts as the fetal neck develops.

2. Brachial clefts form in the fourth to eighth weeks of gestation, during embryologic segmentation.

   a. Four pairs of branchial arches form in the cervicofacial region of the embryo, with clefts expressed externally and pouches expressed internally.

   b. Branchial clefts and their adult derivatives:

      (1) Cleft I becomes the eustachian tube and a portion of the external auditory canal (EAC).

      (2) Cleft II is obliterated without a distinct adult counterpart.

      (3) Cleft III migrates inferiorly to form the inferior parathyroid glands and the thymus.

      (4) Cleft IV migrates inferiorly, but stops above the final level of cleft III, and forms the superior parathyroid glands and thyroid C-cells.

B. Clinical features

1. Although these are congenital anomalies and are thus present at birth, not all are recognized immediately.

2. Individual cleft remnants may form cysts, sinuses, fistulas, and cartilaginous remnants.

   a. Cleft I remnants occur along the angle of the mandible, and sinuses/fistulas may extend to the EAC.

   b. Cleft II remnants occur along the anterior border of the sternocleidomastoid muscle, and may communicate with the tonsillar fossa. They are the most common form.

   c. Cleft III and IV remnants communicate between the piriform sinus and the glands they form, or the neck lower than second-cleft remnants. They are rare.

3. A very small number may harbor malignancy.

C. Diagnosis

1. Diagnosis is purely clinical typically.

2. Sinuses, fistulas, and cartilaginous remnants tend to present early, whereas cysts present later as fluid slowly accumulates.

D. Treatment

1. Complete surgical excision is the only effective treatment.

2. Tract should be free of infection at time of surgery, and if not, antibiotics should be given and surgery postponed.

IV. Thyroglossal Duct Cysts

A. General principles

1. A remnant of the thyroglossal duct; the path of downward migration of the thyroid gland from the base of the tongue to its adult location.

2. Found mainly in the midline and may contain nests of thyroid tissue.

B. Clinical features

1. Cysts develop when the thyroglossal duct fails to obliterate following migration of the thyroid gland from the foramen cecum on the base of the tongue to the neck.

2. Cysts may occur anywhere along the path of the thyroglossal duct.

3. Ectopic thyroid tissue along the duct may develop into papillary adenocarcinoma.

4. The duct passes through the central portion of the hyoid bone in its descent.

5. In rare cases, may contain the patient's only functional thyroid tissue.

C. Diagnosis

1. Typical clinical diagnosis by palpation of a mass in the midline between the submental region and the superior aspect of the trachea.

2. The mass may present as a midline abscess in the neck if there is communication with the base of the tongue, with resultant contamination by oral flora.
3. Noninfected cysts are soft, smooth, and nontender.
4. Cysts may move with swallowing, or protrusion of the tongue.
D. Treatment
1. To prevent recurrence or the possibility of ectopic thyroid carcinoma (less than 1%), the entire thyroglossal duct tract should be excised.
   a. Excision should include the cyst, its tract, and the entire central portion of the hyoid bone.
   b. Dissection is carried up to the foramen cecum at the base of the tongue.
2. If thyroid tissue is present in the resected specimen, thyroid function tests should be performed to rule out postresection hypothyroidism.

CHEST

I. Chest Wall Deformity

A. General principles
1. Represents deformity in development of the supportive architecture of the chest
2. Functional impairment
   a. Rarely affects cardiopulmonary function
   b. Frequently causes psychosocial impairment due to being "different," especially during puberty
B. Clinical features
1. Ribs are formed by segmental somites that advance ventrally toward the sternum. The sternum develops from two mesodermal bands that eventually fuse in the center. The costal cartilages link the developing ribs to the sternum.
2. A wide variety of deformities exist, most of them rare. They include pectus excavatum, pectus carinatum, and sternal cleft.
   a. Pectus excavatum
      (1) The most common chest wall deformity, this condition is present in 1 of 300 to 400 live births.
      (2) The deformity is due to abnormal growth regulation of the costal cartilages.
      (3) If deformity is severe, with compression of the heart, an echocardiogram should be obtained. CT or plain radiographs may help delineate the defect.
      (4) Surgical correction is typically for cosmetic purposes primarily.
   b. Pectus carinatum
      (1) From the Latin "pectus" for chest and "carina" for keel.
      (2) This deformity is characterized by a protrusive appearance with outward displacement of the sternum, which tends to become more pronounced in adolescence.
      (3) Surgical correction is purely cosmetic.
   c. Sternal cleft
      (1) This deformity occurs when the sternal bars of mesoderm fail to completely fuse during development. It may be associated with exstrophy of the heart.
      (2) Part of the pentalogy of Cantrell: sternal cleft, omphalocele, diaphragmatic defect, pericardial defect, and intracardiac defect.
      (3) Surgical correction
         (a) Reapproximation of the cleft in the midline is curative.
         (b) If incomplete, the cleft must be divided completely to allow proper healing.

II. Pulmonary Sequestration

A. General principles
1. This abnormal lung tissue develops without normal communication with the trachea, or a bronchus with an aberrant blood supply.

2. Arterial blood supply is systemic, from the aorta, and venous drainage is either pulmonary or systemic.

3. Pathogenesis is not completely understood, but is thought to arise as a result of an accessory lung bud separate from the main lung, arising from the primitive foregut, with angiogenesis occurring from the aorta instead of the pulmonary circulation.

B. Intralobar and extralobar sequestrations

  1. Intralobar sequestrations are always within the chest, and are invested by visceral pleura.

    a. They tend to be located in the medial, posterior segments of the lower lobes.

    b. Majority are fed by vessels arising from the infradiaphragmatic aorta, and running through the inferior pulmonary ligament.

  2. Extralobar sequestrations are not invested by pulmonary pleura, and may occur within the chest, the diaphragm, or the retroperitoneum.

    a. 4:1 male-to-female predominance.

    b. Often associated with other congenital anomalies, and discovered incidentally during workup.

    c. Rarely may have communication with the foregut.

    d. Almost uniformly left-sided.

C. Clinical features, diagnosis, and treatment

  1. Intralobar sequestrations

    a. Clinical features. Although no distinct bronchus is present, there are usually microcommunications with the airways that can lead to infection of the sequestrum.

    b. Diagnosis

      (1) Typical history is that of recurrent pneumonias beginning early in childhood.

      (2) Diagnostic "gold standard" is arteriography, but contrast CT or MRI have largely replaced this.

      (3) Chest x-ray may reveal an inferiorly located consolidation.

      (4) Frequently, aeration shows on imaging studies.

      (5) Advanced imaging study is essential to delineate blood supply prior to resection.

    c. Treatment

      (1) Treatment is surgical resection of the sequestrum in symptomatic patients.

      (2) Frequently, complete lobectomy is necessary due to inability to distinguish sequestration from surrounding pulmonary lobe.

  2. Extralobar sequestrations

    a. Clinical features: aeration is rare, unless there is communication with the foregut.

    b. Diagnosis: typically, diagnosis occurs by CT obtained to evaluate another congenital anomaly.

    c. Treatment

      (1) Typical treatment is observation.

      (2) Surgical resection is indicated if there is communication with the foregut with resultant infection, or if there is extrinsic compression of the gastrointestinal (GI) tract.

III. Esophageal Atresia/Tracheoesophageal Fistula

A. General principles

  1. Esophageal atresia: congenital disruption of esophageal development, resulting in blind-ending esophagus with obstruction.

  2. Tracheoesophageal (TE) fistula: abnormal fistulous tract between the trachea and esophagus, that usually occurs in conjunction with esophageal atresia.

  3. Five anatomic variants of esophageal atresia/TE fistula (Fig. 13-1):

    a. Type 1: blind-ending proximal and distal pouches without TE fistula (6%).

    b. Type 2: proximal TE fistula with distal blind pouch (2%).

FIGURE
13-1 Variants of tracheoesophageal fistula. **A.** Atresia without fistula (5–7% of cases). **B.** Proximal fistula and distal pouch (<1% occurrence). **C.** Proximal pouch with distal fistula (85–90% of cases). **D.** Atresia with proximal and distal fistulas (<1% of cases). **E.** Fistula without atresia (H-type) (2–6% occurrence).

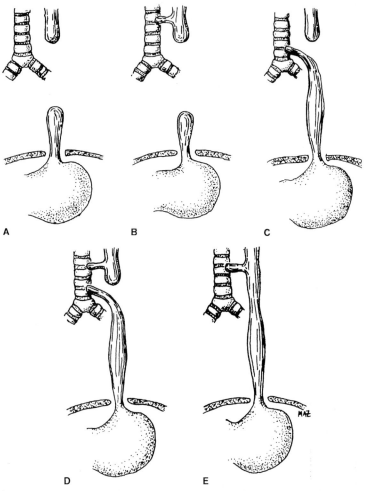

A   B   C

D   E

(Reprinted, with permission, from *The Washington Manual of Surgery*, 3rd ed. Baltimore: Lippincott Williams & Wilkins; YEAR?:642.)

    c. Type 3: proximal blind pouch with distal TE fistula (85%).

    d. Type 4: proximal and distal pouches with TE fistula (1%).

    e. Type 5: pure TE fistula without esophageal atresia H-type fistula (2%).

  4. Frequently occurs with a constellation of other abnormalities known as the **VACTERL** syndrome:

    a. V = vertebral anomalies.

       A = anorectal malformation.

       C = cardiac abnormalities.

       TE = tracheoesophageal fistula.

       R = renal anomalies.

       L = limb deformity.

    b. One, several, or all anomalous features may be present.

 B. Pathogenesis

  1. The trachea and esophagus are derived from a common embryologic tube, the laryngotracheal tube, which forms during the fourth week of gestation.

  2. The lateral walls of the tube invaginate to form the tracheoesophageal septum, which eventually divides the trachea from the esophagus.

  3. Incomplete division of the esophagus and trachea results in esophageal atresia and TE fistula.

C. Diagnosis
 1. Majority are diagnosed at birth by excessive oral secretions and inability to pass a nasogastric tube.
 2. Once diagnosed, patients should also undergo diagnostics to rule out VACTERL syndrome.
   a. Imaging of the chest and spine.
   b. Echocardiogram.
   c. Renal ultrasonography.
   d. Examination of anus and limbs.
   e. Genetic workup.
D. Treatment
 1. Treatment is surgical division of the TE fistula, with anastomosis of the esophageal pouches.
 2. Surgery may be accomplished as a single procedure for short-gap atresia.
 3. Long-gap atresia may require a staged procedure.
   a. Multiple operations have been described.
     (1) Stretching of upper and lower pouches by serial bougienage.
     (2) Fistulization along a surgically placed rod, or suture connecting the pouches.
     (3) Circular esophagomyotomy with primary anastomosis.
     (4) Cervical spit fistula of proximal pouch, with sequential lengthening down the neck.
   b. All staged procedures require a gastrostomy for feeding until anastomosis can be performed.

IV. Congenital Diaphragmatic Hernia
A. General principles
 1. Congenital diaphragmatic hernia (CDH) is a congenital defect in the development of the diaphragm that allows peritoneal contents into the chest, leading to pulmonary hypoplasia.
 2. Left-sided defects are much more common due to earlier closure of the right pleuroperitoneal membrane, and the protective mass effect of the liver under the right side.
 3. CDH carries a mortality rate of 30% to 40%.
 4. Two distinct types
   a. Bochdalek: most common type, located in the posterolateral position.
   b. Morgagni: rare, located anteromedially behind the sternum.
B. Pathogenesis
 1. The primordial diaphragm is formed by the pleuroperitoneal membranes, over which the lateral body wall musculature grows inward to create the muscular diaphragm.
 2. Failure of the pleuroperitoneal membranes to close leads to CDH.
C. Clinical features
 1. Presenting symptoms include marked respiratory distress and cyanosis at birth.
 2. Mild cases may be asymptomatic, or present with mild chronic respiratory disease, pneumonia, feeding difficulty, or bowel obstruction.
D. Diagnosis
 1. Presenting symptoms are diagnostic.
 2. CDH is typically diagnosed by prenatal ultrasound.
   a. Polyhydramnios (80%).
   b. Seen as abdominal contents in the thoracic cavity.
 3. A chest x-ray usually confirms the diagnosis.
E. Treatment
 1. In-utero surgery (fetal surgery) is being performed in select centers.
 2. CDH requires treatment in an advanced neonatal intensive care unit.
 3. Pulmonary support in the immediate postnatal period is critical.

    a. Extracorporeal membrane oxygenation

    b. High oscillation ventilation

    c. Partial liquid ventilation

    d. Inhaled nitric oxide and exogenous surfactant

4. Reduction of the abdominal contents to the peritoneal cavity with repair of the defect is the mainstay of treatment.

5. Pulmonary hypoplasia may be so extensive as to preclude cure, and thus survival has not improved significantly despite advanced techniques for cure.

ABDOMINAL WALL

I. Gastroschisis

  A. General principles

    1. Gastroschisis, or "split stomach," is a misnomer for a condition that is actually a division of the anterior abdominal wall musculature.

    2. Infants are born with their intestine protruding through the abdominal wall defect into the amniotic cavity (Fig. 13-2).

    3. Gastroschisis is more common in males.

    4. The risk of associated congenital or genetic anomalies is low.

  B. Etiology. No uniform cause known, but environmental and drug exposures are thought to play a role.

    1. The condition becomes much more frequent when the mother is under 20 years of age.

    2. Use of cigarettes, alcohol, and recreational drugs increases risk.

    3. Use of aspirin, ibuprofen, and pseudoephedrine increases risk.

  C. Clinical features. The intestine is typically shortened, thickened, and matted or stuck together at birth.

  D. Diagnosis and treatment

    1. Diagnosis

      a. Gastroschisis is easily diagnosed by prenatal ultrasound.

      b. If it is discovered prenatally, the patient should be referred for delivery at a facility with neonatal intensive care, pediatric surgery, and high-risk obstetrics coverage.

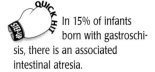 Gastroschisis occurs almost exclusively to the right side of the umbilicus, which is always spared.

 In 15% of infants born with gastroschisis, there is an associated intestinal atresia.

FIGURE 13-2 Gastroschisis. The defect is to the right of the normal umbilicus, and the bowel is thickened and inflamed.

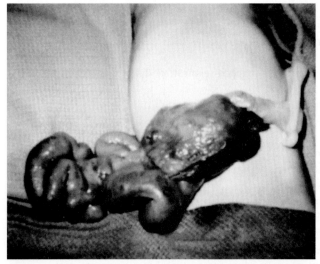

(Reprinted, with permission, from Mulholland MW, Lillemoe KD, et al. *Greenfield's Surgery: Scientific Principles and Practice,* 4th ed. Baltimore: Lippincott William & Wilkins; 2006:1878.)

2. Treatment
   a. Immediately postdelivery, the intestine should be covered in a moist, sterile dressing, a nasogastric tube should be placed to keep the intestine decompressed, intravenous access should be obtained, and broad-spectrum antibiotics should be initiated.
   b. Reduction of the abdominal contents into the peritoneal cavity, and surgical closure of the abdominal defect is curative.
   c. If adequate reduction of the intestine is not possible, placement of a silo bag, with sequential tightening, can be used until intestines are reduced back and abdominal wall closure can be performed without much tension.
   d. Patients will almost uniformly have a prolonged postoperative ileus.
      (1) Patients should be maintained on total parenteral nutrition (TPN) until bowel function is initiated.
      (2) Liver function should be monitored closely while on TPN, because cirrhosis, portal hypertension, and liver failure can occur.

II. Omphalocele

A. General principles
   1. Abdominal wall defect in which viscera extrude through the umbilicus and are encased in a peritoneal and amniotic sac (Fig. 13-3).
   2. High association with genetic and congenital abnormalities.
      a. Associated with trisomy 13, 18, and 21.
      b. Cardiac, musculoskeletal, and gastrointestinal anomalies are common.
      c. Beckwith–Wiedemann syndrome: *E*xomphalos (omphalocele), *M*acroglossia, *G*igantism, and hyperinsulinemia hypoglycemia.
   3. There are 1 in 5,000 live births with omphalocele and herniation of intestine, and 1 in 10,000 live births with omphalocele and herniation of intestine and solid organs.

FIGURE

13-3 **Omphalocele. The herniated intestines and liver are visible inside the sac. The umbilical cord attaches to the sac.**

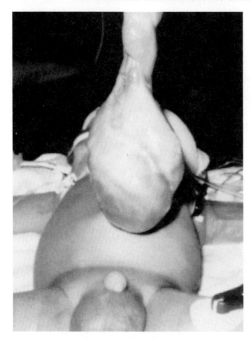

(Reprinted, with permission, from Mulholland MW, Lillemoe KD, et al. *Greenfield's Surgery: Scientific Principles and Practice*, 4th ed. Baltimore: Lippincott William & Wilkins; 2006:1878.)

QUICK HIT

The inner lining of the omphalocele sac is peritoneum, while the outer covering is epithelium of the umbilical cord, derived from the amniotic sac.

B. Pathogenesis
   1. Between the sixth and tenth weeks of normal gestation, the abdominal contents herniate into the umbilicus, and undergo a series of coordinated rotations before returning to the peritoneal cavity, after which the abdominal wall closes.
   2. Omphalocele occurs when the intestine fails to return to the abdominal cavity.
C. Diagnosis and treatment
   1. Typically diagnosed by prenatal ultrasound.
   2. Pre- and postnatal care is essentially the same for omphalocele as for gastroschisis.
   3. Workup for associated anomalies should be undertaken.

III. Exstrophy of the Bladder
A. General principles
   1. Defect in the infraumbilical abdominal wall with failure of the median inferior portion to close, resulting in exposure and protrusion of the posterior wall of the urinary bladder through the defect.
   2. In males, almost uniformly associated with epispadias.
   3. In females, almost uniformly associated with bifid clitoris.
   4. Occurs 1 in every 10,000 to 40,000 live births.
B. Pathogenesis
   1. During the fourth week of gestation, mesenchymal cells migrate into the space between the cloaca and ectoderm of the primitive abdomen.
   2. Failure of this migration leads to no development of abdominal musculature in this position.
   3. Eventually the thin epidermis and anterior wall of the bladder rupture, allowing wide exposure of the mucous membrane of the bladder.
C. Diagnosis and treatment
   1. Diagnosis is clinical by inspection.
   2. Surgical correction consists of closure of the bladder plate, and concurrent repair of epispadias in boys. Surgical repair should proceed within 72 hours of birth with favorable outcomes.

IV. Umbilical Hernia
A. General principles
   1. A defect in the connective tissue around the umbilicus present at birth.
   2. The most common abdominal wall defect in the newborn.
   3. Tends to occur more commonly in African-American infants than in Caucasian infants.
B. Pathogenesis
   1. Failure of complete closure of the linea alba at the umbilicus.
   2. The umbilicus is reinforced by the paired umbilical ligaments (umbilical artery remnants), the round ligament (umbilical vein remnant), the urachus (remnant of the primitive allantois), and the transversalis fascia.
   3. Weakness or failure of any of the reinforcing structures can predispose to umbilical hernia.
C. Diagnosis and treatment
   1. Diagnosis is clinical by inspection and palpation.
   2. In most cases of congenital umbilical hernia, the defect will close spontaneously during the first 3 years of life.
   3. If the hernia persists at 5 years of age, surgical closure is indicated.

V. Congenital Inguinal Hernia/Hydrocele
A. General principles
   1. Inguinal hernia: due to failure of processus vaginalis to close, and allowing herniation of abdominal contents into the inguinal ring, and possibly the scrotum.
   2. Hydrocele: collection of fluid around the testicle within tunica vaginalis.

3. Predisposing factors include prematurity.
4. Represents the most common indication for surgery in the infant population.

B. Pathogenesis
1. The testes develop intra-abdominally and migrate along a path created by gubernaculums.
2. The testis descends into the scrotum through the processus vaginalis, a canal that protrudes through the abdominal wall into the inguinal canal.
3. After descent of the testis, the processus vaginalis closes, and is obliterated.
   a. Failure of the processus vaginalis to close, allowing herniation of intra-abdominal contents, results in a congenital inguinal hernia.
   b. Partial closure of the processus vaginalis with resultant collection of fluid, results in hydrocele.

C. Diagnosis and treatment
1. Diagnosis is clinical
   a. Typical history is of a groin bulge that enlarges with crying or straining with hernias, or a stable scrotal or groin swelling for hydrocele.
   b. Most reduce spontaneously or with gentle pressure.
   c. Hydrocele will transilluminate on examination.
2. Treatment
   a. Surgical treatment is indicated at the time of diagnosis for inguinal hernias and communicating hydrocele, which have a tendency to develop into true hernias.
   b. Noncommunicating hydrocele may be observed as they tend to resolve spontaneously during first 2 years of life.

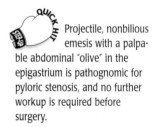

Hydrocele may be **communicating,** in which a small opening in the proximal processus vaginalis remains open, that allows fluid passage but not herniation; or **noncommunicating,** in which proximal closure of the processus vaginalis occurs with distal fluid collection.

ABDOMEN

I. Hypertrophic Pyloric Stenosis
A. General principles
1. Obstruction of the gastric outlet due to hypertrophy of the pyloric muscle
2. Results in narrowing of the pyloric lumen
3. Occurs in 1 in 150 live births of males and 1 in 750 live births of females

B. Pathogenesis
1. This is incompletely understood, but is now thought to result from a deficiency of nitric oxide synthase in the pylorus, resulting in inability of pyloric muscle to relax, resulting in muscular hypertrophy.
2. Maximum narrowing occurs between the fourth and eighth weeks postpartum.

C. Diagnosis
1. Classic history is of projectile, nonbilious emesis beginning in the second to fourth weeks of life.
2. The diagnostic procedure of choice is pyloric ultrasonography that shows a thickened pyloric muscle (4 mm or more) and pyloric channel length (17 mm or more).
3. Contrast upper GI series can be helpful in cases in which physical examination and ultrasonography is not clear.

Projectile, nonbilious emesis with a palpable abdominal "olive" in the epigastrium is pathognomic for pyloric stenosis, and no further workup is required before surgery.

D. Treatment
1. Treatment is surgical pyloromyotomy (Ramstedt) in which the layers, except mucosa, are divided along the entire hypertrophied segment.
2. Preoperatively, IV hydration and correction of serum electrolytes are advised.

II. Duodenal Atresia/Stenosis/Web
A. General principles
1. Obliteration of a segment of duodenum during development that results in a stricture or blind-ending obstruction (atresia)

2. Narrowing of duodenal lumen secondary to annular pancreas (stenosis)
3. Diaphragm, with or without hole, blocking the duodenal lumen (web)
4. Categorized into three types:
   a. Type 1 (92%): intraluminal web or diaphragm with intact mesentery, and intact seromuscular layers in the involved intestinal segment.
   b. Type 2 (1%): fibromuscular cord replaces intestinal segment on an intact mesentery.
   c. Type 3 (7%): complete atretic segment with mesenteric gap, and proximal/distal blind-ending intestinal pouches.
5. Incidence: 1 in 6,000 to 10,000.

B. Pathogenesis
   1. Failure of recanalization
   2. Atresia occurs with vascular disruptions during development
   3. Annular pancreas

C. Clinical presentation
   1. Epigastric fullness
   2. Bilious emesis

D. Diagnosis
   1. Maternal history: polyhydramnios
   2. Birth history: prematurity
   3. Clinical signs: epigastric fullness, bilious emesis
   4. "Double-bubble" sign on x-ray of abdomen (Fig. 13-4)

E. Treatment
   1. IV fluids, antibiotics, and nasogastric or orogastric tube
   2. Surgery
      a. Duodenoduodenostomy
      b. Duodenojejunostomy

III. Intestinal Atresia/Stenosis

A. General principles
   1. Obliteration of a segment of intestine during development that results in a stricture or blind-ending obstruction of the intestine.
   2. Categorized into four types:

FIGURE 13-4 Classic radiographic appearance of duodenal atresia. There is a double bubble of gas in the stomach and proximal duodenum, with no gas in the distal intestinal tract.

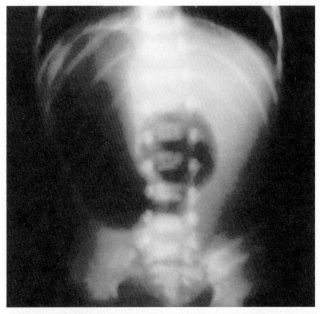

(Reprinted, with permission, from Mulholland MW, Lillemoe KD, et al. *Greenfield's Surgery: Scientific Principles and Practice*, 4th ed. Baltimore: Lippincott William & Wilkins; 2006:1889.)

   a. Type 1: intraluminal web or diaphragm with intact mesentery, and intact seromuscular layers in the involved intestinal segment
   b. Type 2: fibromuscular cord replaces intestinal segment on an intact mesentery
   c. Type 3: two subtypes
      (1) Type 3a: complete atretic segment with mesenteric gap, and proximal/distal blind-ending intestinal pouches.
      (2) Type 3b: complete atretic segment with mesenteric gap, with distal pouch corkscrewed around a single mesenteric vessel.
   d. Type 4: multiple atretic segments in succession with mesenteric gaps (Color Fig. 13-5)
   3. Occurs in about 1 in 500 to 1,500 live births
   4. Occurs in about 15% of cases of gastroschisis
B. Pathogenesis
   1. Fetal intestine develops from the midgut, and undergoes a sequence of elongation, herniation from the coelomic cavity, rotation, return to the coelomic cavity, and fixation to the posterior abdominal wall.
   2. Blood supply is derived from the superior mesenteric artery that arises off of the dorsal aorta during development.
   3. Atresia occur with vascular disruptions during development.
   4. The greater the vascular insult, the more severe the atresia.
C. Clinical features
   1. Bilious emesis
   2. Abdominal distension
   3. Failure to pass meconium
D. Diagnosis
   1. Maternal history: polyhydramnios
   2. Birth history: prematurity
   3. Signs and symptoms: bilious emesis, abdominal distension, failure to pass meconium
   4. Plain abdominal films: dilated proximal intestine and a decompressed distal intestine/colon
   5. Barium enema: microcolon
E. Treatment
   1. Nasogastric suction should be initiated upon diagnosis of atresia.
   2. Correction of any fluid or electrolyte imbalances should be undertaken before surgery.
   3. Surgery may be performed semi-electively after stabilization.
      a. Tapering jejunoplasty
      b. End-to-end anastomosis

IV. Necrotizing Enterocolitis
A. General principles
   1. Necrotizing enterocolitis (NEC) is an intestinal ischemic injury that begins in the mucosa, but may progress to full-thickness necrosis of segments of small bowel and/or colon.
   2. NEC occurs most commonly in premature infants.
   3. The incidence of NEC is increasing, because neonatal intensive care advances allowing younger gestational age infants to survive past delivery.
B. Etiology
   1. The exact cause of NEC is unknown.
   2. The cause is most likely multifactorial. NEC is associated with the initiation of enteral feeding.
      a. It is linked with low blood flow states/hypoxia in the intestine.
         (1) Cardiac defects with shunting
         (2) Respiratory failure
         (3) Hypotension

FIGURE
13-5 Classification of intestinal atresia. Type I, muscular continuity with a complete web. Type II, mesentery intact, fibrous cord. Type IIIa, muscular and mesenteric discontinuous. Type IIIb, apple-peel deformity. Type IV, multiple atresias.

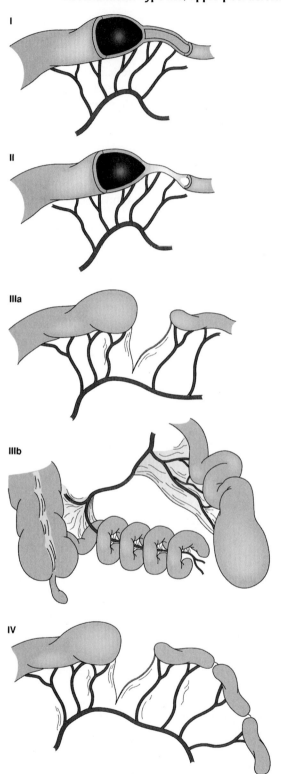

I

II

IIIa

IIIb

IV

(After Grosfeld JL. Jejunoileal atresia and stenosis. In: O'Neill JA Jr., Rowe MI, Grosfeld JL, et al., eds. *Pediatric Surgery*, 5th ed. St. Louis: Mosby; 1998:1145–1158. With permission.)

b. Infectious etiology
(1) Tends to occur in clusters
(2) Association with *Clostridium, Pseudomonas, Klebsiella, Enterobacter,* and *Staphylococcus* species
c. Immunologic factors
(1) Host inflammatory response and free radical damage play a role
(2) May help to propagate and worsen an existing case of NEC

C. Diagnosis
1. Diagnosis and degree of disease is made clinically based on several types of findings
2. Useful findings:
a. Clinical symptoms include abdominal distention, bloody stools, bilious emesis, and intolerance of feedings.
b. Physical examination findings include abdominal distention with tenderness, decreased bowel sounds, blood per rectum, and/or abdominal wall erythema.
c. Laboratory values may show thrombocytopenia, neutropenia, elevated prothrombin time/partial thromboplastin time, metabolic acidosis, and/or hyponatremia.
d. Imaging may reveal diffuse bowel distention/ileus, pneumatosis intestinalis, fixed loops on serial x-rays, and portal venous air/free air.

D. Treatment
1. Most cases of NEC can be managed medically.
a. Nasogastric decompression and bowel rest with TPN.
b. Broad-spectrum intravenous antibiotics.
c. Close monitoring and correction of fluid and electrolyte abnormalities.
d. Proper ventilation and avoidance of hypoxemia.
2. Surgery is indicated in any case of bowel perforation/necrosis with pneumoperitoneum.
a. Abdominal compartment syndrome becoming worse in spite of maximum medical efforts.
b. Goal of surgery is to resect necrotic segments, while maintaining as much viable bowel as possible to avoid short bowel syndrome.
(1) Standard of care is to create an ostomy, rather than to perform primary anastomosis, as the disease process may still progress postoperatively.
(2) Multiple resections and multiple enterostomies may be necessary.
(3) To help preserve intestinal length, marginal areas may be left and re-evaluated at a second-look procedure.

V. Meconium Ileus

A. General principles
1. This is an obstructive condition of the distal ileum in newborn infants with cystic fibrosis, due to thicker-than-normal, inspissated meconium.
2. The presenting symptom in 10% to 20% of patients with cystic fibrosis.
B. Clinical features
1. Cystic fibrosis is a disorder of chloride channels, caused by a single base deletion in the cystic fibrosis transmembrane conductance regulator (CFTR) gene.
2. GI and pulmonary secretions are abnormally thick, due to diminished volume of secretions and increased reabsorption of sodium chloride via normal sodium-potassium pump function, leading to further dehydration of the secretions.
3. Patients typically present with failure to pass meconium, abdominal distention, and bilious vomiting.
4. Death typically occurs by age 30 due to progressive pulmonary disease.
C. Diagnosis
1. Presence of cystic fibrosis, with a family history of the disease

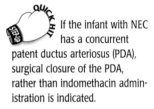

QUICK HIT During the acute inflammatory phase of NEC, contrast studies can worsen the condition and are contraindicated. If the diagnosis is in question, serial abdominal radiographs should be obtained.

QUICK HIT If the infant with NEC has a concurrent patent ductus arteriosus (PDA), surgical closure of the PDA, rather than indomethacin administration is indicated.

QUICK HIT

A classic finding on abdominal x-ray is Neuhauser or "soap bubble" sign, in which there is a ground-glass appearance meconium mixed with air in the right lower quadrant.

QUICK HIT

From 60% to 70% of meconium ileus cases resolve with conservative management.

QUICK HIT

The dense attachments between the body wall and cecum in incomplete rotation are known as Ladd bands; they pass anterior to the small intestine, and may serve as a point of obstruction.

2. Abdominal x-ray: dilated loops of small bowel
3. Contrast enema: a small diameter to the colon

D. Treatment
   1. Treatment of meconium ileus is conservative initially
      a. Saline enemas/irrigation
      b. Gastrografin enemas
      c. Dilute N-acetylcysteine enemas
   2. In refractory cases, surgery may be required
      a. Laparotomy, with enterotomy and manual removal meconium.
         (1) Simple enterotomy with primary closure is the procedure of choice.
         (2) If any nonviable or marginal bowel noted, segmental resection with primary anastomosis may be required.
      b. Temporary surgical enterostomy with continued irrigation may be necessary.
      c. T-tube placement into terminal ileum for continued irrigation may also be used.
   3. Complicated cases may involve segmental volvulus, ischemia, stenosis/ atresia, or perforation, and require segmental resection and anastomosis.
   4. Postoperatively, the continued irrigation of the bowel with dilute N-acetylcysteine via nasogastric tube, or enema to keep meconium and stool soluble for easier passage, may be required.

VI. Malrotation

A. General principles
   1. This abnormal anatomic position of the bowel is due to aberrant or absent embryologic rotation of the gut between the fifth and tenth weeks of gestation.
   2. The result is a malpositioned, shortened intestine with abnormal attachments to the peritoneal wall.
   3. Three main types of malrotation:
      a. Nonrotation: very shortened small intestine on the right, duodenum does not cross midline, cecum at midline, and colon on left.
      b. Incomplete rotation: small intestine mostly on the right, colon on the left with cecum in the left upper quadrant, densely affixed to the right posterior body wall.
      c. Mesocolic hernia: incomplete rotation, resulting in essentially normal length of bowel, but with nonfixation of the right or left colon, allowing for potential space for internal herniation of bowel to occur.

B. Pathogenesis
   1. Normal midgut rotation occurs along the axis of the superior mesenteric artery (SMA) with a 270-degree counterclockwise rotation resulting in an anteriorly located colon and posteriorly located small intestine.
   2. Rotation occurs during physiology herniation outside of the coelomic cavity between weeks 5 and 10 of normal gestation, and is associated with a significant lengthening of the jejunoileal segment during this time.
   3. The failure or cessation of rotation and fixation due to unknown causes is the source of malrotation.

C. Clinical features: patients typically present by 1 month of age with bilious emesis, due to duodenal obstruction due to Ladd bands, or midgut volvulus due to nonfixation.

D. Diagnosis
   1. Many patients remain asymptomatic, and may be discovered incidentally due to studies performed for other reasons.
   2. The diagnostic study of choice is upper GI series with small bowel follow-through.
      a. If the duodenum does not cross the midline, malrotation is the diagnosis.
      b. The appearance will be of a mostly right-sided small bowel and mostly left-sided colon in malrotation.

E. Treatment
1. Because of the risk for midgut volvulus with complete occlusion of the SMA and full loss of the bowel it supplies, the treatment of choice is emergent laparotomy and repair even in asymptomatic patients.
2. Surgical repair, known as Ladd procedure, includes:
   a. Detorsion of the midgut
   b. Division of Ladd bands
   c. Placement of the cecum in the left upper quadrant, and placement of the small intestine in the right upper quadrant
   d. Passage of a catheter through the duodenum to rule out associated duodenal obstruction
   e. Widening of the mesentery
   f. Appendectomy to prevent future misdiagnosis

VII. Hirschsprung Disease (Congenital Aganglionic Megacolon)

A. General principles
1. A functional, rather than mechanical, obstruction of the colon due to failure of ganglion development in a segment of the colon
2. Results in failure of colonic peristalsis and obstruction

B. Pathogenesis
1. During the fifth to seventh gestational weeks, neural crest cells migrate (craniocaudal migration) into the wall of the colon, forming the Auerbach myenteric plexus and Meissner submucosal plexus.
2. Failure of the migration of neural crest cells into the colon wall, or subsequent failure of microenvironmental support and development of neural crest cells that have migrated into the colonic wall, leads to Hirschsprung disease.
3. Exact cause is unknown, but several genes, including the *RET* proto-oncogene, endothelin 3 gene, and endothelin B receptor gene, have been implicated.
4. Varying degrees of aganglionosis occur, but always occur in distal to proximal fashion.

C. Clinical features
1. Patients may present with bilious emesis, abdominal distention, and a history of infrequent bowel movements/constipation.
2. In neonates, a delayed passage of meconium (greater than 24 hours) may occur.

D. Diagnosis. A diagnostic pathway includes:
1. Anorectal examination to rule out anorectal anomaly.
2. Abdominal x-ray to rule out other sources of obstruction.
3. Barium enema to identify the transition zone.
4. Anorectal manometry.
5. Suction-assisted rectal biopsy with absence of ganglion cells confirms the diagnosis.
6. Full-thickness rectal biopsy.

E. Treatment
1. Surgical correction is curative
2. Typically requires temporary colostomy proximal to the transition zone
3. Definitive procedure is performed at age 6 to 12 months
4. Definitive procedures:
   a. Duhame–Martin procedure: resection of aganglionic segment, with colorectal anastomosis of normal colon posteriorly to aganglionic remnant of rectum anteriorly (retrorectal colonic pull-through)
   b. Soave procedure: division of the colon at the transition point with transanal mucosal proctectomy, and transrectal pull-through (endorectal pull-through) excision of aganglionic segment, with colorectal anastomosis
   c. Laparoscopic-assisted pull-through

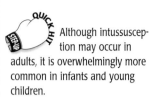

Although intussusception may occur in adults, it is overwhelmingly more common in infants and young children.

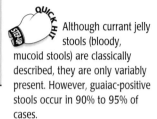

Although currant jelly stools (bloody, mucoid stools) are classically described, they are only variably present. However, guaiac-positive stools occur in 90% to 95% of cases.

VIII. Intussusception

A. General principles
   1. Invagination or "telescoping" of a segment of bowel into itself, resulting in mechanical obstruction
   2. May occur in any segment of intestine, but ileocolic is the most common
B. Etiology
   1. The exact cause is unknown, but thought to occur due to a "lead point" at which the intussusceptum initiates and peristalsis propagates.
   2. Lead points may be lymphoid hyperplasia due to viral infections, Meckel diverticulum, polyps, lymphoma, or other space-filling lesions in the intestine.
C. Clinical features
   1. Typical presentation of a young child with severe colicky abdominal pain, alternating with periods free of pain.
   2. Other symptoms and signs include bilious vomiting, abdominal distention with a sausage-shaped right lower quadrant mass, and "currant jelly stools" on rectal examination.
D. Diagnosis
   1. The presence of clinical features is diagnostic
   2. The diagnostic procedure of choice is contrast enema, which is also therapeutic in roughly 60% of cases
E. Treatment
   1. Hydrostatic reduction with contrast enema is the initial therapeutic procedure.
   2. If hydrostatic reduction fails, pneumatic reduction with air-contrast enema may be attempted.
      a. Pressures are 80 mm Hg for infants, and 120 mm Hg for young children.
      b. This is successful in 90% of patients.
   3. Surgery is indicated for peritonitis/shock or with failure of nonoperative means.
      a. Manual reduction on exploratory laparotomy (open or laparoscopic) is usually sufficient in uncomplicated cases.
      b. Resection may be required if bowel necrosis or a worrisome lead point is observed.
      c. Most surgeons perform an appendectomy to prevent future misdiagnosis.
   4. Patients should be kept in the hospital postreduction. Approximately 12% of intussusceptions recur.
   5. Recurrent intussusceptions in older children warrant exploratory surgery to rule out tumors as a causative lead point.

IX. Imperforate Anus

A. General principles
   1. Failure of the anorectal orifice to develop, which can result in communications between the rectum and urogenital systems anywhere in the pelvis.
   2. Classified as low or high types.
      a. Low: located distal to the puborectalis muscle.
         (1) Does not require colostomy.
         (2) Frequently presents with perineal meconium fistula.
      b. High: located above the puborectalis muscle.
         (1) Requires colostomy.
         (2) Typically with fistulization to urethra, bladder, or vagina.
B. Etiology
   1. Imperforate anus occurs due to abnormal development of the urorectal septum, which results in incomplete division of the fetal cloaca into urogenital and anorectal portions
   2. Associated anomalies
      a. VACTERL syndrome
      b. Urogenital abnormalities (in up to 50%), such as vesicoureteric reflux, solitary kidney, pelviureteric junction obstruction, megaureter, and undescended testis, as well as urinary incontinence

    c. Skeletal abnormalities (in up to 30–40%), such as spinal and vertebral anomalies

    d. Cardiovascular abnormalities (in up to 30%), such as atrial septal defect (ASD), ventral septal defect (VSD), and PDA

    e. Gastrointestinal abnormalities (in up to 10–15%), such as TE fistula and duodenal obstruction

C. Diagnosis

  1. Diagnosis is by physical examination, with close attention paid for possible fistula

  2. Plain x-ray of the pelvis 24 hours after birth (to allow distal passage of swallowed air), with the infant held head down, helps reveal the level of involvement

D. Treatment

  1. Low type: primary repair with perineal approach and pull-through

  2. High type:

    a. Colostomy in infancy, followed by posterior sagittal anorectoplasty at age 4 to 8 months

    b. Laparoscopic-assisted anorectoplasty

X. Biliary Atresia

A. General principles

  1. Obliteration of the biliary tract in infants, resulting in neonatal cholestasis and jaundice

  2. Classified into two types:

    a. Intrahepatic: also known as biliary hypoplasia, a rare condition consisting of a patent but narrow-caliber biliary system.

    b. Extrahepatic: more common form that involves obliteration of the extra-hepatic bile ducts and gallbladder.

      (1) Type I: obliteration of the common bile duct.

      (2) Type II: obliteration of the proper hepatic duct with cystic dilation of the porta hepatic.

      (3) Type III: atresia of the left and right hepatic ducts, extending up to the level of the porta hepatic (most common type).

  3. Untreated, this will progress to cirrhosis and hepatic failure.

B. Etiology

  1. Etiology is unknown, but biliary atresia is thought to occur as a result of inflammatory process in the biliary ductal system after birth.

  2. There is no clear causative factor, but viral infection or toxin exposure in the ductal system may play a role.

  3. The condition is extremely rare in premature or stillborn infants, suggesting a postgestational cause.

C. Clinical features: neonatal jaundice lasting greater than 2 to 4 weeks, icteric urine, and acholic, clay-colored stools.

D. Diagnosis

  1. Clinical symptomatology is suggestive

  2. Elevated direct bilirubin is suggestive

  3. α1-Antitrypsin with Pi typing, to rule out deficiency of this enzyme, and sweat chloride test to rule out cystic fibrosis as sources for cholestasis

  4. Definitive studies

    a. Hepato-iminodiacetic acid (HIDA) scan showing rapid liver uptake with no excretion of radiotracer into bowel.

    b. Liver ultrasound, showing increased liver echogenicity and biliary dilation with a small, shrunken gallbladder.

    c. Liver biopsy

      (1) Considered the most important diagnostic test.

      (2) High sensitivity in a suggestive clinical picture.

      (3) May perform intraoperative cholangiogram via gallbladder cannulation at time of surgery.

d. Endoscopic retrograde cholangiopancreatography (ERCP).
   (1) Until recently, small enough scopes did not exist.
   (2) Likely to be a more utilized diagnostic study in the future.
E. Treatment
   1. Intrahepatic form requires orthotopic liver transplant for survival.
   2. Extrahepatic form can be treated with portoenterostomy.
      a. Described by Kasai in the 1950s.
      b. Involves resection of the atretic ductal system, and anastomosis of a Roux-en-Y limb to the porta hepatic.
         (1) Level of resection determined by frozen section to assess duct diameter adequacy.
         (2) Cholangitis is a frequent postoperative complication.
      c. From 25% to 35% of patients have a 10-year survival without liver transplant, and the remaining two-thirds require transplant.

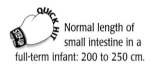

QUICK HIT

Normal length of small intestine in a full-term infant: 200 to 250 cm.

XI. Short Bowel Syndrome

A. General principles: short bowel syndrome (SBS) is the need for TPN for more than 42 days after bowel resection, or a residual small bowel length of less than 25% expected for gestational age.
   1. Anatomic: less than 75% of intestinal resection
   2. Functional: failure to thrive in spite of adequate length
   3. Etiology
      a. NEC: 32%
      b. Atresia: 20%
      c. Volvulus: 17%
      d. Gastroschisis: 17%
      e. Aganglionosis: 6%
      f. Other: 8%
B. Clinical features
   1. Initial period: extreme fluid and electrolyte loss (1 to 2 weeks)
      a. Dehydration secondary to diarrhea
      b. Electrolyte abnormality
      c. Weight loss
   2. Intestinal adaptation (48 hours up to 2 years)
      a. Mucosal hypertrophy: increased villi height, and increased crypt depth
      b. By removing specific portions of small bowel, such as in a jejunectomy, the ileum takes over all the absorptive function of jejunum and gastric hypersecretion, due to jejunal resection.
      c. Ileal resection
         (1) Decreased transit time
         (2) Loss of bile salts leads to cholelithiasis and malabsorption of fat, leading to vitamin deficiency (A, D, E)
         (3) Hyperoxaluria leads to nephrolithiasis
C. Treatment
   1. Medical and nutritional management
      a. TPN is required to maintain nutritional support and continued growth.
      b. Continued enteral feeding is required for the intestinal adaptation.
         (1) Volume should be increased gradually.
         (2) Enteral feeding should be increased, and TPN should be reduced relatively, as per patient tolerance.
         (3) If fluid losses increase by greater than 50% in 24 hours, do not increase enteral feeds.
         (4) Once the balanced combination of enteral and parenteral nutrition is stabilized, TPN should be changed from around the clock to cycling nighttime infusion.

c. Pharmacotherapy
    (1) Nutritional supplement
        (a) Glutamine
        (b) Medium-chain fatty acids
        (c) Pectin
        (d) Soy polysaccharide
    (2) Decrease the gastric secretion
        (a) H_2 blocker
        (b) Protein pump inhibitor
    (3) Increase the intestinal transit time
        (a) Opioid: codeine
        (b) Diphenoxylate
        (c) Loperamide
        (d) Cholestyramine
        (e) Somatostatin and octreotide (severe refractory diarrhea)

2. Surgical management: functions and options
  a. Increased transit time
    (1) Intestinal valves
    (2) Reverse segments
    (3) Recirculatory loop
    (4) Colon interposition
  b. Functional improvement
    (1) Tapering enteroplasty
    (2) Stricturopathy
  c. Increase in intestinal length (increased mucosa surface area)
    (1) Bianchi procedure
    (2) Serial transverse enteroplasty (STEP)
    (3) Kimura procedure (Iowa)
    (4) Intestinal transplant

3. Complications
  a. TPN-induced liver disease
  b. Bacterial overgrowth leading to sepsis
  c. Secretory diarrhea
  d. Vitamin deficiencies
  e. Failure to thrive
  f. Central line infections

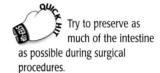 **QUICK HIT** Try to preserve as much of the intestine as possible during surgical procedures.

ABDOMINAL CYSTS

I. Mesenteric Cysts
  A. The majority of these cystic intra-abdominal masses involve the short segment of mesentery.
  B. Clinical features include pain and vomiting.

II. Duplication Cysts
  A. Cyst walls have all three layers of intestine. They can present anywhere along the GI tract.
  B. Types
    1. Tubular (communicating)
    2. Cystic (noncommunicating)
  C. Diagnosis
    1. X-ray of abdomen
    2. Ultrasonography and CT of abdomen
  D. Treatment. Surgical therapy involves excision of cyst with or without bowel resection, depending on extent of lesions.

III. Omental Cysts

A. Cysts are lymph-filled.
B. Symptoms and signs include pain, tenderness, and abdominal distention depending on size.
C. Treatment involves laparoscopic or open operation.

IV. Hepatic Cysts

A. May be single or multiple
 1. Congenital
 2. Acquired
B. Symptoms include abdominal pain
C. Diagnosis
 1. Ultrasound of the abdomen
 2. CT scan of the abdomen
 3. HIDA scan to rule out biliary connectors
D. Treatment: surgical
 1. Noncommunicating cyst: laparoscopic or open marsupialization
 2. Communicating cyst: Roux-en-Y drainage

V. Choledochal Cysts

A. Cystic malformation of biliary tree
B. Types
 1. Saccular or diffuse dilatation of extrahepatic bile duct
 2. Diverticulum of extrahepatic bile duct
 3. Choledochocele
 4. Multiple cysts of extrahepatic or intrahepatic bile duct
 5. Single or multiple intrahepatic bile duct
C. Clinical features
 1. Obstructive jaundice
 2. Abdominal pain and mass
 3. Acholic stools
 4. Signs and symptoms of cholangitis
D. Diagnosis
 1. Conjugated hyperbilirubinemia
 2. Ultrasound and CT of the abdomen
 3. HIDA scan
 4. ERCP in older patients, which may be helpful
E. Treatment: cyst excision with Roux-en-Y hepaticojejunostomy

VI. Lymphangiomas

A. Mostly retroperitoneal intraoperatively
B. Lymph-filled cyst
C. Symptoms and signs: pain and tenderness
D. Treatment: laparoscopic or open operation (partial or near-total removal)

VII. Urachal Remnants

A. Midline swelling of the lower abdomen, which can be found anywhere from urinary bladder to umbilicus, along the course of urachus
B. Clinical features
 1. Abdominal mass
 2. Discharge from the umbilicus
 3. Urinary complaints
C. Diagnosis
 1. Ultrasound of the abdomen and pelvis
 2. Voiding cystourethrogram
D. Treatment: exploration of umbilical region, and excision of urachus remnant with repair of urinary bladder, if required

ONCOLOGY

Although leukemia and lymphoma represent the most common cancer diagnoses in children, their management is generally medical, and beyond the scope of a surgical text. This section will therefore focus on the most common solid tumors of infancy and childhood, where general pediatric surgical therapy is a mainstay of treatment.

I. Neuroblastoma
A. A solid tumor arising from primitive neural crest cells
B. Epidemiology
   1. Incidence: 1 in 7,500 to 10,000
   2. Age of onset: more than 50% present within 2 years of birth
   3. Relative frequency: 10% of childhood tumors, which represents the most common extracranial solid tumor in children
C. Sites. Locations tend to be in the distribution of derivatives of neural crest cells
   1. Adrenal gland (50%)
   2. Paraspinal (25%)
   3. Mediastinum (20%)
   4. Neck (5%)
   5. Pelvis (less than 5%) pelvic organ of Zuckerkandl
D. Etiology
   1. Associated with the N-myc oncogene
   2. Associated genetic abnormalities of deletions on the p arm of chromosome 1, and gain of DNA on the q arm of chromosome 17, both of which confer a worse prognosis
E. Clinical features
   1. Typically appears as highly cellular, uniform tumor with varying degrees of stroma within the tumor on microscopy
   2. Graded on the Shimada scale
      a. Favorable factors are tumor rich in stroma, young age, and a low mitosis/karyorrhexis index (MKI)
      b. Unfavorable factors are nodular pattern, greater age at diagnosis, poor differentiation, and high MKI
      c. MKI assesses the number of mitoses and karyorrhexis per 5,000 cells in the tumor
   3. Typically present as a cervical, abdominal, or pelvic solid mass
      a. Cervical neuroblastoma
         (1) Rarely obstruct the airway
         (2) Arise from the cervical sympathetic chain, and result in a Horner syndrome on the involved side
         (3) Nodal involvement common, distant metastasis rare
      b. Abdominal neuroblastoma
         (1) Most common presentation
         (2) Fixed hard mass arising in the abdomen, crossing the midline, arising from the adrenal medulla or midline sympathetic chain
         (3) Nodal involvement along the aorta, or in the mediastinum is common
      c. Pelvic neuroblastoma
         (1) Often found by parent by palpation
         (2) May lead to obstructive symptoms in the bowel or ureter
         (3) May involve sacral nerves, mandating close physical examination of lower extremity motor function and anal sphincter tone
   4. Associated signs/symptoms
      a. Periorbital ecchymosis due to venous congestion/rupture with metastasis to the eyes
      b. Myoclonus, due to antitumor antibody cross-reaction with Purkinje fibers in the cerebellum
      c. Secretory diarrhea syndrome, due to secretion of vasoactive intestinal peptide

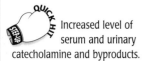

Increased level of serum and urinary catecholamine and byproducts.

F. Diagnosis
1. Imaging with contrasted CT or MRI will show tumor extent
2. Metaiodobenzylguanidine (MIBG) scan
3. Serum and urinary marker
4. Biopsy is the mainstay of diagnosis and staging
G. Treatment
1. Low-risk tumor can be treated with resection alone
2. High-risk tumor should be treated with resection and central venous access device placement for chemotherapy and radiation

II. Nephroblastoma (Wilms Tumor)

A. General principles
1. A tumor of primitive metanephric blastema cells
2. The most common pediatric renal tumor and the fifth most common pediatric cancer
B. Etiology
1. Sporadic form results from two allele loss in a specific tumor suppressor gene
2. *WT1*, an oncogene located on chromosome 11 involved in development of Wilms tumor
3. Associated with other clinical syndromes
   a. Denys–Drash syndrome: Wilms tumor, pseudohermaphroditism, glomerulonephropathy
   b. WAGR syndrome: **W**ilms tumor, **A**niridia, **G**enitourinary malformation, and mental **R**etardation
   c. Beckwith–Wiedemann syndrome
   d. Hemihypertrophy
C. Clinical features
1. Typically presents with a palpable abdominal or flank mass, with or without abdominal pain
2. Other signs include hematuria, hypertension, and/or tumor necrosis with associated fever
D. Diagnosis
1. Imaging
   a. Renal ultrasound is often the initial study obtained to assess renal mass and renal vascular involvement
   b. CT of the chest, abdomen, and pelvis allows assessment of tumor, differentiation from neuroblastoma of the adrenal, assessment of the opposite kidney, and nodal or distant metastasis
2. Staging, which requires surgical resection
   a. Stage 1: tumor confined to kidney and completely resected
   b. Stage 2: tumor completely excised, but with extension beyond renal capsule, or biopsy of confined tumor with local spillage
   c. Stage 3: tumor incompletely excised, positive lymph nodes, or peritoneal implants, or intra-abdominal tumor spillage
   d. Stage 4: hematogenous or lymph node metastasis beyond the abdominal cavity
   e. Stage 5: simultaneous bilateral involvement, with each side staged 1 to 3 separately
E. Treatment
1. Surgical resection is required for treatment and staging
2. Chemotherapy is required for all patients with Wilms tumor diagnoses, and consists typically of doxorubicin, dactinomycin, and Vincristine
3. Radiation therapy is used for stage 3 to 5 disease
4. If found to be unresectable by CT scanning, surgery can be delayed until after cytoreductive chemotherapy

III. Hepatoblastoma

A. General principles

1. Hepatoblastoma is the most common liver malignancy in the pediatric population

2. A relatively rare tumor, with an approximate incidence of 1 in 1,000,000 per year (more frequent 6 months to 3 years of age)

3. Associated with Beckwith–Wiedemann syndrome and familial adenomatous polyposis

B. Pathology. Several histologic variants occur

1. Epithelial

a. Fetal (31%)

b. Embryonal (19%)

c. Macrotrabecular (3%)

d. Anaplastic (3%)

2. Mixed epithelial/mesenchymal (44%)

C. Diagnosis

1. Most patients present with a palpable abdominal mass, with or without abdominal swelling, pain, irritability, gastrointestinal disturbances, fever, pallor, and/or failure to thrive

2. Alpha-fetoprotein levels are significantly elevated with hepatoblastoma (greater than 90%)

3. Imaging

a. Abdominal x-ray may show hepatomegaly

b. CT reveals a heterogenous mass, and is the imaging procedure of choice to assess metastasis but is less sensitive than MRI for primary diagnosis.

c. MRI is the imaging procedure of choice

4. Staging requires resection

a. Stage 1: complete surgical resection

b. Stage 2: microscopic positive margins without regional spread, confined to one lobe of the liver

c. Stage 3: partially resected tumor, spillage of tumor at time of surgery, involving two lobes of the liver with positive lymph nodes

d. Stage 4: distant metastasis

D. Treatment

1. Typically neoadjuvant chemotherapy with doxorubicin and cisplatin prior to surgical resection is used

2. Following cytoreduction, surgical resection with hepatic lobectomy is the procedure of choice, though in rare instances, a wedge resection may be used for small, peripherally located tumors

3. Liver transplantation (up to 6% of patients)

Orthopedic Surgery

Walter Samora, MD
Felix Cheung, MD

FRACTURES

I. General Principles

A. History and physical examination

1. A thorough history and physical are essential to make the diagnosis. Important aspects of the history include the mechanism of injury, as well as the overall health status of the patient.
2. The injury must first be suspected in order to ensure proper imaging is obtained.
3. Distracting injuries may be present. Always inspect and palpate the entire body to ensure injuries are not missed.
4. In trauma patients, always follow Advanced Trauma Life Support (ATLS) protocol.

B. Classification

1. Basis for classification: location
2. Fracture type: open or closed

II. Open Fractures

A. General principles

1. Open fractures are usually caused by high-energy trauma.
2. The mechanism may be from the outside-in, as in a penetrating trauma, or from the inside-out, as in a bone spike that ruptures the skin.
3. Regardless of the mechanism, open fractures are a surgical emergency, and require prompt diagnosis and treatment. Irrigation and debridement, with stabilization of the fracture, are necessary.

B. History and physical

1. The mechanism of the injury, as well as the timing of the injury and where it occurred, are important parts of the history.
2. The history is usually consistent with a high-energy trauma such as a motor vehicle crash or fall from height. Open fractures in the elderly or those with osteoporotic bone may occur with a low-energy trauma.
3. The tetanus status of the patient should be obtained.
4. Important aspects of the physical examination include inspection of the entire involved extremity. In many cases, an obvious deformity is noted, but some open fractures may be subtle.
5. All abrasions and lacerations should be probed to see if they communicate with the fracture. Exposed bone should be placed back in the skin to prevent pressure necrosis.

C. Imaging

1. Standard x-rays of the involved extremity should be obtained as soon as possible. In some instances, "scout" films can be taken in the trauma bay to allow prompt diagnosis before the complete ATLS workup has been completed.
2. Remember to obtain two views of the involved extremity. Most cases require the first responder to hold the extremity to obtain suitable x-rays.

QUICK HIT

Diagnosis is made primarily by radiography. At least two x-rays of the bone/joint taken at right angles to each other are necessary to assess the fracture type.

QUICK HIT

The first responder to the injury should have a camera. Once an open fracture has been identified, a picture is taken to avoid removal of sterile dressings. Redressing the wound in the emergency department carries a threefold to fourfold increase in the infection rate.

QUICK HIT

If the patient has been transferred to your facility, always inspect the skin, even in known closed fractures, because sharp bone fragments may pierce the skin during transport, or small breaks in the skin may have been missed.

QUICK HIT

Always obtain an x-ray of the joint above and the joint below a known fracture/injury.

3. In most cases, splints should be taken off to minimize the risk of inadequate films. If the patient has come from the scene and x-rays can be taken quickly, it is appropriate to provisionally splint the extremity with a pillow or other device and wait until after the x-rays have been taken to splint the patient.

D. Classification

1. The most commonly used classification system is the Gustilo and Anderson system.

2. There are three major types, based on the mechanism of injury, degree of soft-tissue damage, configuration of the fracture, and the amount of contamination.

   a. Type I fractures involve a skin opening of 1 cm or less. Soft-tissue damage is usually minimal.

   b. Type II fractures involve a skin opening of more than 1 cm. Soft-tissue damage is more extensive than type I fractures.

   c. Type III fractures involve extensive skin and soft-tissue damage. The type III fractures are divided into three different subgroups.

   (1) IIIA fractures have sufficient soft tissue to provide adequate bone coverage.

   (2) IIIB fractures require skin grafts or flaps in order to provide coverage.

   (3) IIIC fractures involve vascular injury requiring repair.

E. Treatment

1. Early treatment involves rapid intravenous antibiotics and tetanus prophylaxis, stabilization of the fracture and wound management, followed by aggressive rehabilitation.

2. Surgical options vary, depending on the type of fracture and the area of the body.

   a. For types I, II, and some IIIA open fractures, definitive surgical stabilization can be carried out, usually in the form of intramedullary devices or plates and screws.

   b. For types IIIB and IIIC fractures, external fixation is usually required, with subsequent trips to the operating room for repeat irrigation and debridement before closure.

   c. For types IIIB and IIIC fractures, plastic surgery is usually consulted for skin closure with flaps or grafts, because the wounds require definitive closure 7 days from the time of injury to prevent secondary colonization of bacteria.

3. Antibiotics are given based on the classification and the amount of contamination. They are typically given every 4 hours before surgery, and then every 8 hours after surgery for a duration of 48 to 72 hours.

   a. Type I and II fractures require a first-generation cephalosporin, typically cefazolin.

   b. Type III fractures require a first-generation cephalosporin and an aminoglycoside, usually gentamicin.

   c. For farmyard contamination, as well as vascular compromise and extensive soft-tissue crush injuries, penicillin is added.

III. Fractures of the Cervical Spine

A. General principles

1. Fractures of the cervical spine are usually caused by high-energy trauma such as motor-vehicle crashes and falls from heights.

2. The first responders to the scene (emergency medical technicians [EMTs]) will place a cervical collar (c-collar) on the patient to protect the cervical spine. The patient will also be placed on a backboard to protect the remainder of the spine, and to facilitate the transport of the patient to the emergency department.

3. ATLS protocol includes a lateral x-ray of the cervical spine as well as anteroposterior (AP) x-rays of the chest and pelvis. However, many institutions are foregoing the lateral spine x-ray for a CT scan of the cervical spine.

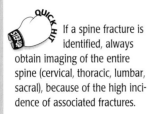

QUICK HIT

If a spine fracture is identified, always obtain imaging of the entire spine (cervical, thoracic, lumbar, sacral), because of the high incidence of associated fractures.

B. History and physical
   1. Important aspects of the history include the age of the patient, mechanism of injury, and associated medical conditions.
   2. Important symptoms include c-spine pain, numbness, paresthesias, or paralysis.
   3. A complete neurologic examination should be documented, including rectal tone, upper and lower extremity reflexes, clonus, and Babinski tests.
C. Imaging
   1. C-spine x-rays (complete c-spine films) include an AP film and open-mouth AP film. (As part of the ATLS protocol, a lateral x-ray of the cervical spine is obtained in the trauma bay.)
   2. Additional imaging of the cervical spine includes a CT scan with reformatted imaging to include sagittal and coronal plane images.
D. Classification
   1. Upper cervical spine fractures
      a. Fractures of the upper cervical spine are grouped into occipitoatlantal fractures, and fractures of the atlas and axis.
      b. Fractures of the occipitoatlantal region include occipital condyle fractures, with or without subluxation, or dislocation of the occipitoatlantal junction.
      c. Fractures of the atlas are usually due to an axial load. These include isolated anterior/posterior arch fractures, and burst fractures. The classic Jefferson fracture is a four-part burst fracture of the atlas.
      d. Fractures of the axis (odontoid) are usually classified using the system of Anderson and D'Alonzo.
         (1) Type I fractures are through the tip of the odontoid.
         (2) Type II fractures occur at the base of the odontoid, at the junction of the odontoid process, and the body of the second cervical vertebrae.
         (3) Type III fractures extend through the body of C2.
      e. Fractures of the axis (pars interarticularis) are known as hangman fractures.
         (1) Type I fractures are nondisplaced.
         (2) Type II fractures show displacement of more than 3 mm, and include ligamentous injury.
         (3) Type III fractures include bilateral pars fractures, and an associated dislocation of one or both facets at C2-C3.
   2. Lower cervical spine fractures
      a. The Denis classification divides the vertebrae into columns.
         (1) The anterior column includes the anterior longitudinal ligament (ALL) and the anterior two-thirds of the vertebral body.
         (2) The middle column includes the remaining one-third of the vertebral body and the posterior longitudinal ligament (PLL).
         (3) The posterior column includes the posterior bony arch and the interconnecting posterior ligamentous structures.
      b. Fractures of the lower cervical spine are classified based on the anatomic location of the fracture. These include fractures of the anterior column, fractures of the facet or lateral mass, and fractures of the posterior column.
      c. Fractures of the anterior column include compression or avulsion fractures of the vertebral body, with or without ligamentous injury, flexion teardrop fractures from flexion or extension injuries, traumatic retrolistheses, burst fractures of the vertebral body (includes middle column), as well as disc and ligamentous injuries.
      d. Fractures of the facet or lateral mass include unilateral or bilateral facet fracture fractures with or without facet dislocation.
      e. Fractures of the posterior column include isolated fractures of the spinous process, lamina, pedicle, or transverse process, as well as ligamentous injuries.

E. Treatment
1. Upper cervical spine fractures
   a. Nondisplaced fractures of the occipital condyles can usually be treated nonoperatively in a c-collar.
   b. Fractures of the occipital condyles with occipitoatlantal dislocation are usually fatal injuries. However, prompt recognition of the fracture pattern (via CT scan) allows for adequate treatment, which is usually a posterior spinal fusion from the occiput to C3, followed by placement in a halo vest.
   c. Isolated anterior/posterior arch, as well as burst fractures with minimal displacement, can be treated with a c-collar for 6 to 10 weeks.
   d. Burst fractures, including Jefferson fractures with more than 7 mm of displacement are treated with halo traction, followed by placement in a halo vest.
2. Lower cervical spine fractures
   a. The goal of treatment is to protect the spinal cord from further trauma, and to stabilize the cervical spine.
   b. Stable fractures of the cervical spine can usually be treated with a c-collar or cervical-thoracic brace for 6 to 8 weeks.
   c. Stable fractures include vertebral body compression fractures, avulsion of the ALL, extension teardrop fractures, mild PLL injuries, and isolated fractures of the posterior elements.
   d. Isolated facet or pedicle fractures without subluxation or dislocation can be treated with a c-collar for 6 to 8 weeks. However, careful follow-up is recommended to ensure the fracture has not displaced.
   e. Flexion teardrop fractures of the cervical spine are usually associated with neurologic injury, and are assessed by the degree of posterior element instability. Initial treatment is typically with traction via Gardner-Wells tongs. Stable fractures require placement in a halo vest for 12 to 16 weeks. Unstable fractures require corpectomy, with anterior decompression and fusion with an anterior plate. Alternative treatment includes a posterior approach with lateral mass fixation if decompression of the spinal canal is not needed.
   f. Patients with traumatic retrolisthesis without neurologic symptoms may be treated in a c-collar. Patients with neurologic symptoms typically require Gardner-Wells traction, followed by anterior decompression and fusion with an anterior plate.
   g. Burst fractures of the cervical spine are assessed by the amount of posterior element stability. Neurologic symptoms, loss of vertebral body height, amount of canal compromise, and degree of kyphosis are important in determining treatment options. Stable burst fractures can be treated with halo vest immobilization for 10 to 12 weeks. Unstable fractures require operative stabilization, usually with a corpectomy, anterior decompression, and fusion with an anterior plate.
   h. Facet fractures (unilateral or bilateral) with subluxation or dislocation are best treated with closed reduction, followed by operative fixation, usually via a posterior approach with either wiring or lateral mass fixation.

IV. Fractures of the Thoracolumbar Spine
A. General principles
1. Thoracolumbar fractures are typically caused by high-energy trauma such as motor vehicle, motorcycle crashes, and falls from height. However, fractures in the thoracolumbar spine may occur with minimal trauma in elderly patients with osteoporosis.
2. The thoracic spine is more stable than the lumbar spine due to the protective effect of the ribs.
3. The spinal cord typically ends at the conus medullaris at the L1-L2 disc space.

 The thoracolumbar junction (T11-L2) is more susceptible to injury than any other part of the spine due to the lack of rib protection, the stress riser effect of the stiffer thoracic segment on the more flexible lumbar segment, and the change in the morphology of the lumbar vertebrae.

B. History and physical
   1. Important aspects of the history include the age of the patient, the mechanism and timing of the injury, medical comorbidities, and associated symptoms.
   2. Important symptoms include thoracolumbar spine pain, numbness, paresthesias, or paralysis.
   3. A complete neurologic examination should be documented, including rectal tone, upper and lower extremity reflexes, clonus, and Babinski tests.
C. Imaging. Current ATLS protocol does not include standard imaging of the thoracolumbar spine. However, the thoracolumbar spine is included in the CT scan of the chest/abdomen and pelvis.
D. Classification
   1. As discussed previously, the Denis classification divides the vertebrae into three columns: anterior, middle, and posterior.
   2. Compression fractures are usually caused by a flexion or axial loading mechanism. By definition, they involve only the anterior column of the vertebrae.
   3. Burst fractures are typically caused by the same mechanism as that of the compression fracture, but usually require higher energy than the compression fractures. In this injury, both the anterior and middle columns are involved.
      a. Important radiographic signs include widening of the pedicles in the AP view, loss of vertebral body height, and amount of kyphosis due to the fracture.
      b. Additionally, amount of canal compromise (usually seen on the axial CT scan) is also important to document.
   4. Flexion-distraction injuries (Chance fractures) can occur through bone, soft tissue, or a combination. The main mechanism is the flexion-distraction forces through the middle and posterior columns, usually leaving the anterior column intact.
      a. Fractures through the vertebral body of one level are typically referred to as bony Chance fractures, whereas fractures involving purely ligamentous structures are referred to as soft-tissue Chance fractures.
      b. Injuries may also occur in which both ligamentous damage as well as bony involvement occur.
   5. Fracture-dislocations of the thoracolumbar spine are typically caused by compression, tension, rotation, or shear forces. In this injury, all three columns are affected, which contributes to the instability of the fracture. Three different injury patterns are recognized.
      a. Flexion-rotation fracture of Holdsworth: all three columns are disrupted, either at the level of the vertebral body, or disc.
      b. Shear-type fracture dislocation: this usually occurs through the disc space, and causes anterolisthesis of the more cephalad vertebrae.
      c. Bilateral facet dislocation injury: this is thought to be a progression of the Chance fracture involving the anterior column as well as the middle and posterior columns, as is seen in Chance fractures.
E. Treatment
   1. Compression fractures are treated depending on the age of the patient, the stability of the fracture, and the amount of pain the patient experiences with weight bearing.
      a. Nonoperative treatment. Radiographic parameters suggestive of nonoperative treatment include loss of vertebral body height of less than 40%, and kyphosis of less than 30 degrees with minimal to moderate pain. Nonoperative treatment usually entails bracing, typically with a thoracolumbosacral orthosis (TLSO). X-rays are obtained with the patient standing in the brace to ensure that the fracture pattern does not worsen with weight bearing.
      b. Operative treatment. Treatment of compression fractures in the elderly is usually performed secondary to pain. Two procedures, vertebroplasty and kyphoplasty, are used to try to maintain vertebral body height.

QUICK HIT

Burst fractures are better tolerated by patients at or below the L2 level due to the absence of the spinal cord. The nerve rootlets are better able to accommodate encroachment by vertebral body segments and disc material than the spinal cord.

(1) Vertebroplasty: a cannula is inserted posteriorly through the pedicle, and cement is injected into the vertebral body.

(2) Kyphoplasty: similar to vertebroplasty, except that a balloon is inserted into the vertebral body, and inflated to try to increase vertebral body height before the cement is injected.

2. Treatment of burst fractures depends on both radiographic parameters and patient symptoms.

    a. Nonoperative treatment. Radiographic parameters suggestive of nonoperative treatment include loss of vertebral body height of less than 40%, kyphosis of less than 30 degrees, and canal compromise of less than 40% to 50%. The absence of neurologic deficits is also important in determining nonoperative treatment. The nonoperative treatment of choice is typically bracing with a TLSO. As with compression fractures, weight-bearing x-rays are obtained with the patient in the brace.

    b. Operative treatment. Such treatment usually involves posterior instrumentation of one to two levels above and below the level of the fracture. Care must be taken to avoid propagating a dural tear, which may occur in up to 50% of burst fractures treated operatively. If significant canal compromise exists that requires extensive decompression of the spinal canal, an anterior approach may be used, particularly if coupled with minimal kyphotic deformity. Significant canal compromise, coupled with a severe kyphotic deformity necessitates both anterior and posterior approaches.

3. Flexion-distraction injuries

    a. Those that occur solely through bone (bony Chance fractures) without neurologic deficits may be treated nonoperatively in a TLSO, or hyperextension cast for 12 to 16 weeks.

    b. Unstable injuries require operative fixation, usually with posterior instrumentation one level above, and below the level of injury.

4. Fracture-dislocations have a high incidence of neurologic deficit and usually require surgical stabilization. Decompression with posterior instrumentation and fusion is preferred, but combined anterior decompression with posterior instrumentation and fusion may be necessary for significant canal compromise associated with a neurologic deficit.

V. Fractures of the Proximal Humerus

A. General principles

    1. These fractures account for approximately 2% to 3% of all fractures of the upper extremities.

    2. The typical patient is a female older than 60 years of age.

B. History and physical

    1. Important aspects of the physical examination, include a thorough neurovascular examination, because the axillary nerve is vulnerable to injury.

    2. The clavicle, the humeral shaft, and elbow must also be thoroughly examined for associated injuries.

    3. Vascular damage to the lateral ascending branch of the anterior circumflex artery may lead to avascular necrosis of the humeral head.

    4. Associated rotator cuff injuries may be difficult to evaluate due to the pain of the fracture.

C. Imaging. A trauma series of the shoulder includes an anteroposterior view, a scapular "Y" view, and an axillary view. The axillary view is necessary to evaluate the glenohumeral joint to ensure that an associated dislocation did not occur.

D. Classification

    1. The Neer system is the most commonly used classification system.

    2. In this system, the proximal humerus is divided into four segments, which consist of the head, shaft, and the greater and lesser tuberosities.

    3. Each segment is considered significant if it is displaced more than 1 cm, or is rotated more than 45 degrees.

 It is imperative to ensure that there is no middle column involvement in compression fractures treated with vertebroplasty or kyphoplasty, because of the risk of extrusion of cement into the spinal canal.

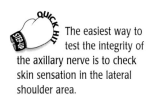 The easiest way to test the integrity of the axillary nerve is to check skin sensation in the lateral shoulder area.

E. Treatment
1. Treatment is based on the fracture type, the quality of bone, as well as the general health of the patient.
2. Most proximal humerus fractures are treated nonoperatively. The mainstay of nonoperative treatment is early protection combined with immobilization. Most patients can be placed in a sling for 1 to 2 weeks, followed by a formal physical therapy program.
3. Surgery is usually reserved for active, healthy patients. It usually consists of either closed reduction and percutaneous pinning, or open reduction and internal fixation (ORIF).
4. Elderly patients with severely comminuted fractures may opt for prosthetic replacement of their proximal humerus.

VI. Fractures of the Distal Radius
A. General principles
1. Fractures of the distal radius are very common. They include a wide spectrum of fractures, ranging from simple fractures requiring minimal treatment, to complex fractures requiring ORIF.
2. Fractures of the distal radius have a bimodal distribution, occurring commonly in children from 6 to 10 years of age and in adults from 60 to 69 years of age.
B. History and physical
1. Important aspects of the history include the age of the patient and their associated medical conditions, the mechanism of the injury, as well as previous injuries to the wrist.
2. Important aspects of the physical examination include a thorough inspection of the skin and associated deformities, as well as the neurovascular status of the involved extremity.
3. The radial nerve can be tested by asking the patient to give you a "thumbs up" (extensor pollicis longus muscle), as well as by testing the sensation of the radial side of the thumb.
4. The median nerve can be tested by asking the patient to perform the "A-OK" sign (opponens pollicis muscle), as well as testing the sensation on palmar surface of the index finger.
5. The ulnar nerve can be tested by asking the patient to abduct the fingers (dorsal interossei muscles), as well as testing the sensation on the ulnar side of the small finger.
C. Imaging
1. Imaging of the upper extremity should include anteroposterior and lateral x-rays of the wrist, as well as x-rays of the forearm and elbow.
2. Radiographic parameters in the normal wrist include the radial inclination (normally 23 degrees), the radial height (normally 12 mm), as well as the volar tilt (normally 11 degrees).
3. Radiographic signs in the fractured wrist include the level of the fracture (distance from the radiocarpal joint), loss of radial height, amount of dorsal comminution, extension of the fracture into the radiocarpal joint, and loss of volar tilt (resulting in dorsal tilt).
D. Classification
1. Numerous classification systems exist for fractures of the distal radius. For simplicity, and the ability to describe the injury to a co-worker, an anatomic description, as well as a description of the radiographic signs is most commonly used.
2. Eponymous descriptions are still widely used, and include Colles, Smith, Chauffer, and Barton fractures.
3. Colles fractures are transverse, extra-articular fractures of the distal radius. The distal fragment is displaced dorsally, resulting in the classic "dinner fork" deformity.

4. Smith fractures are reverse Colles fractures, in that the displacement of the distal fragment is volar (palmar).

5. Chauffer fractures are intra-articular fractures of the radial styloid.

6. Barton fractures are intra-articular fractures that result from a shearing force and are best seen in the lateral x-ray. Barton fractures are classified as either dorsal or volar depending on which cortex the fracture extends into.

E. Treatment

1. Treatment options are based on the fracture pattern and the stability of the fracture. Factors that influence operative treatment over nonoperative treatment based on the initial injury x-rays are age (greater than 60 years), extension into the radiocarpal joint, loss of radial height (greater than 0.5 cm), amount of dorsal comminution, and loss of volar tilt (dorsal tilt greater than 20 degrees).

2. Nonoperative distal radius fractures can be treated with closed reduction and casting in the emergency department.

a. Options for anesthesia include reduction without anesthesia, oral/intravenous analgesia, hematoma block, bier block, conscious sedation, and general anesthesia. Typically, a hematoma block augmented with oral analgesia is used.

b. Based on the stability of the reduction, patients can usually be maintained in a short-arm cast with a three-point mold. Unstable fractures require a long-arm cast to prevent pronosupination at the distal radioulnar joint.

3. Operative interventions vary, depending on the experience of the surgeon. The two main methods include (i) ORIF (with a volar or dorsal plate) and (ii) and external fixation.

VII. Fractures of the Femur

A. General principles

1. It is estimated that the incidence of hip fractures (femoral neck and intertrochanteric fractures) is more than 300,000 per year in the United States alone. The risk of falling doubles between the ages of 65 and 85. Combined with the increased incidence of osteoporosis in this age group, the risk of sustaining an associated hip fracture increases 100-fold.

2. Fractures in elderly patients

a. Significant low-energy injuries may result from osteoporosis or neoplasm.

b. Although subtrochanteric, femoral shaft, and distal femoral fractures may occur in elderly patients due to low-energy trauma, usually high-energy trauma such as a fall from height or an automobile, motorcycle, or all-terrain vehicle crash is necessary.

B. History and physical

1. Important aspects of the history include the patient's age, the mechanism of injury, and associated medical comorbidities.

2. Important aspects of the physical examination include a thorough neurovascular examination, because some patients may sustain injuries to the sciatic nerve or develop compartment syndrome as a result of bleeding from the fracture site.

C. Imaging

1. Most fractures of the proximal femur, including femoral head/neck fractures and intertrochanteric and subtrochanteric fractures, can be seen in the AP pelvis x-ray obtained in the trauma bay.

2. Additional x-rays can be obtained if necessary.

D. Classification

1. Fractures of the femur are generally classified based on the anatomic location. The different locations are the femoral head, neck, intertrochanteric region, subtrochanteric region, shaft, and distal femur.

2. Femoral neck fractures are typically classified using the Garden classification.

a. Grade I fracture is valgus impacted.

b. Grade II fracture is nondisplaced.

     c. Grade III fracture is incompletely displaced in varus alignment.

     d. Grade IV is completely displaced, with no contact between the fracture fragments.

3. Intertrochanteric femur fractures are more difficult to classify.

     a. Most systems classify the fracture patterns as stable or unstable, with special attention placed on reverse obliquity patterns.

     b. The stability of the fracture is generally based on the integrity of the posteromedial cortex (calcar femorale), which allows native bone to withstand compressive loads after reduction and fixation.

4. Subtrochanteric femur fractures are generally unstable fractures, based on the location of the fracture and the muscle forces pulling on the proximal fragment. Subtrochanteric fractures are best classified based on the location, extension into the intertrochanteric region or down the shaft of the femur, the fracture pattern, and the amount of comminution.

5. Fractures of the femoral shaft are usually best classified based on the location of the fracture, the fracture pattern, and the amount of comminution.

     a. The location is usually give in terms of which third of the femoral shaft contains the fracture.

     b. The fracture pattern is usually a descriptive term based on the radiologic appearance, such as transverse, oblique, or spiral.

     c. The amount of comminution ranges from a large butterfly fragment of less than 50% of the width of the bone, to segmental comminution with no bone contact between the proximal and distal fragments.

6. Fractures of the distal femur are also best classified using descriptive terminology.

     a. The three main groups of fractures include extra-articular fractures, fractures of either the medial or lateral condyle, or bicondylar fractures.

     b. As with femoral shaft fractures, the fracture pattern as well as the amount of comminution is important.

E. Treatment

1. Treatment of femur fractures are based on the age of the patient, the patient's comorbidities, the quality of the patient's bone, and the preinjury level of activity.

2. For treatment purposes, fractures may be classified as Garden I/II and Garden III/IV.

     a. Garden I and II fractures, as well as any femoral neck fracture in a young adult, are usually treated with closed reduction and percutaneous pinning of the fracture. Usually, three screws are placed into the femoral head from the lesser trochanter.

     b. Garden III and IV fractures are usually treated with a unipolar hemiarthroplasty, a bipolar hemiarthroplasty, or a total hip arthroplasty with or without cement.

3. Intertrochanteric femur fractures can be fixed with a variety of implants, based on the surgeon's preference. Common implants include a compression hip screw with a side plate, intramedullary sliding hip screws, and 95-degree angled plates.

4. Reverse obliquity intertrochanteric fractures are considered unstable fractures and require more stable fixation methods. These include long intramedullary sliding hip screws, or 95-degree angled plates.

5. Subtrochanteric fractures are unstable fractures, and require stable fixation methods. These include long compression hip screw with a side plate, long intramedullary sliding hip screws, or long 95-degree angled plates.

6. Femoral shaft fractures are best secured with intramedullary devices, or a plate and screws.

7. Extra-articular fractures of the distal femur may be fixed using a retrograde intramedullary device, a plate and screw device, or a 95-degree angled plate device. Fractures involving the articular surface must be anatomically

---

QUICK HIT Femoral neck fractures are intracapsular hip fractures, and the greatest risk associated with fixation of the fracture is avascular necrosis of the femoral head.

QUICK HIT The compression hip screw with a side plate is contraindicated in reverse obliquity intertrochanteric femur fractures, because the sliding hip screw does not promote interfragmentary compression because of the orientation of the fracture plane.

QUICK HIT The proximal fragment will be flexed and externally rotated (from the pull of the iliopsoas muscle inserting into the lesser trochanter), as well as abducted (from the pull of the gluteus medius inserting into the greater trochanter).

reduced, in order to prevent the early onset of post-traumatic arthrosis. Fixation devices include plate and screw constructs as well as 95-degree angled plate devices.

VIII. Fractures of the Ankle

A. General principles
1. The ankle is one of the most frequently injured areas of the body.
2. There is a continuum from sprains to fractures based on the mechanism of the injury and the amount of energy involved.

B. History and physical
1. Important aspects from the history are the energy and mechanism of the injury, previous injuries to the same area, and the associated medical comorbidities.
2. Important aspects of the physical examination are the condition of the skin, associated swelling or bruising, and a detailed examination of the nerves, arteries and muscles that cross the ankle.

C. Imaging
1. The Ottawa ankle rules determine the appropriateness of obtaining ankle x-rays. These rules state that x-rays are indicated if there is pain in the malleolar zone of the ankle, and one or more of the following is present: age greater than 55, bone tenderness at posterior edge of distal 6 cm, tip of medial or lateral malleolus, or the inability both to weight bear immediately after injury and walk four steps.
2. Three views of the ankle are required to accurately assess fractures. Standard films include AP, lateral, and mortise views.

D. Classification
1. There are several ankle classification systems, including the AO-OTA and the Lauge–Hansen classifications. However, the most common practical classification system is based on a description of the fracture pattern involving the three malleoli of the ankle: lateral, medial, and posterior malleoli.
   a. Fractures of the lateral malleolus are classified based on the level of the fracture (Weber classification), with a Weber A fracture being below the level of the distal tibiofibular joint, a Weber B fracture being at the level of the joint, and a Weber C fracture being above the level of the joint.
   b. Fractures of the medial malleolus are usually described by the fracture pattern and the amount of displacement.
   c. Fractures of the posterior malleolus are described based on the amount of joint space involvement and the amount of articular step-off.
2. Fractures of more than one malleolus are called bimalleolar and trimalleolar ankle fractures, with descriptions of the fracture pattern of each malleolus involved.
3. Medial clear space widening of greater than 4 mm is indicative of ligamentous instability on the medial aspect of the ankle, and is considered an "equivalent" fracture of the medial malleolus. Therefore, an isolated Weber B lateral malleolus fracture with medial clear space widening is described as a "bimalleolar equivalent fracture."

E. Treatment
1. Treatment of ankle fractures is based on restoration of the normal anatomy of the tibiotalar (ankle) joint.
2. Isolated fractures of the lateral malleolus (Weber A or B) are usually treated nonoperatively. Small avulsion fractures of the tip of the lateral malleolus can be treated with an Aircast. Weber B fractures usually require a short leg walking cast. Before placement in a cast, however, always ensure that the tibiotalar joint is anatomically reduced based of the mortise view.
3. Isolated Weber C fractures are typically unstable and require ORIF.
4. Isolated medial malleolus fractures may be treated nonoperatively if the fracture is nondisplaced. However, the treatment is a short leg cast with non-weight bearing for several months.

5. Bimalleolar and bimalleolar equivalent fractures usually require ORIF. For bimalleolar fractures, the lateral malleolus is initially fixed (to restore length of the ankle joint), usually with a plate and screws. The medial malleolus is then fixed, usually with two screws.

6. For bimalleolar equivalent fractures, the ankle can be given an eversion/inversion stress under fluoroscopy after the lateral malleolus is reduced, to assess the stability of the ankle joint. Stable fractures require no further treatment. However, if the ankle remains unstable after fixation of the lateral malleolus, the syndesmosis requires stabilization, usually with one or two horizontal screws from the fibula to the tibia.

7. Trimalleolar ankle fractures typically require operative treatment. ORIF is used as for bimalleolar fractures. The posterior malleolus is then assessed for articular step-off and amount of joint involvement. Small fractures involving less than 25% to 35% of the joint with minimal incongruity may be left alone. However, larger fragments are usually fixed, usually with a screw from anterior to posterior, capturing the fragment and reducing it to the remainder of the distal tibia.

ORTHOPEDIC SYNDROMES

I. Compartment Syndrome

A. General principles

1. Compartment syndrome is characterized by increased pressure in an enclosed space (fascial compartment) with the potential to cause irreversible damage to its contents.
2. It is an orthopedic emergency, which necessitates prompt diagnosis and treatment.
3. It is usually associated with a fracture of a long bone.

B. Tissue pressure measurements

1. These measurements are usually reserved for polytrauma or obtunded patients.
2. They can be performed using a variety of different measurement systems.

C. Diagnosis

1. The diagnosis of compartment syndrome is either clinical, assuming a conscious and alert patient, or based on a compartmental pressure determined before tissue pressure measurements are conducted.
2. Common values used are 30 mm Hg, or a compartment pressure within 10 to 30 mm Hg of the patient's diastolic pressure.

D. Treatment

1. Compartment syndrome is treated via fasciotomy. Skin, subcutaneous fat, and fascial layers must all be widely decompressed and left open.
2. If compartment syndrome is associated with a fracture, rigid stabilization of the bone is necessary.
3. After the initial insult has subsided, the wounds may be closed primarily, or may require split-thickness skin grafting.

II. Compression Neuropathies: Carpal Tunnel and Cubital Tunnel Syndromes

A. General principles

1. These syndromes are thought to be caused by ischemia/mechanical factors.
2. Decreased epineural blood flow is seen at 20 to 30 mm Hg.
3. Decreased axonal transport is demonstrated at 30 mm Hg.
4. Paresthesias are elicited at 30 to 40 mm Hg.
5. Chronic compression leads to fibrosis of nerve rather than just a vascular insult.

B. History and physical

1. Symptom location, onset, duration, quality, and severity are important to form a differential diagnosis.

QUICK HIT

Remember the Ps: **p**ain out of proportion based on the findings (first clue of impending/established compartment syndrome), **p**ain with palpation of the swollen compartment, **p**ain with passive stretch, **p**aresthesias, **p**ulselessness, **p**aralysis.

2. Sensory testing should be carried out using Semmes–Weinstein monofilaments.
3. Weakness and muscle atrophy on physical examination, usually indicates chronic symptoms and requires prompt treatment.

C. Diagnostic studies
1. Electromyographic (EMG)/nerve conduction studies are considered the "gold standard" for diagnosis.
2. However, in most instances, diagnosis is made based on the history and physical examination.

III. Carpal Tunnel Syndrome

A. General principles
1. This syndrome is the most common compression neuropathy.
2. It is caused by compression of the median nerve at the wrist.

B. History and physical
1. Symptoms include pain and paresthesias on the palmar radial aspect of the hand, often waking the patient from sleep, and exacerbated by repetitive forceful use of the hand.
2. Phalen wrist flexion test and Tinel nerve percussion test are usually positive.

C. Diagnostic studies. Nerve conduction studies usually reveal distal motor latencies of more than 4.5 milliseconds, and distal sensory latencies of more than 3.5 milliseconds.

D. Treatment
1. Nonoperative treatment includes neutral wrist splints, oral anti-inflammatory medication, and steroid injections. Steroid injections offer transient relief in up to 80% of patients whose symptoms have been present less than 1 year.
2. Operative treatment involves decompression of the carpal tunnel.

IV. Cubital Tunnel Syndrome

A. General principles. This condition is caused by compression of the ulnar nerve at the elbow.

B. History and physical
1. Symptoms include numbness along the small and ring fingers, often accompanied by clumsiness and weakness in grip.
2. Examination should include the cervical spine to rule out cervical disc disease, arthritis, or thoracic outlet syndrome.
3. Elbow flexion test and Tinel nerve percussion test are usually positive.

C. Diagnostic studies
1. EMG/nerve conduction studies can help localize the level of the lesion, as well as differentiate other associated neuropathic lesions.
2. The classic finding is a focal slowing in conduction as the ulnar nerve crosses the elbow.
3. The lower limit of normal motor conduction velocity across the elbow is 49 m/sec with the elbow flexed to 135 degrees.

D. Treatment
1. Nonoperative treatment includes rest, avoidance of excessive elbow flexion, and anti-inflammatory medication.
2. Operative treatment includes simple decompression, medial epicondylectomy, or anterior transposition (either subcutaneous or submuscular).

QUICK HIT Systemic conditions such as alcoholism or hypothyroidism may lower the threshold for development of compression neuropathies, and must be addressed in conjunction with the proposed treatment.

ORTHOPEDIC ONCOLOGY

I. General Principles

A. Sarcomas are neoplasms that originate from mesenchymal tissue, as opposed to epithelial tissue (carcinomas).
B. Malignant tumors that primarily originate from the bone are rare (2,500 new cases per year in the United States).

C. Soft-tissue sarcomas (arising from fat, muscle, or tendons) are also rare (10,000 new cases per year in the United States).
D. In contrast, metastatic cancer to the bone is much more common (1.2 million new cases per year in the United States).
E. Many benign lesions affect bone and soft tissue.

II. Benign Lesions of Bone

A. Enchondroma
1. Second most common benign bone tumor
2. Asymptomatic, clear area with speckling in metaphyseal/diaphyseal area
3. Most common in hands and feet, in the humerus, and in other long bones. This may be expansile, but there is no soft-tissue mass.
4. May present with fracture
5. Small (less than 1%) malignant potential to chondrosarcoma
6. Treatment: observation, intralesional excision, and curettage
7. Ollier disease
   a. Nonhereditary multiple enchondromatosis, causing long bone deformation
   b. Malignant potential of 25%
8. Maffucci syndrome
   a. Multiple enchondromatosis, with associated soft tissue angiomatosis.
   b. Malignant potential greater than Ollier disease
B. Osteochondroma (exostosis)
1. Cartilage capped bony projection on the external surface of the bone near metaphysis–diaphysis junction, communicating with medullary canal.
2. Most common benign bone tumor.
3. Pedunculated tumors have stalk, and sessile tumors have no stalk.
4. Small malignant potential (1%) to chondrosarcoma.
5. Treatment includes observation or excision if painful.
6. Multiple hereditary exostosis.
   a. Autosomal dominant condition with many exostosis, causing bone deformation and mechanical joint block.
   b. Malignant potential of 10%.
C. Enostosis (bone island)
1. Found in adult cancellous bone
2. Asymptomatic, often an incidental finding
3. Small (less then 2 cm) sclerotic lesions with thorny borders, which blend into the rest of the bone
4. Bone scans are cold or show only modest activity
5. Treatment is observation
D. Osteoid osteoma
1. Affects ages 5 to 30 years, with a male–to–female ratio of 2 to1
2. Painful, worse at night, relieved with nonsteroidal anti-inflammatory agents
3. Small (less than 1 cm) nidus surrounded by reactive bone in the diaphysis
4. May look like an abscess
5. Self limiting over several years
6. Treatment includes excision or radiofrequency ablation
E. Fibrous cortical defect
1. Affects metaphyseal bone as a growth defect with lucent focus surrounded by sclerotic bone
2. Asymptomatic
3. It will fill in with bone as the child grows
4. Treatment is observation, or curettage and bone grafting if the lesion is large, and a fracture is impending
F. Fibrous dysplasia
1. Affects metaphyseal–diaphyseal bone
2. Can cause bony deformity ("shepherd's crook") and lead to fracture
3. Proliferation of fibroblasts in a disorganized fashion

4. Radiographs show a lytic lesion with a rim of reactive bone, and a classic "ground glass" appearance.
5. Histologically, a proliferation of fibroblasts are seen, producing a dense collagenous matrix.
6. Bone fragments are disorganized, and described as "Chinese letters."
7. McCune–Albright syndrome: Yellow patches of skin, precocious puberty, multiple bone lesions.
8. Treatment includes internal fixation and allograft, if in a high-stress area (e.g., proximal femur).

G. Giant cell tumor of bone
1. A lytic, hemorrhagic, aneurysmal lesion in the metaphyseal–epiphyseal region of bone, that may cause pathologic fracture.
2. Occurs in females more than males between 20 and 40 years of age.
3. Most common around distal femur, proximal tibia, sacrum, distal radius.
4. Histologically, the nuclei of the cells in the stroma will look like the cells in the multiple giant cells.
5. Treatments include curettage, bone grafting, cementation, cryosurgery, and radiation.
6. Local recurrence with curettage, cryosurgery, and cementation is as low as 3%.
7. Although this is a histologically benign lesion, it does have a 2% chance of metastatic spread to the lungs. Resection of lung lesions lead to a 76% disease-free outcome.

III. Malignant Tumors of Bone

A. Osteosarcoma
1. Most common primary malignant tumor of bone (3 per 10,000 new cases per year in the United States).
2. Classically defined as a malignant spindle cell sarcoma that produces new bone.
3. Occurs more frequently in males than females, between 10 and 20 years of age.
4. Cause unknown: genetics, viruses, radiation, alkylating agents are suspected.
5. Most common in metaphyseal bone: distal femur, proximal tibia, humerus.
6. Metastatic lesions to lung and other bones are common at presentation.
7. Clinically presents with a painful soft-tissue mass for 3 or more months, night pain.
8. Alkaline phosphatase and lactic dehydrogenase levels may be elevated.
9. Radiographs show destruction of the trabecular pattern with indistinct borders. "Codman triangles" (elevated periosteum) and a starburst pattern are classical descriptions.
10. Histologically, malignant osteoblasts that are producing osteoid are identified.
11. Treatment centers on neoadjuvant chemotherapy (chemotherapy prior to surgery), wide resection, and limb reconstruction.
12. Survival is around 70% for those who present without metastatic disease.

B. Ewing sarcoma
1. Second most common tumor in children (besides osteosarcoma).
2. Occurs more frequently in males than females, and mostly in white children 5 to 30 years of age. It affects 3 per 1,000,000 white children under the age of 21.
3. Unknown cause, and is associated with translocation t(11:22)(q24;q12).
4. A kind of the primitive neuroectodermal tumor.
5. Located in the diaphysis: femur, pelvis, ribs, vertebra, scapula, clavicle.
6. Clinically presents as limb pain, swelling, occasionally fracture. Fevers, sweats chills, night pains are not uncommon.
7. Laboratory values show an elevated erythrocyte sedimentation rate, alkaline phosphatase, and lactate dehydrogenase.

8. Radiographs show periosteal elevation ("Codman triangle") and onion skinning of the periosteum. MRI is helpful for distinguishing the extent of the lesion.

9. Histology shows a small, round, monotonous, bluish cell. Pseudorosettes may be present. HBA-71 stain helps distinguish it from lymphoma.

10. Treatment consists of neoadjuvant chemotherapy, radiation, wide surgical resection, and limb reconstruction.

C. Chondrosarcoma

1. Second most common malignant tumor of bone.

2. Characterized by malignant chondrocytes, but it is very difficult to distinguish between benign and malignant on histologic examination.

3. Clinical clues for favoring malignant cartilage lesion instead of benign.
   a. Large size.
   b. Central location in bone.
   c. Older age.
   d. Greater number of lesions.
   e. Hot bone scan (benign lesions can be hot, too).
   f. Local recurrence.
   g. Night pain.

4. Radiographs show small round calcific bodies ("popcorn balls"), or speckled calcification.

5. Pathology reveals chondrocytes that show hypercellularity, cellular atypia, pleomorphism, binucleate forms, and invasion of bony trabeculae, and is either high or low grade.

6. Treatment includes wide resection with limb reconstruction. Lesions are not responsive to chemotherapy and radiation.

7. Survival is 60% to 80% for those with high-grade lesions.

IV. Metastatic Disease

A. 1.2 million metastatic to bone cases per year in the United States

B. Half will come from breast, lung, kidney, and prostate

C. Most lesions will go to spine, pelvis, ribs, and proximal limb girdles

D. Clinical presentation includes rest and night pain, and tenderness

E. Biopsy
   1. Not needed if there is a known primary with known metastasis.
   2. Should be done if there is an unknown primary, or if patient was previously thought to be disease free and there is a solitary met.

F. Workup for unknown primary includes radiographs of the lesion, chest x-ray (CXR), CT of chest and abdomen, complete blood count (CBC), serum protein electrophoresis, calcium, and phosphate

G. Mirels scoring system for impending pathologic fracture
   1. Graded 1 to 3.
   2. Location (proximal femur highest score for highest stresses).
   3. Pattern of bony destruction (lytic lesions highest score).
   4. Amount of bony destruction (75% cortical involvement the highest).
   5. Amount of pain (severe highest score).
   6. Sum of factors greater than 10 was high risk for fracture, less than 7 low risk.

H. Goal of surgery is for pain relief, prevention of fracture, early mobilization.

I. External beam radiation is useful to nonoperative sites.

V. Pseudotumors

A. These conditions often mimic sarcomas, but are not neoplastic in nature

B. Stress fractures
   1. Repetitive stress to the tibia, fibula, and metatarsal bones cause a nondisplaced fracture to the trabecular bone, that results in reactive bone formation and periosteal elevation.
   2. Differentiated clinically by history of changes in training regimen, pain with activity.

C. Myositis ossificans
   1. Cause is direct trauma to large muscles, resulting in a hemorrhagic fibrotic mass that will calcify.
   2. Biopsy reveals mature bone, not malignant cells.
D. Osteomyelitis
   1. Low-grade infection of the bone may not cause an elevation in temperature, white count, or erythrocyte sedimentation rate.
   2. Most common organism is *Staphylococcus aureus*, but may be tuberculosis or fungus.
   3. Biopsy reveals white blood cells and/or fungi on stains.
E. Hyperparathyroidism
   1. Increased parathyroid hormone levels from chronic renal failure, or an adenoma can cause lytic lesions that mimic giant cell tumors.
   2. Laboratory studies can help distinguish these two entities.
F. Paget disease
   1. Early lytic phase can appear neoplastic in nature.
   2. Characterized by hot bone scan, and very high alkaline phosphatase.
G. Langerhans cell histiocytosis
   1. Also called histiocytosis X, eosinophilic granuloma, Hand–Schüller–Christian disease, Letterer–Siwe disease.
   2. Originate from CD34 marrow cells, with Birbeck granules under electron microscope.
   3. Causes a lytic lesion with periosteal reaction in the diaphysis, like Ewing sarcoma.
   4. Biopsy should reveal this entity.
H. Hemorrhagic disorders
   1. Repeated bleeds can mimic tumors.
   2. Hemophilia, warfarin use, and scurvy are causes.
I. Bone island
   1. Dense, compact cortical bone forms in cancellous bone.
   2. Cold on bone scan.
J. Bone infarct
   1. Death of a portion of the metaphyseal or epiphyseal bone can mimic enchondroma or chondrosarcoma.
   2. Cold on bone scan, unlike chondrosarcomas.

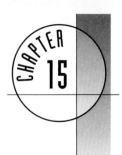

CHAPTER 15

Neurosurgery

Stanley Zaslau, MD, MBA, FACS

CONGENITAL MALFORMATIONS AND DISORDERS OF CEREBROSPINAL FLUID CIRCULATION

I. Hydrocephalus

A. General principles
1. May be congenital or acquired.
2. Caused by an obstruction to the flow of cerebrospinal fluid (CSF). The most common causes are:
   a. Intraventricular hemorrhage in a premature infant.
   b. Stenosis of the aqueduct.
   c. Chiari malformation.
3. The most common type of Chiari malformation is downward herniation of the fourth ventricle and the cerebellar tonsils.

B. Clinical features
1. Patients may present with bulging fontanelles, dilation of scalp veins, and increased head circumference.
2. Parinaud syndrome (altered upward gaze), nausea, vomiting, ataxia, lethargy, and irritability may result.

C. Diagnosis. Computed tomography (CT) scan or magnetic resonance imaging (MRI) confirms the diagnosis.

D. Treatment
1. Shunt placement to divert ventricular fluid is necessary.
2. The most commonly used shunt is a ventriculoperitoneal shunt.
3. Ventriculoatrial shunts may be considered in very small infants, because of the smaller absorptive surface of their peritoneum.

II. Spinal Dysraphism

A. General principles
1. This is a defective fusion of the raphe, with associated physical defects on examination.
2. Findings may include hair tufts, nevus, lipoma, abnormal blood vessels, gluteal cleft, or dimples.
3. Examples include spina bifida, meningocele, and myelomeningocele.
   a. Spina bifida results from failure of fusion of the arches of the vertebrae.
   b. Meningocele is a sac-like midline herniation of the dura.
   c. Myelomeningocele is herniation of the dura and neural elements.

B. Clinical features
1. Patients with spina bifida and meningocele can be asymptomatic.
2. Neurological defects are common with myelomeningocele.

C. Diagnosis. Physical examination, and CT or MRI confirm the diagnosis.

D. Treatment. Therapy for the associated congenital abnormalities may be required, such as for the cosmetic defects associated with each condition.

INTRACRANIAL BLEEDING

I. Epidural Hematoma
A. General principles
1. This condition is seen in patients with head trauma with associated skull fracture.
2. Fracture involves laceration of the middle meningeal artery leading to laceration and expansile hematoma formation.
3. Increased intracranial pressure produces brain compression, and can lead to herniation.

B. Clinical features
1. Loss of consciousness without obvious neurologic deficits may occur.
2. Patient loses consciousness in a rapid and progressive fashion.
3. Consciousness should be assessed with the Glasgow Coma Scale (GCS).
   a. Patients with severe injuries, and a GCS of less than 8, require airway protection with endotracheal intubation.
   b. Immediate neurosurgical evaluation is compulsory.

C. Diagnosis. CT scan indicates the diagnosis.

D. Treatment
1. Emergency decompression is performed for patients with problems in the following areas: airway control, altered and decreased level of consciousness, and a depressed skull fracture.
2. Creation of a burr hole over the area of hematoma removes the blood clot, and lowers the intracranial pressure.
3. The dura is fixed to bone to prevent hematoma reaccumulation. The bleeding middle meningeal artery is ligated.

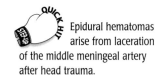

Epidural hematomas arise from laceration of the middle meningeal artery after head trauma.

II. Subdural Hematoma
A. General principles
1. Subdural hematoma is a low-flow, low-pressure cause of intracerebral bleeding.
2. Bleeding is secondary to either spontaneous or traumatic bleeding of bridging veins that drain the superior sagittal sinus.
3. Consider this diagnosis in an elderly patient with known cerebral atrophy, taking oral anticoagulants such as warfarin.

B. Clinical features
1. Patients present with headache, drowsiness, and hemiparesis.
2. Patients rarely have seizures or papilledema.

C. Diagnosis. CT scan confirms the diagnosis.

D. Treatment. Burr hole decompression is required in patients with a significant mass effect and neurologic deficits.

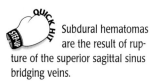

Subdural hematomas are the result of rupture of the superior sagittal sinus bridging veins.

III. Subarachnoid Hemorrhage
A. General principles
1. The most common cause is trauma. However, this hemorrhage may be secondary to arteriovenous malformation (AVM) or aneurysm.
2. Blood fills the subarachnoid space instead of CSF.
3. Development may be spontaneous.
4. 15% of patients have multiple aneurysms.
5. 15% of patients have no angiographic evidence of subarachnoid hemorrhage.

B. Clinical features
1. Sudden onset of severe headache is characteristic. Nausea, vomiting, stiff neck, photophobia, and altered mental status can occur.
2. Third nerve palsy results from aneurysm of the posterior communicating artery.
3. Monocular visual field cuts result from aneurysm of the internal carotid-ophthalmic vessels.

C. Diagnosis
1. CT scan reveals the diagnosis in nearly 90% of cases.
2. If the CT scan is negative and does not reveal mass effect, lumbar puncture may establish the diagnosis.
D. Treatment. Therapy involves surgical clipping and resection of the aneurysmal defect.

IV. Arteriovenous Malformation
A. General Principles
1. Arteriovenous malformations (AVMs) are congenitally abnormal connections between arteries and veins, without intervening small vessels to decrease pressure and flow.
2. This allows high flow and high pressure arterial blood to rupture the AVM.
3. AVMs are located in the brain parenchyma and can cause intracerebral hematoma.
B. Clinical features
1. Neurologic presentation depends on location of the AVM.
2. Aphasia and contralateral arm and/or leg hemiplegia can result from intracerebral hematoma.
3. Visual field defects can result from occipital hematomas.
C. Diagnosis
1. CT scan reveals an intracerebral hematoma.
2. Angiography may reveal smaller AVMs.
D. Treatment
1. Patients with elevated intracranial pressure and evidence of herniation require surgical evacuation of the hematoma.
2. Small AVMs diagnosed by angiography may be observed initially, but definitive removal is recommended.
3. Radiosurgical techniques may be feasible for AVMs less than 3 cm, and in locations of the brain that are difficult to approach surgically.

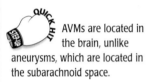
AVMs are located in the brain, unlike aneurysms, which are located in the subarachnoid space.

DISEASES OF THE SPINE: SPINAL CORD INJURY

I. General Principles
A. Spinal cord injuries may result from vertebral fracture, subluxation, or hyperextension of the cervical spine.
B. Penetrating injuries from gunshot or stab wounds can also result in these injuries.
C. Patients with head injury should be immobilized and placed on a backboard, with immobilization and stabilization of the cervical spine.
D. Next, a complete evaluation and radiologic assessment must be completed.

II. Clinical Features
A. Patients may have tenderness of the spine upon palpation.
B. Numbness, paresthesias, respiratory distress, and hypotension may be present and suggest possible spinal cord injury. Hypotension can occur with lesions above T5.
C. In complete lesions, loss of all motor and sensory function occurs below the lesion. This may include areflexia and autonomic paralysis.
D. Incomplete spinal cord lesions can present with ipsilateral motor paralysis, loss of position/vibration sensation, and contralateral loss of pain and temperature sensation below the level of injury. This is known as the Brown–Séquard syndrome.
E. With cord injury above C3, complete loss of respiratory function occurs. Spinal cord injury can lead to ileus and gastric distension.

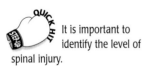
It is important to identify the level of spinal injury.

III. Diagnosis
A. Hemodynamic stability must be achieved.
B. Patients with a cervical collar need complete imaging of the cervical spine.
C. Complete imaging studies include CT scans, MRI, and myelography.

IV. Treatment
A. The goal of treatment is correction of spinal alignment, protection of normal neural tissues, and achievement of spinal stability.
B. Cervical dislocation is corrected with closed or open reduction techniques.
C. Thoracic and lumbar are treated with immobilization. Surgery may be required at a later date.

BENIGN AND MALIGNANT CNS TUMORS

I. Ependymoma
A. General principles
   1. These well-circumscribed lesions occur near the ventricles.
   2. They are spread via CSF pathways.
   3. Median survival approaches 5 years.
B. Clinical features
   1. Elevated intracranial pressure is characteristic.
   2. Nausea, vomiting, and lethargy often occur.
C. Diagnosis. A CT scan or MRI reveals an irregularly enhancing lesion with well-defined borders near the ventricle.
D. Treatment
   1. Aggressive surgical resection.
   2. Radiation therapy.

II. Medulloblastoma
A. General principles
   1. This malignant tumor of the fourth ventricle or vermis occurs due to a maturation arrest of neuroectodermal cells during development.
   2. It is most common before age 20, and more common in males.
   3. The 10-year survival approaches 30%, but can be improved with total mass resection and postoperative radiotherapy.
B. Clinical features
   1. Cerebellar and brain-stem dysfunction occur due to increased intracranial pressure.
   2. Lesions are most common in the midline or lateral cerebellar hemisphere.
C. Diagnosis. CT scan or MRI reveal a nonhomogeneous mass that enhances with contrast, and is located near or in the fourth ventricle.
D. Treatment
   1. Surgical resection and radiotherapy.
   2. CSF seeding is possible.
   3. Chemotherapy is used in young children, whereas radiotherapy is reserved for older individuals.

III. Astrocytoma
A. General principles
   1. This slow-growing tumor has a peak incidence in the fourth decade of life.
   2. Prognosis relates to a variety of factors, including patient age, neurologic status, and tumor histopathology.
   3. Patients with low-grade astrocytomas have a median survival of 5 years, whereas those with anaplastic astrocytomas survive approximately 2 years. Survival is worst with glioblastoma, which has a 1-year median survival rate.
B. Clinical features. Patients may present with seizures, headaches, and focal neurologic defects.

C. Diagnosis. CT scan or MRI reveal an irregular nonhomogeneous enhancing mass with a zone of edema surrounding the lesion.
D. Treatment
1. Aggressive and complete surgical resection
2. Radiotherapy
3. Possible boost radiation therapy to the tumor bed. Brachytherapy may also be considered.
4. Chemotherapy

IV. Meningioma
A. General principles
1. These lesions account for 15% of intracranial neoplasms.
2. They are near the dura with a well-circumscribed border.
3. They often contain calcium, which leads to edema and corresponding cerebral compression.
4. Prognosis relates to the location of the lesion as well as its size.
B. Clinical features. Headache, focal neurologic defects, and seizures may occur.
C. Diagnosis. CT scan and MRI may reveal a homogeneous, contrast-enhancing mass with a well-circumscribed border.
D. Treatment
1. Surgical excision
2. Radiation therapy
3. Chemotherapy for malignant lesions

V. Acoustic Neuroma
A. General principles
1. This lesion arises from the vestibular portion of cranial nerve VIII.
2. Prognosis relates to size of tumor and extent of resection.
B. Clinical features
1. Patients present with tinnitus, hearing loss, and balance disturbance.
2. Hearing loss is gradual. Ability to discriminate speech affected first.
3. Physical examination may reveal facial weakness, and loss of corneal reflex.
4. Nystagmus and gait ataxia are seen with lesions that compress the cerebellum.
C. Diagnosis
1. CT and MRI reveal a mass in the internal auditory meatus.
2. Brain stem-evoked potentials and audiometric evaluation may reveal cranial nerve VIII defects.
D. Treatment
1. Surgical resection
2. Stereotactic radiosurgery

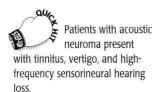 Patients with acoustic neuroma present with tinnitus, vertigo, and high-frequency sensorineural hearing loss.

VI. Metastatic Tumors
A. General principles
1. The most common sources include tumors of the lung, breast, kidney, prostate, and skin (malignant melanoma).
2. 20% of cancer patients develop brain metastasis.
3. Patients with a single metastasis can survive at least 1 year.
B. Clinical features. Increased intracranial pressure, obstructive hydrocephalus, neurologic deficits, and spontaneous cerebral bleeding are seen.
C. Diagnosis
1. CT or MRI reveals a well circumscribed, contrast-enhancing mass surrounded by cerebral edema.
2. Multiple cerebral lesions are common.
D. Treatment
1. Surgical resection should be considered for solitary lesions.
2. Whole-brain radiotherapy may be considered.
3. Corticosteroids may be used.

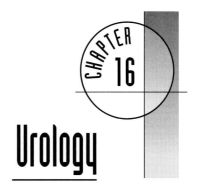

CHAPTER 16

Urology

Susan E. Saunders, MD
Stanley Zaslau, MD, MBA, FACS

KIDNEY

I. Development

A. Three kidney systems are formed embryologically in cranial to caudal sequence: first is the vestigial pronephros in the fourth week of gestation, second is the mesonephros, and third is the metanephros in the fifth week of gestation, which is considered the definitive kidney (Table 16-1). Embryologic abnormalities of kidney formation are shown in Table 16-1.

B. Nephrons are formed from the metanephric mesoderm, and consist of the glomeruli and the excretory tubules (i.e., the proximal convoluted tubule, the loop of Henle, and the distal convoluted tubule).

C. The collecting system of the permanent kidney arises from the ureteric bud, an outgrowth of the mesonephric duct.

D. The ureteric bud penetrates the metanephric tissue, and then dilates to form the renal pelvis and splits into the calyces.

II. Anatomy

A. General principles
1. The kidneys are bean-shaped bilateral structures in the retroperitoneum.
2. They are encased in Gerota fascia.

B. Arterial supply
1. The arterial supply of the kidney is branched with four or more segmental vessels (five is most common). The renal arteries are found posterior to the renal veins.
2. The right renal artery leaves the aorta and then travels behind the inferior vena cava.
3. The left renal artery is shorter than the right renal artery and originates directly from the aorta.
4. The segmental arteries come from the main renal artery.
   a. These then branch into lobar arteries, as they course deeper into the renal parenchyma. These further branch into interlobar arteries, arcuate arteries, interlobular arteries, and afferent arterioles of the glomerulus.
   b. After entering the glomerulus, they branch into efferent arterioles, and then filter into the vasa recta capillary system.

C. Venous supply
1. The venous system begins at the capillaries of the nephron, and drain into progressively larger parts of the venous system. In order, these are the interlobular veins, arcuate veins, lobar veins, and the segmental veins.
2. The right renal vein is short and enters the inferior vena cava directly.
3. The left renal vein crosses anterior to the aorta. It receives three other veins prior to draining into the inferior vena cava. These include the lumbar vein, left gonadal vein, and the left adrenal vein.

TABLE 16-1	Embryologic Abnormalities of Kidney Formation
Embryological Abnormality	**Description**
Pelvic kidney	As the kidneys ascend from the pelvis, they sometimes cannot pass through the umbilical arteries and remain in the pelvis.
Horseshoe kidney	While ascending from the pelvis, the kidneys sometimes get pushed together as they pass through the umbilical arteries and then they fuse at the lower poles. They usually get trapped at the lower lumbar vertebrae by the inferior mesenteric artery.
Renal agenesis	May be unilateral or bilateral. Bilateral agenesis is not compatible with life. It is termed Potter syndrome and is diagnosed by fetal oligohydramnios and absent kidneys on prenatal ultrasound. Renal agenesis is usually secondary to either a failure of the ureteric bud to form or an absence of the nephrogenic ridge.

III. Physiology

A. The kidneys receive 20% of the resting cardiac output, and filter the plasma to remove waste, toxins, and metabolites. The plasma is filtered by the renal tubules.

B. Bowman capsule filters 20% of the plasma.

C. The proximal convoluted tubules absorb 70% of the filtrate.

D. The loop of Henle receives the solute, and concentrates the urine to a certain osmolality.

E. The renin-angiotensin system is an important regulator of blood pressure.

    1. Renin is an enzyme released from the juxtaglomerular apparatus in the kidney. It regulates blood pressure by responding to the changes in the pressure of the afferent arteriole.

    2. Renin acts on angiotensinogen to produce angiotensin I, and then angiotensin II.

    3. Angiotensin II is a potent vasoconstrictor, and it also affects the release of aldosterone from the adrenal cortex.

IV. Diseases of the Kidney

A. Polycystic kidney disease

    1. Autosomal dominant polycystic kidney disease.

      a. This disease is commonly called adult polycystic kidney disease.

      b. The incidence is about 1 in 1,000 people.

      c. It always occurs bilaterally, and causes the kidneys to become massive in size and full of cysts. It accounts for 10% of chronic renal failure.

      d. Symptoms include hematuria, flank pain, hypertension, and proteinuria.

      e. Between 10% and 30% of patients have cerebral Berry aneurysms.

    2. Autosomal recessive polycystic kidney disease.

      a. This rare disorder of bilateral kidney disease presents in infants and young children.

      b. The kidneys are fairly smooth on the outside, but are enlarged by multiple dilated collecting ducts.

      c. The liver is usually cystic as well, and can cause hepatic fibrosis.

      d. Death is secondary to renal failure and congenital hepatic fibrosis.

B. Renal cell carcinoma (RCC) (Fig. 16-1)

    1. 3% of all visceral cancers, and 85% of all renal cancers, are RCC.

    2. The male:female ratio is 2 to 1.

    3. Histologic patterns include clear cell (70%), chromophobe RCC (5%), and papillary RCC (15%).

    4. RCC usually occurs in patients in their 50s and 60s.

    5. An important risk factor is tobacco smoking.

    6. 10% of patients have the classic symptom triad, which includes hematuria, dull flank pain, and a palpable mass.

FIGURE
16-1 Abdomen axial CT. Left renal cell carcinoma (*straight arrows*). The mass lesion is solid, and its border with the normal kidney (*curved arrow*) is poorly defined.

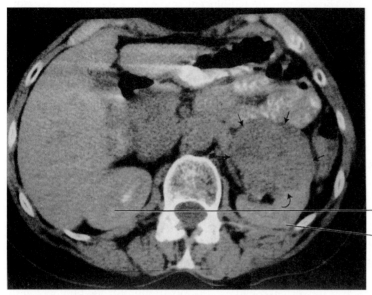

Normal right kidney

Normal portion left kidney

(Reprinted, with permission, from Erkonen WE, Smith WL. *Radiology 101: The Basics and Fundamentals of Imaging*, 2nd ed. Baltimore: Lippincott Williams & Wilkins; 2005.)

7. Diagnosis is made by computed tomography (CT), or magnetic resonance imaging (MRI).
  a. There is no role for percutaneous biopsy, because of the high rate of false-negative results.
  b. Definitive diagnosis is made after surgical removal of the mass.
8. Treatment is surgical, and the standard of treatment is radical nephrectomy if the contralateral kidney is normal.
  a. Laparoscopic radical nephrectomy has shown to have similar survival in the literature, and has less recovery time for the patient.
  b. Nephron-sparing partial nephrectomy is indicated in a solitary kidney, bilateral kidney tumors, and von Hippel–Lindau disease.
    (1) Relative indications for partial nephrectomy include a small tumor (4 cm or smaller) with a normal contralateral kidney.
    (2) Local recurrence is less than 10%.
    (3) There is a high incidence of urinary fistula, which is treated with conservative management including a ureteral stent and Foley catheter drainage.
    (4) RCC sometimes invades the inferior vena cava.
9. Chemotherapy for RCC has limited success. Two adjuvant therapies used are interleukin-2 and interferon.
10. Metastatic renal cell carcinoma may still be managed surgically if there are solitary metastasis or for purposes of cytoreduction. RCC is thought to metastasize via both the lymphatics and hematogenous spread.
11. Recurrence of RCC is rare for patients with stage T1 and T2 tumors. 5-year survival for patients with stage T3 tumors is about 40%.
12. Follow-up after surgical removal of RCC is performed at 6-month intervals, and includes liver function testing, chest x-ray (CXR), urinalysis, and CT scan of the abdomen and pelvis.

V. Urinary Tract Calculi
  A. Incidence is 20 in 10,000, and more common in males.
  B. Types of kidney stones:
    1. Calcium oxalate (60%).
    2. Calcium phosphate (10% to 20%).

3. Struvite (10%). These stones form in the presence of urease-producing infectious organisms.

4. Uric acid (10%). These stones are radiolucent, and cannot typically be seen on plain films, but can be seen on CT scan.

5. Cystine (1%).

C. Kidney stones typically become lodged and cause obstruction at one of the following anatomic places:

  1. Ureteropelvic junction.

  2. Mid to distal ureter at the location that the iliac vessel crosses the ureter.

  3. Ureterovesical junction.

D. Clinical features

  1. Flank pain, is colicky in nature, with nausea and vomiting.

  2. Hematuria may occur.

E. Diagnosis

  1. CT scan without contrast is the most common test ordered in the emergency department for flank pain. This test also shows whether or not a stone causes obstruction and hydronephrosis (Fig. 16-2).

  2. Ultrasound: this test is not optimal for calculi, but will show whether or not there is hydronephrosis. Sometimes stones can be visualized as well.

  3. X-rays of the kidneys, ureter, and bladder (plain x-ray of the abdomen and pelvis).

    a. Advantages: it is inexpensive, and a good way to monitor the progression of a stone.

    b. Disadvantages: it does not show all stones (especially the radiolucent stones such as uric acid or cystine stones), and it does not typically show hydronephrosis.

  4. Urinalysis: may reveal microscopic hematuria.

  5. Creatinine: reveals acute renal insufficiency from obstruction secondary to stones.

F. Treatment

  1. Medical management

    a. Patients may be given a trial of passage of the stone. Typically, stones less than 5 mm can be passed.

     (1) The patient is given pain medication, and instructed to drink plenty of water and strain their urine.

FIGURE 16-2 Urolithiasis. Computed tomographic scan of a patient with right renal collecting system calculus.

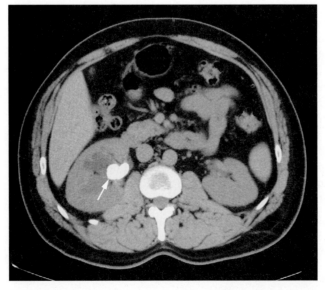

(Reprinted, with permission, from Zaslau S. *Blueprints Urology*. Baltimore: Lippincott Williams & Wilkins; 2004.)

(2) Any stones passed should be kept and analyzed for their organic composition.

b. Patients who are frequent stone formers should have serum parathyroid hormone and calcium levels taken to evaluate for hyperparathyroidism. They should also have citrate levels and uric acid levels as well as a 24-hour urine study.

2. Surgical management

a. Extracorporeal shock wave lithotripsy (ESWL) is a method in which focused high-pressure shock waves are aimed at the stones with the use of fluoroscopy or ultrasound. The stones are then broken into smaller fragments, so that the patient can pass them.

(1) Complications of ESWL include transient hypertension, subcapsular renal hematoma, failure to completely break stones, urosepsis, and Steinstrasse syndrome. Steinstrasse syndrome is a large quantity of stone fragments with may accumulate, and block the ureter.

(2) Contraindications include inability to localize the stone secondary to the stone being radiopaque, pregnancy, and bleeding disorders.

b. Ureteroscopy is a method in which a small-caliber instrument called a ureteroscope is advanced into the ureter and into the kidney. The stone can then be retrieved with a basket or grasper and endoscopically removed from the urinary tract.

(1) If the stone is too large to safely remove manually, it may be broken into smaller fragments with a laser and then removed.

(2) Complications include damage to the ureter including perforation, strictures, avulsion, and sepsis.

c. Percutaneous nephrolithotripsy is a method for stone removal that is usually reserved for patients with a staghorn calculus, a significant stone burden, or any stones that the surgeon is unable to remove with the aforementioned methods.

(1) The patient has a nephrostomy access placed.

(2) Next, a scope is advanced into the renal pelvis and the stones are removed manually.

(3) If the stones are too large to remove manually, then they may be broken up with laser fibers prior to removal.

d. Open surgery for stone retrieval has largely fallen out of favor, secondary to the invasive nature of this procedure. It is still performed occasionally for large complete staghorn calculi.

BLADDER

I. Development

A. The bladder is formed during the fourth to seventh weeks of development. It is formed by the division of the cloacae into an anal canal posteriorly, and a urogenital sinus anteriorly. The largest portion of the urogenital sinus becomes the bladder.

B. The apex of the bladder is connected to the urachus during development. The urachus eventually becomes the median umbilical ligament.

II. Anatomy

A. General principles

1. The bladder sits atop of the prostate in the male. It is anterior to the vagina in the female.

2. Three layers of muscle make up the bladder: the inner longitudinal layer, the middle circular layer, and the outer longitudinal layer. The inner layer is covered by transitional epithelium.

3. The inside view of the bladder includes the lateral walls of the bladder, dome of the bladder, and the triangular base of the bladder which is known as the trigone.

4. The ureteral orifices are the two holes in which the ureters are connected to the bladder. They enter the bladder on either side of the trigone at the base of the bladder.

B. Vascular blood supply of the bladder
   1. The arterial supply of the bladder is supplied by the inferior vesical and superior vesical artery. Both are arteries are branches of the internal iliac artery.
   2. Venous drainage of the bladder terminates in the internal iliac veins.

C. Innervation of the bladder
   1. Sympathetic innervation of the bladder originates from T10 to L2 spinal nerves.
   2. Parasympathetic innervation of the bladder comes from S2 to S4 spinal nerves.

III. Transitional Cell Carcinoma

A. General principles
   1. Transitional cell carcinoma (TCC) comprises 90% of all bladder cancers.
   2. The tumors can be papillary, sessile, or ulcerative.
   3. TCC is newly diagnosed in about 53,000 people in the United States annually.
   4. TCC of the bladder is a slow-growing tumor. However, it is often recurrent. About 50% of low-grade cancers recur, and 80% to 90% of high-grade cancers recur.
   5. Factors that cause TCC include smoking, exposure to cyclophosphamide, or industrial exposure to arylamine.

B. Clinical features
   1. The most common presentation for TCC of the bladder is gross or microscopic hematuria. This is the presenting symptom in about 90% of patients with newly diagnosed TCC.
   2. Patients may also have irritative voiding symptoms, also known as lower urinary tract symptoms. These include urgency, frequency, and dysuria.

C. Diagnosis
   1. A voided urine specimen may be sent for cytology to screen for malignant cells.
   2. Imaging studies may find a suspicious bladder wall thickening, or a large bladder mass. Imaging modalities include CT scan, ultrasound, and MRI.
   3. The standard for diagnosis of a bladder cancer is cystoscopy. Cystoscopy can be performed under local anesthesia. A flexible cystoscope or a rigid cystoscope may be used to enter the bladder. Masses are found by direct visualization.

D. Treatment
   1. Initial staging of the bladder cancer must be determined by transurethral resection of the bladder tumor (TURBT).
      a. This procedure is performed by inserting a resectoscope through the urethra, and into the bladder.
      b. The tumor is then resected off of the bladder wall using cautery.
      c. The tissue is then sent to pathology to diagnose the extent of invasion.
      d. Complications include bladder wall perforation.
   2. If the TCC is stage T1, management includes surveillance cystoscopy with TURBT for any recurrence. The patient should have surveillance cystoscopy every 3 months for 2 years, then every 6 months for 2 more years, and then every year thereafter.
   3. Bacillus Calmette–Guérin therapy is performed by intravesical infusion of an attenuated strain of *Mycobacterium bovis*. This exerts an antitumor effect by an unknown mechanism. This is a very effective therapy for patients with carcinoma *in situ* to prevent recurrence.
   4. Other chemotherapeutic agents include mitomycin C (Thiotepa) and doxorubicin.
   5. Partial cystectomy is a procedure for removing the part of the bladder that is affected by the tumor. It is reserved for tumors that cannot be resected via TURBT secondary to bladder wall thinning at that region. An example would be a tumor inside of a bladder diverticulum.

UROLOGY

6. Radical cystectomy is the standard of care for muscle invasive TCC of the bladder.
   a. This procedure includes removal of the prostate and seminal vesicles in men and removal of the uterus, cervix, and ovaries in women.
   b. A lymph node dissection is also performed at the time of cystectomy.
   c. The ureter drainage must be diverted. There are many methods of diversion; including continent diversions, as well as the more common noncontinent urostomies such as the ileal conduit. The ileal conduit is the most common choice for urinary diversion in the United States.
      (1) In this diversion, a piece of the ileum that is about 20 cm from the ileocecal valve is utilized to bring a urostomy to the skin.
      (2) The ureters are implanted to the ileal pouch, and then drain the urine into an ostomy bag.

IV. Neurogenic Bladder

A. General principles
   1. Neurogenic bladder is the loss of normal function of the bladder secondary to damage to part of the nervous system.
   2. Causes include any disease process that can damage the nerve fibers that innervate the bladder. These include traumatic spinal cord injury, spinal cord neoplasm, spina bifida, stroke, multiple sclerosis, cerebral palsy, Parkinson disease, and others.
B. Clinical features. Symptoms include urinary incontinence, urinary retention, frequent urinary tract infections, pyelonephritis, urinary urgency, and urinary frequency.
C. Diagnosis
   1. Tests should be performed to locate the neuroanatomic lesion. These tests include CT or MRI of brain, electroencephalography, and films of the spine.
   2. The standard test for diagnosis of neurogenic bladder is cystoscopy with complex urodynamics.
      a. The urodynamics procedure is performed by inserting a urethral catheter, and placing electrodes on the perineum to assess the contractions of accessory muscles and the detrusor contraction, during filling as well as voiding.
      b. Urodynamics can detect detrusor hyperreflexia, as well as sphincteric dysfunction.
D. Treatment
   1. Behavioral therapy
      a. Clean intermittent catheterization is an excellent way of managing a patient with urinary retention, and neurogenic bladder. Patients are instructed to void on their own, and then to catheterize themselves to remove the postvoid residual urine in their bladder.
      b. Scheduled voiding can be used for patients with urinary incontinence. This decreases the amount of episodes of incontinence during the day.
   2. Medical management
      a. Anticholinergic therapy is used to decrease the bladder contractility, and thus to decrease the amount of involuntary bladder contractions.
         (1) This treatment works by inhibiting the postganglionic parasympathetic receptors in the bladder smooth muscle.
         (2) The agents do have significant side effects for the patient including dry mouth and constipation.
      b. Prophylactic antibiotics may be considered for patients with recurrent urinary tract infections.
   3. Surgical management
      a. Bladder augmentation is performed to increase the bladder size with accessory tissues.
      b. Paralytic agents such as botulinum toxin may be injected to relax the urethral sphincter.

V. Interstitial Cystitis

A. General principles

1. Interstitial cystitis (IC) is a constellation of symptoms including pelvic pain, urgency, frequency, dyspareunia, and severe dysuria.
2. The female to male ratio is 8 to 1.
3. Findings at cystoscopy include glomerulations (submucosal hemorrhages) on the bladder mucosa. The patients also may have diffuse cystitis.
4. Patients with symptoms consistent with IC must be evaluated for urinary tract infection, cancer, or other urinary tract disorders prior to the diagnosis of IC.
5. The etiology of IC is not known. Many theories have been proposed. These include the presence of a fastidious infectious organism, and that the condition results from an autoimmune disfunction. The current theory is that the condition results from a defect in the glycosaminoglycan layer of the bladder mucosa. This defect is proposed to leave the bladder mucosa permeable to small molecules such as potassium. These molecules are thought to irritate the bladder mucosa, and cause bladder mast cells to secrete inflammatory mediators. Nerve stimulation and detrusor muscle depolarization also occur.

B. Diagnosis

1. IC is a diagnosis of exclusion. Urine cultures should be negative, and urine voided cytology should be negative for malignant cells.
2. An upper urinary tract study is warranted to evaluate the possibility of upper urinary tract disease causing the symptoms. Such a study should consist of either an ultrasound of the kidneys, or a CT scan of the abdomen and pelvis.
3. Cystoscopy should be performed to evaluate the bladder mucosa. Often times, patients with IC have evidence of cystitis cystica (inflammation of the bladder) or glomerulations of the bladder mucosa.

C. Treatment

1. Medical management
   a. Tricyclic antidepressants are frequently utilized to stabilize the mast cells and block histamine receptors. They also treat neuropathic pain.
   b. Anticholinergic therapy may be used to treat the symptoms of urgency and frequency by inhibiting parasympathetic receptors.
   c. Sodium pentosanpolysulfate (Elmiron) is a heparin-like glycosaminoglycan. It is partially excreted in the urine.
      (1) It is given orally, and has been shown to have some effect on pelvic pain associated with IC.
      (2) It takes 3 to 6 months for a patient to experience a significant response.
   d. Intravesical dimethyl sulfoxide is a treatment administered into the bladder. It acts as an anti-inflammatory agent and also modulates the immune system.

2. Surgical management
   a. There is no role for cystectomy in patients with IC.
   b. Sacral neuromodulation is a surgical therapy that is gaining popularity for refractory cases of urgency/frequency.
      (1) This is a procedure in which an electrode is inserted into the S3 sacral nerve foramen.
      (2) A stimulator is connected to an implantable battery pack placed under the skin. The stimulator sends impulses that stimulate the S3 nerve root.
      (3) It is thought that the electrical stimulation excites the pudendal nerves, and then modulates a reflex to stabilize the bladder contractions. Preliminary results are promising.
   c. Hydrodistention of the bladder is an effective method that provides temporary relief of symptoms of IC.
      (1) During this procedure, the bladder is distended above its capacity under anesthesia.
      (2) This provides temporary relief from frequency for up to 6 to 8 months.

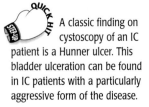

A classic finding on cystoscopy of an IC patient is a Hunner ulcer. This bladder ulceration can be found in IC patients with a particularly aggressive form of the disease.

PROSTATE

I. Development
A. The urogenital sinus develops from the cloaca at the 28th day of gestation.
B. The prostate gland forms as an outgrowth of the urethra. The stimulus for this development is testosterone secreted from the testes and dihydrotestosterone (DHT).

II. Anatomy
A. General principles
1. The prostate is a bilobed firm glandular structure covered by a capsule.
   a. It is found between the bladder neck and the verumontanum, next to the external sphincter.
   b. It is bordered posteriorly by the rectum, and thus is palpable in men on digital rectal examination (DRE).
2. The zones of the prostate include the peripheral zone, the central zone, and the transition zone.
3. The urethra runs through the center of the prostate.
4. The prostate emits a molecule called prostate-specific antigen (PSA). The function of this molecule is to liquefy the seminal coagulum after ejaculation.
B. Blood supply
1. Arterial supply is from the prostatic artery, that originates from the inferior vesical artery, which comes from the internal iliac artery.
2. Venous drainage is via the hypogastric veins.

III. Prostate Cancer
A. General principles
1. The incidence of adenocarcinoma of the prostate is about 180,000 new cases per year. It is one of the most common cancers among men.
2. Prostate cancer is more likely to occur at the peripheral zone of the prostate.
3. The cause of prostate cancer is unknown. It is more likely to occur in a patient who has a first degree relative with prostate cancer, and it is more likely in African-Americans.
4. Prostate tumors spread by direct extension into the seminal vesicles, or by extracapsular extension via the periprostatic nerve routes. Lymphatic metastasis also occurs. Most distant metastasis occurs in the bones.
5. Prostate cancer is a slow-growing cancer. The patients who have low-grade disease, and are treated for their disease have a less than 10% chance of cancer-related mortality in 10 years.
6. Gleason grading is a system of tumor grading that takes into account the glandular differentiation of the cancer. The scores range from 2 to 10, with the higher numbers representing increasingly more aggressive tumors.
B. Clinical features
1. Patients with prostate cancer often report no symptoms. They may have symptoms of urinary obstruction, hematuria, and bone pain if distant metastasis has occurred.
2. DRE may reveal a prostate nodule. Absence of a nodule does not exclude the presence of cancer, and presence of a nodule does not automatically mean that the patient has disease.
C. Diagnosis
1. PSA is the most useful laboratory test. The American Cancer Society recommends that serum PSA and yearly DRE be performed in men over the age of 50. The cutoff for an abnormal PSA is any value above 2.0 ng/mL. Acid phosphatase is another serum marker.
2. Prostate needle biopsy is a transrectal, ultrasound-guided procedure to obtain prostatic tissue for pathologic diagnosis. Several cores are obtained from each lobe of the prostate, as well as at the transitional zone. This procedure is often performed under local anesthesia in the office setting.

3. Bone scans are used to assess for distant bone metastasis.
4. CT and MRI are utilized to view the potential of local invasion and lymph node metastasis.

D. Treatment
1. Radical prostatectomy is the standard of therapy for a patient that is expected to survive greater than 10 years, and has organ confined disease.
   a. This surgical procedure is usually performed open via retropubic approach, or using a robotics approach to assist in dissection.
   b. It is common practice to perform nerve-sparing procedures to help reduce the amount of postoperative erectile dysfunction.
   c. Approximately 6% of patients also experience significant urinary incontinence from the procedure.
2. Brachytherapy is a less invasive therapy for organ-confined prostate disease. This procedure consists of ultrasound-guided placement of radioactive seeds into the prostate that emit radiation to destroy prostatic tissue.
   a. Results are better for prostate cancer with a lower Gleason score.
   b. Some side effects include urinary retention, urethritis, and irritative voiding symptoms.
3. External beam radiation therapy is the treatment preferred for T3 disease with extracapsular extension.
   a. Complications of this therapy include radiation cystitis, hematuria or hemorrhagic cystitis, and erectile dysfunction.
   b. The side effects are decreasing, as techniques are improving to protect the bladder from stray radiation.
4. Bilateral orchiectomy is removal of the testicles. This procedure is performed for advanced prostate cancer to remove all androgens. Because prostate cancer is receptive to androgens, ablating the androgens causes about 40% of the tumors to regress. Side effects include hot flashes and loss of libido, as well as erectile dysfunction.
5. Medical castration has the same principle as surgical castration, which is to remove all androgen activity. This is accomplished medically by administering luteinizing, hormone-releasing hormone (LHRH) agonists. LHRH agonists cause an initial increase in testosterone followed by a decrease in the receptors.
   a. The medication is administered either monthly, or every 3 to 4 months.
   b. Side effects are the same as those caused with surgical castration.

IV. Benign Prostatic Hyperplasia
A. General principles
1. Benign prostatic hyperplasia (BPH) is caused by benign growth in prostate tissue as men age. Up to 50% of men older than 50 years of age have BPH, but it is not usually clinically significant.
2. Causes of BPH are not fully understood. According to some theories, BPH is caused by increasing estrogen levels in men as they age.
3. BPH forms in the transitional zone of the prostate, which is the zone that encircles the urethra. This often causes obstructive voiding symptoms in patients who suffer from BPH.

B. Clinical features
1. Patients who have BPH often complain of a decreased urine stream, urinary hesitancy, frequency, urgency, and straining to void.
2. Patients can have episodes of urinary retention.

C. Diagnosis
1. Serum PSA may be slightly elevated in patients with BPH.
2. Imaging studies such as renal ultrasound are sufficient to evaluate the kidneys and ureters for hydronephrosis. Hydronephrosis is usually bilateral if caused by BPH.
3. Cystoscopy is the standard for evaluating a patient with obstructive voiding symptoms, and possible BPH.

    a. Because the prostate can be visualized while advancing the cystoscope through the prostatic urethra, cystoscopy is an excellent way to visualize the size of the prostate, and the amount of bladder outlet obstruction the prostate is causing.

    b. Other findings on cystoscopy include thickening of the bladder wall musculature, known as trabeculations, which is caused by a bladder that is constantly straining to achieve micturition.

4. Postvoid residual (PVR) is a useful study that can be performed by having the patient empty his bladder, and then using an ultrasound bladder scanner to assess the amount of urine that remains after micturition. This value can also be obtained with a simple straight catheterization of the bladder. Patients with BPH often have a PVR greater than 50 to 100 mL.

5. Urodynamics is a useful study that can rule out other causes of voiding dysfunction for a patient with obstructive voiding symptoms and possible BPH. This also measures the flow rate during voiding, which is often markedly decreased in patients with BPH.

D. Treatment

1. Medical management

    a. Alpha blockers are often used to treat patients with BPH. These medications work on the alpha-1-adrenoreceptors found in the prostate and bladder. The blockade of alpha receptors causes a decrease in the amount of alpha–receptor-moderated muscle tone in the prostate and bladder.

      (1) Treatment with these medications results in improved urinary flow rate and symptom scores.

      (2) Side effects include hypotension, dizziness, and retrograde ejaculation.

    b. 5-Alpha reductase inhibitors such as finasteride and dutasteride are competitive selective inhibitors of 5-alpha reductase.

      (1) These agents decrease the amount of prostatic DHT, which then causes a decrease in the size of the prostate.

      (2) Side effects include loss of libido and ejaculatory dysfunction.

2. Surgical management

    a. The most common method of resection of BPH is transurethral resection of the prostate (TURP). This method utilizes electrocautery to remove excess prostatic tissue. This is performed using a resecting endoscope inserted through the penis.

      (1) Patients may have significant hematuria, erectile dysfunction, or even urinary incontinence after the procedure.

      (2) Another risk is transurethral resection syndrome, caused by absorption of the hypotonic irrigating solution that is infused into the bladder during the procedure. This can cause hypervolemia and hyponatremia, which leads to confusion, visual disturbances, and cardiac arrhythmias.

    b. Laser TURP is a relatively new variation of TURP. This utilizes the same principle as traditional TURP. However, a laser is used to resect the prostatic tissue as opposed to electrocautery. Advantages of this procedure are a decreased amount of hematuria after the procedure, and a decreased risk of transurethral resection syndrome.

    c. Open prostatectomy is utilized when the prostate is too large (over 100 grams) to remove transurethrally.

V. Prostatitis

A. General principles

1. Prostatitis can be broken down into three groups.

    a. The first group is less common, and is called acute bacterial prostatitis. This type of prostatitis is caused by a severe urinary tract infection, and causes significant pain as well as fevers and chills. A bacterial organism is cultured from the prostatic secretions of the urine.

b. The second group is chronic bacterial prostatitis. This type of prostatitis causes symptoms such as chronic pelvic, perineal, or low back pain. Patients may also have pain after ejaculating or irritative voiding symptoms. Recurrent bacterial organisms can be cultured in the urine or prostatic secretions.

c. The third group, the most common group, is called chronic abacterial prostatitis. The symptoms are the same as chronic bacterial prostatitis. However, no organisms can be cultured.

B. Diagnosis
   1. Diagnosis of prostatitis is usually based upon history.
   2. Patients often experience reproduction of their pelvic pain upon DRE.
   3. Attempt to culture an organism is made using either the voided urine specimen, or by milking prostatic secretions and culturing the secretions.

C. Treatment
   1. Treatment is via medical management. Patients are usually given 6 weeks of antibiotics, as well as nonsteroidal anti-inflammatory drugs, such as ibuprofen. Some patients require chronic prophylactic antibiotics.
   2. Complications of prostatitis include prostatitic abscess. This can be diagnosed with transrectal ultrasound, and can be drained by percutaneous drainage.

PENIS

I. Development
A. The external genitalia in the male develops at 10 weeks of age.
B. The phallus elongates, and pulls the urethral folds together until they form the urethral groove.
C. During the third month of gestation, the urethral folds close over the urethral plate to form the penile urethra.

II. Anatomy
A. General principles
   1. Three tissue bodies comprise the penis. These include the paired erectile corpora cavernosa and the corpus spongiosum, which contains the urethra.
   2. Sexual desire and parasympathetic stimulation causes erection by causing relaxation in the cavernosal arterial smooth muscles. Arterial engorgement of the corpora cavernosa prevents venous outflow from the corpora to cause erection.
B. Arterial supply to the penis comes from the internal pudendal artery. The deep artery of the penis runs through the center of the erectile body. Superficial blood supply is supplied by the external pudendal artery.
C. Venous drainage comes from the deep dorsal vein of the penis.

III. Priapism
A. General principles
   1. Priapism is defined as a painful erection that lasts over 4 hours. This erection is not relieved by orgasm. This condition is a urologic emergency, because it can damage the erectile tissue and cause impotence.
   2. There are two types of priapism: high flow (nonischemic), and low flow (ischemic priapism).
      a. High-flow priapism can be idiopathic or as a result of trauma.
      b. Low-flow priapism can be idiopathic, can occur as a result of prescription or recreational drug abuse (especially cocaine), or as a result of sickle cell disease or leukemia.
B. Diagnosis
   1. History taking is important when evaluating a patient with priapism. This is to identify a cause for the problem, including drug abuse or past medical history.

2. Physical examination often reveals a firm penis with a flaccid glans. The penis is often very tender to palpation.
3. Laboratory values that must be obtained include a drug screen, a CBC, hemoglobin electrophoresis if sickle cell anemia is suspected, and a cavernosal blood gas.
   a. In high-flow priapism, the blood gas taken from the cavernosa is similar to that of the arterial blood gas (ABG) obtained peripherally.
   b. In low-flow priapism, the corporal blood gas usually reveals a pH of less than 7.25 and a PCO_2 of over 60.
4. Ultrasound of the cavernosa can be performed to determine if the priapism is high flow or low flow.

C. Treatment
1. Low-flow priapism
   a. The initial treatment includes corporal aspiration and irrigation.
   b. After aspiration and irrigation, corporal injection of alpha agonists should be performed.
      (1) The alpha agonists that should be injected include epinephrine and phenylephrine. The patient should be on a cardiac monitor while these medications are being injected.
      (2) If the penis does not reach detumescence, then the injection of epinephrine or phenylephrine may be repeated every 5 minutes up to three times.
   c. If the penis is still erect, then a distal cavernosal shunt (Winter shunt) may be performed.
   d. If the condition recurs, then a proximal cavernosospongiosal shunt may be performed.
2. High-flow priapism
   a. Treatment begins with a pelvic angiogram with embolization or observation. Embolization may be repeated if the penis is still erect.
   b. Failure of embolization can be treated with surgical management as discussed above.

IV. Peyronie Disease
A. General principles
1. Peyronie disease is defined as an idiopathic curvature of the penis that is acquired, and commonly presents in men age 40 and over.
2. It is caused by scarring or fibrosis of the tunica albuginea, and causes a fibrous plaque. Causes of the disease are thought to be secondary to microtrauma to the penis.
3. The incidence is less than about 2% of the male population, and is more common in Caucasian men.
4. The disease has been associated with patients who also have Dupuytren contracture of the hands.

B. Diagnosis
1. Patients with Peyronie disease often complain of curved, painful erections, and a palpable plaque on the shaft of the penis.
2. Physical examination usually reveals a palpable fibrous plaque.
3. Ultrasound is not necessary, but may be utilized when the examination findings are not impressive enough to make the diagnosis.

C. Treatment
1. Medical management
   a. Potassium para-aminobenzoate to reduce pain and improve curvature.
   b. Vitamin E supplements.
   c. Nonsteroidal anti-inflammatory agents.
   d. Calcium-channel blockers.
2. Surgical management. Surgery, including plaque excision with graft to the excised portion of tunica albuginea is the most effective treatment for refractory cases of Peyronie disease, that cause impotence or severe deformity.

V. Erectile Dysfunction

A. General principles

1. It is estimated that up to 25 million American men suffer from erectile dysfunction (ED).

2. There are many causes of ED. Its origins may be vasculogenic, psychogenic, neurogenic, endocrine, or iatrogenic.

   a. Vasculogenic causes include diabetes mellitus, atherosclerosis, or thromboembolic disease.

   b. Psychogenic causes include anxiety, depression, and posttraumatic stress disorders.

   c. Neurogenic causes include diabetic neuropathy, and any disease that causes lesions in either the peripheral or central nervous system (e.g., multiple sclerosis or spinal cord injury).

   d. Endocrine causes include any disease that causes primary or secondary hypogonadism (e.g., Prader-Willi syndrome, Kallmann syndrome).

   e. Iatrogenic causes include drugs such as alcohol, and selective serotonin reuptake inhibitors.

B. Diagnosis

1. A careful history should be taken to attempt to determine the cause of the ED.

2. Physical examination should be performed to assess the neurologic, vascular, and genitourinary systems.

3. Laboratory values necessary to evaluate a patient for ED include prolactin level, testosterone level, fasting blood sugar, and even cholesterol studies.

4. Nocturnal penile tumescence testing measures the ability of a patient to achieve erection while sleeping. The normal number of erections is four or more per night.

C. Treatment

1. Medical management

   a. Phosphodiesterase inhibitors include sildenafil, vardenafil, tadalafil.

      (1) These agents work by inhibiting the enzyme phosphodiesterase to achieve elevated levels of cyclic GMP. Cyclic GMP then causes an increase in nitric oxide which in turn causes engorgement of the corpora cavernosa.

      (2) Side effects include headache, visual disturbance, flushing, and hypotension. These drugs may not be used in patients taking nitrates secondary to risk of hypotension.

   b. Intracavernosal injection therapy is with prostaglandin E1, an injectable agent that the patient must inject into the corpora cavernosa prior to intercourse. It is very effective. However, side effects include burning and pain, as well as corporal fibrosis.

   c. Vacuum erection devices are mechanical treatments that involve using a pump to create a pressure gradient that causes filling of the cavernosa.

   d. If a patient has low testosterone, topical testosterone cream may assist with increasing the patient's libido.

2. Surgical management

   a. Surgical management is reserved for refractory cases. This treatment involves placement of a penile prosthesis. There are several types of penile prostheses, including mechanical, inflatable, and malleable devices.

      (1) Malleable rods are paired implants that are placed into the corpora cavernosa. The patient has a constant semirigid penis.

      (2) Inflatable devices are placed and allow the patient to pump the penis to the erect state prior to intercourse.

   b. Complications of penile prosthesis include infection, erosion, and device malfunction requiring revision.

VI. Penile Cancer

A. General principles

1. The incidence is about 1 in 100,000.

2. Risk factors include uncircumcised phallus, balanitis, Bowen disease, poor hygiene, and human papilloma virus.

3. The 5-year survival rate is 65% to 80% for patients without palpable adenopathy, and 20% to 50% for patients with palpable adenopathy.
4. The most common pathologic type of penile cancer is squamous cell carcinoma.

B. Diagnosis
   1. Diagnosis is by physical examination of the penis and foreskin, which reveals an abnormal skin lesion.
   2. Biopsy is necessary for pathological diagnosis.
   3. CT scan or MRI is needed to assess lymph node involvement.

C. Treatment
   1. If lesion is confined to prepuce, circumcision is indicated.
   2. Tumors of the glans or penile shaft should be resected surgically, with partial or total penectomy (removal of penis) with at least a 2-cm margin.
   3. Patients with palpable inguinal lymphadenopathy require inguinal lymph node dissection.

URETHRA

I. Development and Anatomy

A. Development. The urethral folds close over the urethral plate to form the penile urethra during the third month of gestation.

B. Anatomy.
   1. General principles.
      a. The male urethra is divided into four parts, which include (from proximal to distal): the prostatic urethra, the membranous urethra, the bulbar urethra, and the penile urethra.
      b. The type of epithelium in the urethra changes from transitional epithelium to squamous epithelium at the distal portion.
   2. Blood supply. The urethra obtains arterial blood supply from the internal pudendal artery, and its venous drainage goes to the internal pudendal vein.

II. Hypospadias

A. General principles
   1. Hypospadias is a congenital malformation in which the urethral meatus opens onto the ventral side of the penis. This results from incomplete fusion of the urethral folds in utero.
   2. Incidence is 1 in 300 live male births
   3. There are five classifications of hypospadias:
      a. Coronal, in which the meatus is at the coronal sulcus.
      b. Glandular, in which the meatus is on the proximal glans penis.
      c. Meatal opening on the penile shaft.
      d. Scrotal hypospadias, when the meatus is at the base of the penis at the scrotal level.
      e. Penoscrotal hypospadias, when the meatus opens onto the perineum.
   4. Significance
      a. Hypospadias does not usually cause any problems for an infant.
      b. It becomes problematic as the child ages, and is unable to urinate with a straight stream.
      c. Associated with chordee (curvature of the penis), which can make intercourse difficult once the patient becomes mature.

B. Diagnosis: Based on physical examination findings of the above classification of hypospadias.

C. Treatment
   1. Surgical correction is the only treatment for hypospadias.
   2. Hypospadias can be surgically corrected after 4 months of age, but should be done prior to the child entering school. The child should not be circumcised prior to surgical correction of hypospadias.

3. There are many different methods of surgical correction. The repair usually involves straightening the penis by removing the chordee, and urethral reconstruction utilizing a graft that usually comes from the excess foreskin.
4. Complications of hypospadias repair include urethrocutaneous fistula in up to 30% of patients. This is repaired surgically.

SCROTUM

I. Development and Anatomy
A. Development. The male bilateral scrotal swellings fuse at the scrotal septum during development.
B. Anatomy
   1. General principles.
      a. The scrotum houses the testicles and epididymis.
      b. The scrotal sac consists of skin, dartos muscle, external spermatic fascia, cremasteric muscle, internal spermatic fascia, and tunica vaginalis.
   2. Blood supply
      a. The anterior scrotum derives its blood supply from the external pudendal artery.
      b. The posterior scrotum derives its blood supply from the cremasteric and testicular arteries.

II. Hydrocele
A. General principles
   1. Hydroceles are a collection of fluid between the parietal and visceral layers of the tunica vaginalis.
      a. In infants, they are caused by a patent processus vaginalis that allows peritoneal fluid to enter the scrotum.
      b. In adults, they are thought to be from a secretory imbalance in the tunica vaginalis.
   2. Hydroceles present as a scrotal swelling that transilluminates.
      a. In infants, they are usually painless.
      b. In adults, they can become large enough to cause discomfort or pain.
B. Diagnosis
   1. Hydroceles present as a scrotal swelling that transilluminates to light on physical examination.
   2. Ultrasound of the scrotum can be performed to confirm the diagnosis.
C. Treatment
   1. In infants, hydroceles can be monitored until 1 year of age. This is unlike inguinal hernias, which should be fixed as soon as possible; secondary to a risk of incarceration of the hernia sac. Many hydroceles spontaneously resolve by 1 year of age.
   2. In infants older than 1 year of age with continued hydrocele, surgical management is indicated. Hydrocelectomy is performed to ligate the patent processus vaginalis.
   3. In adults, surgical management is indicated only if the hydrocele is large enough to bother the patients' daily life or if the hydrocele is painful.

III. Fournier Gangrene
A. General principles
   1. Fournier gangrene was first described by a French physician named Fournier in the late 1800s.
   2. This condition is defined by a necrotizing fasciitis of the scrotum that travels up the lower abdomen. This is a urologic emergency with mortality rates up to 50%.
   3. Symptoms include a painful, erythematous scrotum that rapidly progresses within hours, and can travel up the abdomen. Crepitance of the erythematous region can be palpated if the offending organism is a gas-forming bacteria.

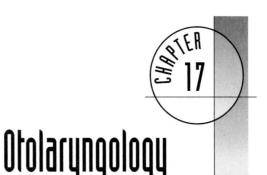

Otolaryngology

Adam Cassis, MD
Matthew Oliverio, MD

COMMON OTOLARYNGOLOGIC CONDITIONS

I. Acute Sinusitis

A. General principles

1. Infection of the paranasal sinuses for less than 4 weeks.
2. Usually results from upper respiratory infection (about the second week of the upper respiratory infection [URI]).
3. Minimal mucosal inflammation can obstruct the drainage of the sinuses, leading to bacterial infection of retained sinus secretions.
4. Most common pathogens are *Streptococcus pneumoniae*, *Haemophilus influenzae*, and *Moraxella catarrhalis*.

B. Clinical features

1. Nasal congestion, facial pain, headache, and anosmia.
2. Postnasal drip and purulent drainage.

C. Diagnosis

1. Laboratory studies: HIV and immunoglobulin serologies are useful if there is any evidence of an immunocompromised state.
2. Endoscopic evaluation: visualize purulent drainage, as well as septal deviation, nasal polyps, and other obstructing features that may cause blockage of sinus drainage.
3. Imaging
   a. Computed tomography (CT) scan: method of choice, and can assess bony structures, as well as evaluate for air–fluid levels and mucosal thickening.
   b. Magnetic resonance imaging (MRI): does not image bone as well as CT, but good for differentiating soft-tissue masses from retained mucus.

D. Treatment

1. Medical management
   a. Prevention
      (1) Nasal saline or nasal steroids.
      (2) Allergy management (antihistamines, environmental control, immunotherapy).
      (3) Oxymetazoline spray: causes vasoconstriction of nasal mucosa, and can cause rebound swelling, therefore, short use (less than 3 days) is recommended.
   b. Antibiotics
      (1) Cornerstone of treatment of acute sinusitis.
      (2) First-line: amoxicillin or trimethoprim-sulfamethoxazole for 10 to 14 days.
      (3) Second-line: amoxicillin/clavulanic acid or fluoroquinolones.
2. Surgical management. Surgery is considered an option after 4 to 6 weeks of failure of maximum medical therapy.

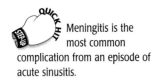

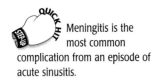

Meningitis is the most common complication from an episode of acute sinusitis.

a. Functional endoscopic sinus surgery aims to open the natural sinus ostia, while preserving as much of the sinus mucosa as possible.

b. Open sinus surgery.

3. Complications: orbital infection, brain abscess, meningitis, cavernous sinus thrombosis.

II. Bacterial Pharyngitis

A. General principles

1. Inflammation/irritation of the pharynx (oropharynx most commonly) has many causes: bacterial or viral infection, carcinoma, reflux disease, postnasal drip, environmental exposures.

2. Bacterial pharyngitis accounts for 5% to 10% of cases of pharyngitis.

3. This pharyngitis commonly affects the palatine tonsils, uvula, soft palate, and posterior pharyngeal wall.

B. Clinical features

1. Sore throat, odynophagia, fever, chills, malaise, headache, neck stiffness, and anorexia.

2. Cervical adenopathy, pharyngeal erythema and edema, gray-white tonsillar exudates, and petechiae on the soft palate.

3. Cough absent.

4. Pharyngitis can lead to rheumatic fever, scarlet fever, post-streptococcal glomerulonephritis.

C. Diagnosis

1. History and physical examination (Centor criteria): fever, adenopathy, tonsillar exudates, absent cough.

2. Rapid antigen test (80–90% sensitivity, less than 95% specific).

3. Antistreptolysin titers are not helpful in diagnosis of acute pharyngitis.

D. Treatment

1. Medical management. Antibiotics include:

a. Penicillin

b. Erythromycin for penicillin-allergic patients

2. Surgical management. Tonsillectomy is appropriate for those patients with recurrent bacterial pharyngitis, whose episodes do not decrease with appropriate antibiotic therapy.

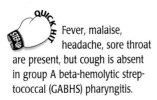

Fever, malaise, headache, sore throat are present, but cough is absent in group A beta-hemolytic streptococcal (GABHS) pharyngitis.

III. Epiglottitis

A. General principles

1. Highest prevalence in children 3 to 6 years of age.

2. Most common pathogen associated with this disease is the *Haemophilus influenzae* B (HIB).

3. Incidence has decreased 90% since the introduction of the HIB vaccine.

B. Clinical features

1. Fever, drooling, and sore throat with severe odynophagia.

2. Patients are usually sitting up in the bed and drooling.

3. Biphasic stridor is a late sign.

C. Diagnosis

1. Lateral neck x-ray: thumbprint sign (thickened epiglottis).

2. Direct visualization in the operating room, with anesthesia nearby for intubation.

D. Treatment

1. Medical management

a. Antibiotics: second- or third-generation cephalosporins (ceftriaxone/cefuroxime).

b. Corticosteroids.

2. Surgical management. If the patient develops respiratory arrest during examination in operating room, a tracheotomy may be needed to maintain the airway.

IV. Laryngeal Trauma

A. Blunt injury

1. Causes include motor vehicle accidents, all-terrain vehicle accidents, assaults, strangulation, and clothesline injuries.

2. Larynx is necessary for airway, so trauma to this structure is life threatening.

B. Penetrating injury

1. Causes include stabbings and gunshot wounds.

2. Mass and velocity determine damage to neck.

3. Often have damage to surrounding structures in the neck.

C. Intubation injury

1. Intubation can cause glottic edema, ulceration, and pressure necrosis of the larynx/trachea. This can lead to granulation tissue with subsequent fibrosis, and stenosis in the healing process.

2. Can also cause arytenoid dislocation from laryngoscope/endotracheal tube, or removal of endotracheal tube with cuff inflated.

D. Clinical features

1. Hoarseness, pain, dysphagia, odynophagia, and dyspnea.

2. Hemoptysis, stridor, and crepitus over laryngeal cartilage.

3. Damage to surrounding structures (esophagus, vessels): hematemesis, subcutaneous emphysema, expanding hematoma, and bruit.

E. Diagnosis

1. Flexible laryngoscopy: check for vocal cord movement and arytenoids symmetry. Can also evaluate for granulation tissue or stenosis, suggesting intubation trauma.

2. Plain films of neck may show air around trachea or chest that may compromise airway.

3. CT scan: best radiographic tool to evaluate for laryngeal injury, especially when physical examination is normal.

F. Treatment

1. Airway, breathing, and circulation (ABC).

   a. Secure the airway.

   b. Immobilize the cervical spine.

   c. Stabilize the patient hemodynamically, while controlling bleeding.

2. Medical management: can be used on those patients with a stable airway.

   a. Humidified air

   b. Elevate the head of the bed

   c. Voice rest

   d. Antibiotics, if there are any breaks in the mucosa

   e. Serial laryngoscopic examinations

   f. Steroids can be helpful if given within the first few hours of injury

3. Surgical management

   a. Blunt neck trauma

   (1) Lacerations, vocal fold immobility, exposed cartilage, or comminuted fractures necessitate surgical correction.

   (2) Early intervention has shown to have favorable long-term outcome, compared to delayed treatment.

   b. Penetrating neck trauma: depends on zone of involvement.

   (1) Zone I: sternal notch to cricoid cartilage.

   (a) Surgical approach to structures difficult.

   (b) Often obtain preoperative angiography and esophageal studies to assess for injuries.

   (2) Zone II: cricoid cartilage to angle of mandible is usually explored without imaging, unless damage to another neck zone is suspected.

   (3) Zone III: angle of mandible to skull base, where angiography is usually performed with embolization for treatment.

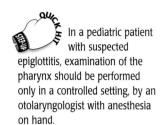 In a pediatric patient with suspected epiglottitis, examination of the pharynx should be performed only in a controlled setting, by an otolaryngologist with anesthesia on hand.

OTOLARYNGOLOGY

CONGENITAL CONDITIONS

I. Branchial Cleft Cysts

A. General principles
1. Caused by failure of branchial clefts to obliterate during the fetal period.
2. Comprise one-third of all congenital neck masses.
3. Most are second branchial cleft cysts (found deep to anterior border of sternocleidomastoid muscle).

B. Clinical features
1. Nontender fluctuant mass
2. Can become inflamed, and form an abscess
3. Dysphagia, dysphagia, and stridor

C. Diagnosis
1. Ultrasound: differentiate between cystic and solid masses.
2. CT: cystic versus solid. Evaluate proximity to surrounding structures.
3. MRI: cystic versus solid. Evaluate proximity to surrounding structures.

D. Treatment
1. Medical management: antibiotics to treat the infection.
2. Surgical management: excision of cyst is the only definitive treatment.
   a. Incision and drainage is best avoided (makes excision more difficult).
   b. Aspiration can be beneficial in decompression of mass.

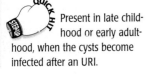
Present in late childhood or early adulthood, when the cysts become infected after an URI.

II. Infantile Hemangioma

A. General principles
1. Most common tumor of infancy, with a 4% to 10% prevalence at 1 year of age.
2. Rapid postnatal growth (8–12 months), followed by slow regression (5–8 years).
3. Appears during first 6 weeks of life, and is not seen in newborn nursery. A subset of congenital hemangiomas is present at birth, and does not have rapid postnatal growth.

B. Clinical features
1. Firm and rubbery with a bright red color, and well-circumscribed
2. Ulceration, bleeding, and infection
3. Visual defects, if they involve periorbital structures
4. Subglottic hemangioma may lead to airway obstruction
5. Heart failure (high-output type)

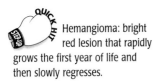
Hemangioma: bright red lesion that rapidly grows the first year of life and then slowly regresses.

C. Diagnosis
1. History and physical
2. Imaging techniques are helpful in assessing the extent of the lesion, and infiltration into surrounding structures
   a. Ultrasound
   b. MRI

D. Treatment
1. Medical management
   a. Watchful waiting
   b. Corticosteroids: oral, intravenous, intralesional (should see a response in 3 to 7 days)
   c. Interferon, vincristine, if lesion is refractory to corticosteroid treatment
2. Surgical management
   a. Removal of residual tissue after involution of lesion
   b. Laser or open resection of lesion, if clinical symptoms result: visual defects, stridor, or congestive heart failure (CHF)

III. Thyroglossal Duct Cysts

A. General principles
1. Comprises one-third of congenital neck masses.
2. Usually seen midline at hyoid bone.

3. Can be found anywhere between foramen cecum and thyroid gland.

4. Up to 45% have thyroid tissue.

B. Clinical features

　1. Usually asymptomatic.

　2. Mild dysphagia.

　3. Infection leading to significant dysphagia and choking.

C. Diagnosis

　1. History and physical.

　2. Ultrasound.

　3. Radionucleotide uptake scan.

D. Treatment

　1. Medical management: Treat infection with antibiotics.

　2. Surgical management: Sistrunk operation (thyroglossal duct cyst excision).

　　a. Small cuff of tissue (including center portion of hyoid bone) is excised.

　　b. A small percentage of cysts contain thyroid carcinoma, therefore they must undergo histologic examination.

> **QUICK HIT** Thyroglossal duct cyst: midline neck mass that elevates with swallowing.

IV. Lymphatic Malformations

A. General principles

　1. Can occur anywhere on body, although head and neck regions (80%) are most commonly affected.

　2. Results from sequestered lymphatics that do not connect to the lymphatic system.

　3. Filled with eosinophilic and proteinaceous fluid. Hemorrhage into lesion is common.

　4. May be present at birth.

B. Clinical features

　1. Can look clear, red, or black, depending if there is hemorrhage into lesion.

　2. Lesions tend to grow in size, and rarely involute on their own.

　3. Microcystic.

　　a. Vesicular lesions commonly found in or near oral cavity.

　　b. Tend to invade local tissues.

　　c. Usually present at birth.

　4. Macrocystic (e.g., cystic hygroma).

　　a. Usually involve the anterior and posterior triangle of the neck.

　　b. Less infiltration into local tissues.

　　c. Lesions are soft and compressible.

C. Diagnosis

　1. History and physical

　2. Macrocystic lesions tend to show sharp demarcations of the cystic areas on imaging, while microcystic lesions are isodense and poorly defined.

　　a. CT

　　b. MRI

D. Treatment

　1. Medical management: sclerotherapy, with intralesional ethanol, sodium tetradecyl sulfate, doxycycline, cyclophosphamide, bleomycin, OK-432.

　2. Surgical management

　　a. Manage airway complications: tracheostomy, gastrostomy

　　b. Laser surgery

　　c. Surgical resection

> **QUICK HIT** Recurrence of lymphatic malformations after surgery is very common, especially if all disease is not removed.

OTITIS

I. Otitis Externa

A. General principles

　1. Inflammatory/infectious process in the External Auditory Canal (EAC)

　2. Most common pathogens:

        a. *Pseudomonas*
        b. *Staphylococcus aureus*
        c. Fungi
    3. Risk factors:
        a. Heat
        b. Humidity
        c. Trauma to skin of the EAC
    4. Malignant otitis externa
        a. Osteomyelitis, involving the skull base, is most frequently found in elderly and diabetic patients as a complication of otitis externa.
        b. Pseudomonas is the most common pathogen implicated.
  B. Clinical features
    1. Otalgia, otorrhea, pruritus, and tenderness to palpation/manipulation of pinna.
    2. Possible hearing loss, depending on the amount of edema of EAC.
    3. Lymphadenopathy and cellulitis of EAC/pinna.
  C. Diagnosis: history and physical
  D. Treatment
    1. Medical management
        a. Cleaning of the EAC
        b. Topical therapy
            (1) Antibiotics: ofloxacin, ciprofloxacin, polymyxin B, neomycin, gentamicin, or tobramycin.
            (2) Steroids: help decrease edema and pain.
        c. Analgesics: nonsteroidal anti-inflammatory agents, opioids, steroids.
    2. Surgical management: patients with malignant otitis externa often need to be taken to the operating room for debridement of affected temporal bone.

II. Acute Otitis Media

  A. General principles
    1. Inflammation of middle ear cavity, most commonly due to bacterial infection, which is usually preceded by viral upper respiratory infection.
    2. Generally due to dysfunction of the eustachian tube.
    3. Incidence peaks about 2 years of age.
    4. Most common bacteria.
        a. *Streptococcus pneumoniae* (40%).
        b. *Haemophilus influenzae* (20–30%).
        c. *Moraxella catarrhalis* (10–20%).
    5. Risk factors are largely environmental and include:
        a. Tobacco smoke exposure.
        b. Day-care exposure.
        c. Breast-feeding.
        d. Seasonal variations of respiratory infections.
  B. Clinical features
    1. Fever
    2. Irritability in infants who pull at ear
    3. Earache in older children
    4. Hearing loss (conductive)
  C. Diagnosis
    1. Pneumatic otoscopy is accepted standard.
        a. Decreased or immobile tympanic membrane.
        b. Thickened hyperemic membrane.
    2. Laboratory results: leukocytosis, bacteremia.
    3. Ear discharge can be cultured in cases in which first-line treatment fails.
  D. Treatment
    1. Medical management
        a. Antibiotics

QUICK HIT

In an elderly patient with diabetes, granulation tissue in the EAC is indicative of malignant otitis externa, which is osteomyelitis of the temporal bone.

(1) Antibiotic therapy is controversial, because most cases resolve spontaneously, which tends to shorten course of illness.

(2) Amoxicillin is first-line therapy, but resistance is developing. There may be a need to add clavulanic acid to antibiotic therapy (Augmentin).

b. Analgesics and antipyretics

2. Surgical management: myringotomy with ventilation tubes is usually used for cases refractory to medical therapy (recurrent or chronic otitis media), or where a complication has occurred).

FRACTURES

I. Temporal Bone Fractures

A. General principles
1. 20% of all skull fractures.
2. Males 21 years of age and under are at high risk for temporal bone fractures.
3. Common causes are motor vehicle accidents, falls, assaults, and motorcycle collisions.
4. Blunt trauma to lateral skull often results in a temporal bone fracture.
5. Two types of temporal bone fractures are longitudinal and transverse. The differentiating factor is that transverse fractures involve the otic capsule.

B. Clinical features
1. Battle sign: postauricular ecchymosis, resulting from bleeding from the postauricular artery.
2. Raccoon eyes: periorbital ecchymosis often associated with a temporal bone fracture.
3. Other findings include cerebrospinal fluid (CSF) leak, otorrhea, facial nerve paralysis, and conductive hearing loss on the side of the fracture.

C. Diagnosis
1. CT scan of head and facial bones.
2. Tuning fork test: Weber test results in sound localizing to the side of the fracture.
3. Audiometry: can be done a few weeks after the injury if ear symptoms persist.

D. Treatment
1. Medical management
   a. Can observe fracture if nondisplaced.
   b. If hemotympanum is present, facial nerve paralysis can be observed, and will sometimes resolve in 2 to 3 weeks.
2. Surgical management
   a. CSF leak that is persistent after a week should be surgically repaired.
   b. Tympanic perforation that persists should be surgically repaired with a tympanoplasty.

II. Midface Fractures

A. LeFort 1 fractures
1. General principles
   a. Separate the palate from the midface.
   b. Involves the pterygoid plates bilaterally.
2. Clinical features
   a. Patient presents with malocclusion.
   b. Patients also have an open bite deformity.
   c. In the most severe cases, patients can be found to have airway compromise.
3. Diagnosis
   a. Diagnosis is by CT scan of the facial bones.
   b. Diagnosis can also be supported by clinical findings (physical examination findings of a stable midface, but mobile palate).

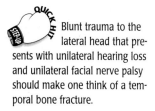

A patient with otitis media, diagnosed 2 days ago, who suddenly experiences the abrupt relief of otalgia, most likely has perforated their tympanic membrane.

Blunt trauma to the lateral head that presents with unilateral hearing loss and unilateral facial nerve palsy should make one think of a temporal bone fracture.

QUICK HIT

Patients with facial trauma, who present with a mobile palate but with a stable midface, should be evaluated for a Le Fort 1 fracture

4. Treatment
    a. The patient needs to be surgically managed by first being placed in class 1 occlusion. This is accomplished by aligning the mesiobuccal cusp of the maxillary first molar with mesiobuccal groove of the first mandibular molar.
    b. The fracture should then be reduced, and plated with titanium miniplates.
    c. If the patient has a relatively nondisplaced fracture, it can be managed with just intermaxillary fixation for 4 to 6 weeks
  B. LeFort 2 fracture
    1. General principles: LeFort 2 fractures involve the pterygoid plates, the frontonasal maxillary buttress, and often the skull base via the ethmoid bone.
    2. Clinical features.
       a. Palatal and upper midface mobility, and other factures and morbidities.
       b. Sometimes CSF leak.
    3. Diagnosis.
       a. Physical examination findings.
       b. Fine-cut CT scan.
    4. Treatment.
       a. Usually requires surgical intervention.
       b. Patients need to be put into occlusion via intermaxillary fixation.
       c. The patient then needs to be plated with a titanium miniplate.
  C. LeFort 3 fractures
    1. General principles
       a. These usually occur with high-energy trauma.
       b. These result in midface mobility.
       c. These fractures involve the pterygoid plates, the frontonasal maxillary buttress, and the frontozygomatic buttress.
    2. Clinical features
       a. Midface mobility.
       b. CSF leak often present.
    3. Diagnosis
       a. CT scan of facial bones.
       b. Use CT to confirm physical examination findings.
    4. Treatment
       a. Patients need a tracheotomy before surgery to secure a definitive airway.
       b. Patients need to be put into intermaxillary fixation.
       c. Patients need multiple surgical approaches to stabilize the facial bones.

QUICK HIT

A patient, who presents with a recent high-velocity trauma and has midface mobility on physical examination should be imaged and evaluated for a LeFort fracture.

III. Mandible Fractures
  A. General principles
    1. Occur in multiple types of traumas.
    2. Patients often present several days after the fracture, due to the fact that they were under the influence of alcohol or illicit drugs at the time of injury.
    3. Mandibular fractures may be nondisplaced or displaced. Nondisplaced fractures are more difficult to manage.
  B. Clinical features
    1. Pain with eating.
    2. Malocclusion.
    3. Numbness in the V3 distribution of the trigeminal nerve.
    4. Fractures of the body, symphysis, and angle are often mobile on physical examination.
    5. Condylar fractures are often difficult to detect.
  C. Diagnosis
    1. Plain x-ray of the face, or CT scan of facial bones, to make diagnosis.
    2. Panorex series can often be beneficial because they can differentiate a condylar fracture from an angle fracture.

QUICK HIT

A patient, who presents with a history of trauma and pain with mastication as well as numbness in the V3 region, should be evaluated for a mandible fracture.

D. Treatment
1. Patients with nondisplaced fractures often need minimal surgical management.
2. Patients with displaced fractures often need to be placed into intermaxillary fixation. This approach requires the patient to have jaw immobilization for 4 to 6 weeks.
3. Open splinting using titanium miniplates allows the patient to resume mastication almost immediately after surgery.
4. The type of repair system often depends on the surgeon, and in some instances, both approaches are used to achieve fixation of the fracture.
5. Patients often require antibiotics postoperatively.

IV. Sinus Fractures
A. General principles
1. Motor vehicle accidents are the most common cause of sinus fractures.
2. Patients are often under the influence of alcohol.
B. Clinical features
1. Patients with sinus fractures often sustain loss of consciousness as the result of the trauma.
2. Patients with sinus fractures can present with facial numbness, crepitus, and step-offs on palpation.
C. Diagnosis
1. CT scans of the head and facial bones are the "gold standard" for making the diagnosis of facial fractures.
2. The CT scan of the facial bones should include axial and coronal series with cuts from 1.5 to 3 mm.
3. Scans can be correlated with physical examination findings to make the diagnosis.
D. Treatment
1. Patients with sinus fractures often require surgical intervention to prevent further complications, and restore the normal contour of the face.
2. Displaced fractures require open reduction.

QUICK HIT Patients, who present with step-offs on physical examination and have multiple facial bone fractures, should be evaluated thoroughly for a sinus fracture.

NEOPLASMS

I. Acoustic Neuroma
A. General principles
1. This is a nerve sheath tumor of the eighth cranial nerve.
2. Acoustic neuromas originate in the medial internal auditory canal or lateral cerebellopontine angle.
3. These tumors interfere with the anatomy in this region, and cause symptoms.
B. Clinical features
1. These patients often present with hearing loss, which can be progressive and is unilateral in most cases.
2. A large group of patients with these tumors often present with tinnitus and disequilibrium.
3. Patients may often also present with facial numbness and numbness in the distribution of the sensory component of the facial nerve. They may also experience effects on the motor component of the facial nerve.
C. Diagnosis
1. MRI with gadolinium contrast along with clinical correlation of symptoms is considered the "gold standard" in securing this diagnosis.
2. CT scan with contrast can be used in situations where MRI is not readily accessible. It is not as sensitive in diagnosing these tumors.
3. A standard auditory evaluation using pure-tone audiometry, speech discrimination score, and acoustic reflex should be used to evaluate patients who present with unilateral hearing loss, unilateral tinnitus, or disequilibrium.

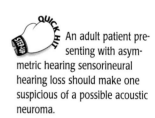

QUICK HIT An adult patient presenting with asymmetric hearing sensorineural hearing loss should make one suspicious of a possible acoustic neuroma.

D. Treatment
1. Patients with an acoustic neuroma can be treated with surgery, observation, or radiation.
2. Patients with an acoustic neuroma often have surgery to resect the tumor.
3. Patients, who are unstable for surgery or have a short-predicted life expectancy, are candidates for radiation or observation.
4. If the growth rate is less than 2 mm a year during the first year after diagnosis, patients can continue to be followed with observation.
5. Radiation to treat acoustic neuromas can be considered with the goal of preventing permanent hearing loss and facial nerve dysfunction.

II. Glomus Tumor
A. General principles
1. These tumors are also referred to as paragangliomas.
2. The most common of these tumors is a carotid body tumor. There are also two glomus tumors in the temporal bone: the glomus tympanicum, which arises in the middle ear, and glomus jugulare, which arises in the jugular foramen.
3. These tumors are most common in Caucasian populations.
B. Clinical features
1. Patients with a paraganglioma in the temporal bone often present with hearing loss and tinnitus.
2. Patients should be evaluated for sympathetic symptoms, such as tachycardia or flushing.
3. Physical examination of the tympanic membrane should reveal a bluish mass behind the tympanic membrane.
C. Diagnosis
1. CT or MRI of the skull base should be done to evaluate these tumors.
2. Magnetic resonance angiography can also be done to evaluate these tumors.
D. Treatment
1. Surgical removal of these tumors using a microsurgical technique is recommended.
2. If patients have vague or mild symptoms, observation and serial imaging studies can be used to manage these patients.

III. Juvenile Nasopharyngeal Angiofibroma
A. General principles
1. These tumors occur primarily in young males.
2. These highly vascular tumors occur in the posterior nasal cavity.
B. Clinical features
1. Nasal obstruction
2. Recurrent epistaxis
C. Diagnosis
1. Nasal endoscopy
2. Possible recurrent epistaxis
D. Treatment
1. Surgical resection
2. Occasionally, radiation is used to treat recurrent disease that cannot be treated surgically.

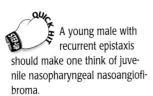
A young male with recurrent epistaxis should make one think of juvenile nasopharyngeal nasoangiofibroma.

IV. Papilloma
A. General principles
1. This rare disease is most common in the larynx of young children.
2. It is caused most commonly by human papilloma virus strains 6 and 11.
B. Clinical features
1. Hoarseness
2. Abnormal cry
3. Dyspnea and stridor with advanced disease

A young child with stridor and dyspnea, who otherwise does not appear to be clinically ill, should make one think of papillomatosis.

C. Diagnosis: microlaryngoscopy with biopsy of the lesion to establish a definitive diagnosis.

D. Treatment
1. Ablation with a CO_2 laser is the most common treatment modality.
2. In the past, surgical approaches were common, but have become less common with the evolution of the CO_2 laser technique.

SQUAMOUS CELL CARCINOMA

I. Squamous Cell Carcinoma of the Oral Cavity

A. General principles
1. The oral cavity contains the anterior two-thirds of the tongue, the buccal mucosa, the floor of the mouth, the hard palate, the alveolar ridge, and the retromolar trigone.
2. More common in males.
3. The probability increases with age.
4. Tobacco and alcohol use are synergistic in the development of squamous cell carcinoma (SCC).

B. Clinical features
1. Patients present with nonhealing ulcers in the oral cavity.
2. Patients also may have areas of leukoplakia or erythema that can be dysplasia, or early-stage disease.
3. Patients can also present with unilateral otalgia that is being referred from the oral cavity.

C. Diagnosis
1. It is important to perform a thorough head and neck examination in any patient with a suspicious lesion of the mouth.
2. CT or MRI or both of the head and neck is appropriate to establish the extent of the lesion as well as to evaluate for lymph node metastasis.
3. Biopsy of the lesion is also needed to establish a histological diagnosis.

D. Treatment
1. Primary resection of the tumor using a surgical technique is the first choice.
2. Radiation therapy can be used postoperatively, or in patients with tumors that are difficult to manage surgically.

> **QUICK HIT** A male patient who presents with a long history of tobacco use and has a nonhealing oral ulcer should be considered at high risk for an oral cavity squamous cell carcinoma.

II. Squamous Cell Carcinoma of the Larynx

A. General principles
1. More than 90% of patients with laryngeal cancer have an extensive history of alcohol and tobacco use.
2. Gastroesophageal reflux disease is also a risk factor.
3. Patients with a history of laryngeal papilloma are at high risk to develop laryngeal SCC.
4. Laryngeal cancers are divided into the supraglottic, glottic, and subglottic.

B. Clinical features
1. Patients present with a mass in the neck.
2. Signs and symptoms include ear pain, dysphagia, hoarseness, and hemoptysis.
3. Physical examination should include an indirect mirror examination in clinic, as well as flexible laryngoscopy, to evaluate the patient for lesions.
4. A thorough neck examination should also be conducted to evaluate for lymph node disease.

C. Diagnosis
1. CT or MRI of the head and neck should be done to evaluate for tumor and lymph node involvement.
2. Laryngoscopy with biopsy of the lesion is necessary.
3. Positron emission tomography (PET) scans are becoming more prevalent in the work up of patients with laryngeal cancer.

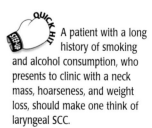

> **QUICK HIT** A patient with a long history of smoking and alcohol consumption, who presents to clinic with a neck mass, hoarseness, and weight loss, should make one think of laryngeal SCC.

D. Treatment
1. Medical management. Radiation and chemotherapy are alternatives to surgery.
2. Surgical management.
   a. Microlaryngoscopy with endoscopic removal is done for small T1 lesions.
   b. Laryngectomy.
      (1) Hemilaryngectomy: this procedure involves vertically removing one half of the larynx. This procedure is appropriate for tumors with subglottic extension below the vocal cord not less than 1 cm, an affected cord that is mobile, and no cartilage invasion or soft tissue invasion.
      (2) Supraglottic laryngectomy: a supraglottic laryngectomy involves removal of the supraglottis or the upper part of the larynx.
         (a) For tumors with a T stage of T1 to T3.
         (b) The vocal cords are not paralyzed.
         (c) Cartilage is not invaded.
         (d) There is no involvement of the anterior commissure.
      (3) Supracricoid laryngectomy: this procedure involves excising the true vocal cords, the supraglottis and thyroid cartilage. The arytenoid and cricoid cartilages are preserved. This procedure is appropriate for cancers in the anterior glottis or in the pre-epiglottic space.
      (4) Near-total laryngectomy: this involves preserving one arytenoid, and making a tracheoesophageal stoma for speech. Patients that meet criteria for this procedure have extensive lesions with one arytenoid uninvolved.
      (5) Total laryngectomy: this involves removing the entire larynx, the thyroid, and cricoid cartilages.
         (a) It is usually reserved for patients with extensive disease.
         (b) Patients have a permanent tracheostomy after this procedure.

III. Squamous Cell Carcinoma of the Nasopharynx
A. General principles
1. More common in Chinese Americans.
2. Associated with Epstein–Barr virus.
3. Smoking increases the risk of disease.
B. Clinical features
1. Cervical adenopathy
2. Unilateral otitis media with effusion
3. Nasal obstruction
4. Epistaxis
C. Diagnosis
1. Nasopharyngoscopy
2. Biopsy of the lesion with endoscopic guidance
3. CT scan to evaluate for involvement of tumor
D. Treatment
1. Patients with nasopharyngeal carcinoma usually undergo radiation therapy.
2. This is the treatment of choice, because it is difficult to obtain surgical margins in the nasopharynx.

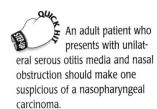

An adult patient who presents with unilateral serous otitis media and nasal obstruction should make one suspicious of a nasopharyngeal carcinoma.

IV. Squamous Cell Carcinoma of the Oropharynx
A. General principles
1. Oropharynx consists of the posterior third of the tongue, tonsillar fossa, soft palate, and the posterior pharyngeal wall.
2. These tumors are often silent and difficult to detect in the early stages of the disease.
3. The chances of occurrence increase with the consumption of alcohol and tobacco.
B. Clinical features
1. Patients present with nonhealing ulcers in the oral cavity.

5. Treatment
    a. For the asymptomatic patient in sinus rhythm with mild MS, treatment is directed at prophylaxis against endocarditis.
    b. For mild symptoms, or evidence of pulmonary hypertension, mechanical relief such as balloon valvotomy is indicated. Balloon valvotomy may be performed if no cuspal or annular calcification, subvalvular chordal fusion and distortion, atrial fibrillation, or clot exists.
    c. Other options are open commissurotomy, mitral valve reconstruction, or replacement.
    d. In those patients with established atrial fibrillation, surgical interventions may be combined with Cox-maze (ablative) procedure to ensure postoperative sinus rhythm.

E. Mitral regurgitation
    1. Etiology. Common causes are myxomatous degeneration of the mitral valve (Barlow syndrome, mitral valve prolapse), collagen vascular disease, infective endocarditis, rheumatic fever, secondary to ischemic disease or nonischemic cardiomyopathy.
    2. Clinical features. Compensated mitral regurgitation may remain asymptomatic, even with exertion, for years.
    3. Physiologic compensation
        a. Mitral regurgitation allows unloading of the left ventricle into the left atrium during systole.
        b. The left ventricle compensates by increasing ejection volume (increased EF).
        c. Eventually the left ventricle is not able to compensate, leading to eccentric cardiac hypertrophy and CHF.
        d. Intervention should be before left ventricular decompensation occurs.
    4. Diagnosis
        a. ECHO allows assessment of mitral regurgitation as well as left ventricular function.
        b. CATH before surgery to evaluate for concomitant CAD.
    5. Treatment
        a. Annual follow-up is indicated for patients with mild mitral regurgitation and no symptoms or cardiac enlargement.
        b. EF should not fall below the normal range before referral for intervention.
        c. Mitral valve repair results in better late outcome, lower operative mortality, and better preservation of left ventricular function and less need for anticoagulation.
        d. During mitral valve replacement, attempt should be made to preserve chordal structures and connections to avoid reduction in mitral regurgitation function.

F. Mitral valve prolapse
    1. This valvular disease is the most common valvular heart disease, affecting 2% to 6% of population.
    2. Some patients with mitral valve prolapse (5% to 10%) develop mitral regurgitation.
    3. Mitral valve prolapse represents the most common cause of mitral regurgitation since the decline of rheumatic fever.
    4. Asymptomatic patients should be evaluated every 3 to 5 years clinically, and by ECHO. More frequent follow-up is indicated if mitral regurgitation arises.
    5. Surgical repair is indicated only for significant mitral regurgitation, changes in left ventricular dimensions, or for flail leaflet due to chordal rupture.

G. Tricuspid regurgitation
    1. The most common cause of tricuspid regurgitation is secondary to mitral valve disease.
    2. Tricuspid regurgitation is usually due to right ventricular dilation, with secondary distortion of the tricuspid valve.

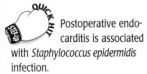

There is a very high rate of thromboembolic complication with mechanical prostheses in the tricuspid position despite adequate anticoagulation.

The now-discontinued anorectic (diet) drugs fenfluramine and phentermine are associated with left- and right-sided valve regurgitation, secondary to valve fibrosis. Prevalence is related to the duration of therapy. Patients who had this treatment should undergo annual cardiovascular physical and ECHO examination.

Endocarditis associated with intravenous drug use is often right-sided, and *Staphylococcus aureus* is often the responsible organism.

Postoperative endocarditis is associated with *Staphylococcus epidermidis* infection.

Perivalvular abscess is associated with *s. aureus* infection and may occur in 20% of cases of endocarditis.

3. Severe tricuspid regurgitation has poor prognosis, due to underlying right ventricular dysfunction.
4. Annuloplasty may be indicated for severe tricuspid regurgitation after correcting the offending left-sided valvar lesion.

II. Endocarditis
A. Epidemiology
1. Endocarditis affects normal or more commonly diseased native or prosthetic valves.
2. It is associated with rheumatic heart disease (24%), congenital abnormality (23%), hypertrophic cardiomyopathy, and mitral valve prolapse.
3. It affects left-side valves more than the right side.
4. Prosthetic valve endocarditis occurs in 1% to 2% of prosthetic valves, and accounts for 15% to 30% of endocarditis.
5. Mortality occurs in 10% to 15% of patients.
B. Etiology: infectious organisms.
1. Endocarditis may be precipitated by any cause of transient bacteremia.
2. Most common causes of endocarditis are *S. aureus* and alpha-hemolytic streptococcal infections (*Streptococcus viridans*).
   a. *S. aureus* is associated with higher morbidity, and more virulent course.
   b. Streptococcal infections can be associated with dental procedures.
3. Infection of a diseased valve tends to have a subacute, indolent course, whereas infection of a normal valve can present with a fulminant course.
4. Culture-negative endocarditis may occur with prior antibiotic treatment, fungal infections, and noninfective endocarditis as seen in systemic lupus erythematosus, otherwise called Libman–Sachs endocarditis.
C. Clinical features. Signs and symptoms of endocarditis are presented in Table 18-2.
D. Diagnosis. Diagnostic studies include ECHO and serial blood cultures.
E. Treatment
1. Medical treatment includes prolonged directed intravenous antibiotics.
2. Indications for surgical intervention include valve regurgitation, CHF, vegetations less than 2 cm, infection unresponsive to antibiotics or fungal endocarditis.
3. Treatment may include excision of the offending valve, debridement of abscess, valve replacement with allograft, valve repair, and tricuspid valve excision (would require replacement for long-term survival).
4. Reinfection after surgery is 1% to 13%.
5. Operative intervention for native endocarditis has 0% to 5% operative mortality, while prosthetic endocarditis has a significantly greater operative mortality.
F. Complications
1. Complications besides valvular regurgitation include perivalvular or intramyocardial abscess, systemic emboli, conduction defects, sinus of Valsalva aneurysms, intrapericardial rupture with pyogenic pericarditis, and septic picture.
2. Fungal vegetations may produce stenosis due to their bulk.

TABLE 18-2 Signs Associated with Endocarditis	
Sign	**Manifestation**
Roth spots	Retinal spots
Osler nodes	Raised painful nodes on soles and palms
Janeway lesions	Flat painless lesions on soles and palms
Splinter hemorrhages	Hemorrhages on fingernails

G. Types of valves
  1. Mechanical valves
     a. Mechanical valves include tilting disc and bileaflet valves.
     b. St. Jude valve is the most commonly used bileaflet valve. Thromboembolic events occur in 2% of patients per year.
     c. Mechanical valves have good long-term durability, but there is a risk of thromboembolism and bleeding secondary to anticoagulation. The most common valve-related morbidity is secondary to anticoagulation (1–3% of patients per year).
  2. Bioprosthetic or tissue valves
     a. Types of tissue valves include porcine and pericardial valves, allograft for aortic or mitral valves, and autograft of pulmonic valve into the aortic position (also called the Ross procedure).
     b. These degenerate over time.
     c. Bioprosthetic valves have about a 40% failure at 10 years.
     d. Aortic allografts have a lower degeneration at 10 years. However, they have limited availability, increased cost, and a technically more complex insertion.
     e. Ross procedure or the pulmonary valve autograft is used when aortic valve replacement is required in a younger patient. This is also used primarily in children to allow growth of the graft, and has an 85% success rate at 20 years.
     f. All tissue valves have low risk of thromboembolism, and do not require anticoagulation after 3 months. However, their failure rates are higher (30–40% at 10 years), especially in younger patients.
H. Cardiac indications for anticoagulation
  1. Mechanical prosthesis
  2. Intracardiac thrombus
  3. Atrial fibrillation with or without previous embolism or cardiomyopathy
  4. Anticoagulation is not indicated for infective endocarditis, aortic valve disease, mitral valve prolapse or disease.

III. Acquired Heart Disease
A. Coronary anatomy. The left and right coronary arteries are the first branches of the aorta originating just above the aortic valve, most commonly in the sinuses of Valsalva.
  1. The left coronary divides into the left anterior descending (LAD) artery and the left circumflex artery.
     a. The branches of the LAD are the septals and diagonal coronary arteries.
     b. The branches of the circumflex are the obtuse marginal arteries.
  2. The right coronary artery arises more anteriorly, and after supplying the sinus node, divides on the inferior surface of the heart into the posterior descending and posterolateral arteries.
  3. The posterior descending artery (PDA) may arise from the left circumflex coronary artery in about 10% of people when it is called a left dominant system. This is important, because the PDA supplies the atrioventricular node and its occlusion can result in heart block.
B. Ischemic heart disease
  1. Etiology and epidemiology
     a. Atherosclerotic plaques are composed of smooth muscle, collagen, lipids, elastin, and other matrix components.
     b. Disruption in the plaque surface results in thrombogenic ulcerations.
     c. Risk factors include age, genetic predisposition, male gender, hypertension, diabetes, hyperlipidemia, and smoking.
     d. This disease is more likely to be underdiagnosed or undertreated in women, and therefore results more often in death and disability.
  2. Pathophysiology
     a. Atherosclerotic disease directly compromises coronary blood flow, resulting in an imbalance of blood supply and myocardial demand.

QUICK HIT
Valve selection is dependent both on size and patient factors. Bioprosthetic valves are indicated for patients over 65 years, those patients in whom anticoagulation is contraindicated or unwilling to take warfarin, and those with a life expectancy less than than 10 years. Mechanical valves are for younger patients who tolerate lifelong anticoagulation.

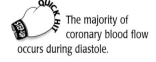

QUICK HIT
The majority of coronary blood flow occurs during diastole.

CARDIOTHORACIC SURGERY

b. Atherosclerotic disease results in decreased ventricular compliance, decreased myocardial contractility, and potential myocardial necrosis and scarring.

3. Clinical features
   a. Continuum of three interrelated ischemic clinical syndromes: angina pectoris, myocardial infarction (MI), and ischemic cardiomyopathy.
   b. May be asymptomatic
   c. Ischemic cardiomyopathy is an atypical presentation, resulting from loss of ventricular function due to myocardial scarring. This is also seen in patients with multiple MIs resulting in heart failure due to loss of ventricular muscle.
   d. Signs and symptoms
      (1) Angina pectoris typically presents as substernal chest pain lasting 5 to 10 minutes.
      (2) Angina may be described as stable, unstable (new onset or increasing frequency), or occurring at rest.

4. Diagnosis
   a. History is vital
   b. EKG may be normal. Abnormal findings include ST-segment changes and T-wave changes.
   c. Exercise stress testing and radionucleotide scans assist in evaluation, and delineating areas of ischemia and infarction.

5. Treatment
   a. Medical management
      (1) Prevention and risk factor reduction is the mainstay of treatment.
      (2) Among the pharmacological agents used to treat are beta-blockers, aspirin, angiotensin-converting enzyme inhibitors, and statins.
      (3) Nitrates are prescribed for symptom management.
   b. CATH
      (1) CATH is an invasive evaluation of coronary vascular anatomy.
      (2) It allows angiography assessment, as well as potential intervention with angioplasty and stent placement, to alleviate myocardial injury.
      (3) Intervention is indicated for patients with intractable symptoms and proximal lesions that put a large amount of myocardium at risk.
      (4) Percutaneous intervention is usually not indicated for lesions in the left main coronary artery, if target vessel is less than 2 mm, and if multiple obstructions are present within the same vessel.
      (5) The advent of newer high-resolution CT angiograms may alter the invasive study of coronary artery disease.
   c. Surgical management: coronary artery bypass graft (CABG).
      (1) Indications: surgical treatment may be indicated in left main disease, triple-vessel disease, double-vessel disease including the LAD, unstable angina, post-MI angina, symptoms uncontrolled with medical therapy and lifestyle, coronary artery rupture, dissection or thrombosis with PTCA, and CAD in patients with diabetes.
      (2) Procedure
         (a) The diseased artery is bypassed, thereby reestablishing blood flow beyond the area of stenosis.
         (b) The internal mammary artery is used most commonly. Radial arteries or greater saphenous veins are also used when additional grafts are needed. Nearly all (95%) of internal mammary arteries and 50% to 60% of vein grafts are patent at 10 years.
         (c) Cardiopulmonary bypass and cardioplegia are used to stop the heart, and achieve a quiet, bloodless field. The surgery can also be performed on a beating heart, otherwise called the off-pump bypass grafting.

QUICK HIT
Cardiac disease must be included in the diagnosis of any presenting complaint from the jaw to umbilicus. Patients with diabetes are at greater risk for silent MI. Women more often have atypical symptoms.

QUICK HIT
All patients with known CAD should take aspirin and lipid-lowering agents in the absence of contraindication.

(3) Complications
    (a) Postoperative complications include MI, arrhythmias, tamponade, infection, hemorrhage, graft thrombosis, sternal dehiscence, stroke, and postpericardiotomy syndrome.
    (b) Operative mortality is greatly dependent on ventricular function.
    (c) The mortality rate for CABG is 1% to 3%.
    (d) Reoperative CABG has a higher mortality rate (5–8%).
    (e) The 5-year survival rate is 90%, and 10-year survival rate is 80%.

  d. Extracorporeal circulation
    (1) Extracorporeal circulation is artificial pumping and oxygenation, allowing removal of blood from the superior and inferior vena cava, and returning it to the aorta allowing cardiac arrest during procedures.
    (2) It provides constant pulsatile or nonpulsatile flow.
    (3) It requires anticoagulation with heparin and is reversed with protamine.
    (4) Heparin rebound is the phenomenon of increased anticoagulation after bypass as heparin returns to circulation from peripheral tissues.
    (5) Atrial fibrillation may occur in one-third of patients after bypass.
    (6) Complications of extracorporeal circulation are presented in Table 18-3.

> **QUICK HIT** Dressler syndrome is pericarditis after MI. Postpericardiotomy syndrome is pericarditis after cardiac surgery. Both are treated with NSAIDs and sometimes steroids.

IV. Cardiac Tumors

A. Epidemiology
  1. The most common cardiac tumors are secondary tumors from lung (men) or breast (women).
  2. Primary tumors are rare, and 80% are benign.

B. Pathology. Types of cardiac tumors include:
  1. Myxoma
    a. Myxoma is the most common tumor of the heart, more common in women, usually in adulthood.
    b. The majority (75%) are found in the left atrium.
    c. Myxoma may present with thromboembolic events, and/or constitutional symptoms.
  2. Rhabdomyoma
    a. Rhabdomyoma is usually found in children.
    b. Mortality is 80% at 1 year (often multiple).

C. Clinical features. Presentation may be embolic, unexplained murmur, CHF, or dysrhythmia.

D. Diagnosis. These tumors are usually diagnosed when ECHO is performed for other indications.

E. Treatment
  1. Treatment is excision.
  2. If resection is not possible, then relief of obstruction may give good long-term results.

> **QUICK HIT** Closure of the pericardium after open-heart surgery facilitates reentry into the sternum, but increases risk of tamponade.

> **QUICK HIT** The most common tumor in all groups is metastasis from a remote organ.

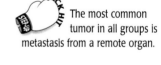

TABLE 18-3 Complications of Extracorporeal Circulation
Trauma to blood elements resulting in hemolysis and platelet destruction
Pancreatitis due to low flow
Heparin rebound
Stroke
Failure to wean from bypass
Systemic inflammatory response syndrome (SIRS)

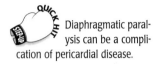

Diaphragmatic paralysis can be a complication of pericardial disease.

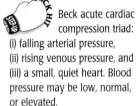

Beck acute cardiac compression triad: (i) falling arterial pressure, (ii) rising venous pressure, and (iii) a small, quiet heart. Blood pressure may be low, normal, or elevated.

V. Pericardial Disease

A. Anatomy of the pericardium
1. The serous and fibrous pericardium together composes the parietal pericardium.
2. The visceral pericardium (epicardium) covers the heart and great vessels.
3. Phrenic nerves lie in the parietal pericardium.
4. Superiorly, it merges with the adventitia of the great vessels.
5. Inferiorly, it attaches to the central tendon of the diaphragm.
6. It normally contains 15 to 50 mL of straw-colored serous fluid.

B. Physiology. Structural functions include mechanical protection and anchoring, prevention of acute cardiac distention, and serving as an infection barrier.
1. Chemical functions include absorption. Mechanoreceptors govern blood pressure and heart rate, and the pericardial fluid has fibrinolytic properties.

C. Cardiac tamponade
1. Cardiac tamponade is a hemodynamically significant cardiac compression due to accumulating pericardial contents.
2. Acute accumulation of 100 to 200 mL may produce tamponade.
3. Chronic effusion may allow accumulation of liters before tamponade occurs.
4. Tamponade usually occurs when pericardial pressures rise to 20 to 30 mm Hg.
5. Clinical features.
   a. Clinical findings include dyspnea and tachycardia.
   b. Pulsus paradoxus is usually present with a fall in systolic blood pressure of 10 mm Hg during inspiration.
      (1) Other causes of pulsus paradoxus include chronic obstructive pulmonary disease, asthma, pulmonary embolism, right ventricular failure or infarction, obesity, and tense ascites.
      (2) Pulsus paradoxus may be absent in the presence of tamponade with left ventricular dysfunction, atrial septal defect, or with positive pressure ventilation.
6. Diagnosis is confirmed through the use of ECHO.
7. Cardiac manometry may reveal equalization of ventricular pressures.
8. Treatment is needle pericardiocentesis or surgical drainage. The approach to the pericardium can be subxiphoid, thoracotomy, or sternotomy.
9. Postoperative tamponade can occur without classic signs, and must be considered in any postoperative patient from any heart surgery with decreased cardiac output of unclear origin. The diagnosis is predominantly clinical.

D. Pericardial constriction
1. The heart is contained by a thickened, fibrotic pericardium.
2. The pericardial space may be obliterated, or effusion filled.
3. Pericardial constriction is progressive over months to years.
   a. The most common etiology is following cardiac surgery.
   b. It may be a late sequela of any acute pericarditis, or due to mediastinal irradiation, amyloidosis, scleroderma, hemochromatosis, neoplastic disease, sarcoidosis, and/or trauma.
4. Clinical features
   a. The clinical picture may include dyspnea, orthopnea, cough, fatigue, pleural effusion, abdominal swelling and discomfort, hepatomegaly, ascites, peripheral edema, fatigue, and pulsus paradoxus.
   b. Kussmaul sign is an increase in jugular venous distention with inspiration.
   c. Pericardial knock is a loud third heart sound produced by rapid diastolic ventricular filling.
   d. Some patients (25%) have atrial fibrillation or flutter.
   e. Some patients (40%) have pericardial calcification (pathognomonic).
5. Treatment is pericardiectomy, or if that is not feasible, multiple pericardotomies.

E. Neoplasia
  1. Metastatic disease is the most common tumor, and the most common cause of pericardial effusion.
  2. Palliative treatment with repeated drainage or sclerosing agents such as doxycycline.
F. Dressler and postpericardiotomy syndrome
  1. Dressler syndrome is pericarditis during the evolution of acute MI, which is present in 3% to 5 % of patients.
  2. Occurrence is similar in 10% to 40% of postcardiac surgery patients.
  3. It develops 10 days to 2 months after surgery.
G. Pericardiocentesis
  1. A long, large-gauge needle with a sheath is inserted just to the left of the xiphoid process, and aiming at a 45-degree angle for the left shoulder. The needle is slowly advanced until fluid is aspirated.
  2. ECHO or fluoroscopy is mandatory for guidance in the absence of an emergency.
  3. Pericardiocentesis is useful for diagnosis of the etiology of effusion or treatment of tamponade.
H. Pericardial biopsy and surgical drainage. Open surgical drainage may be necessary for bloody, purulent, or recurrent effusions.
I. Pericardectomy
  1. Pericardectomy is usually for constrictive pericarditis, chronic malignant effusion, and/or unresponsive effusions.
  2. Care must be taken to preserve both phrenic nerves.

VI. Pediatric Cardiac Disease

A. General principles
  1. Congenital heart disease occurs in 3 in 1,000 live births.
  2. Etiology is usually unknown. However, rubella infection in the first trimester is associated with congenital heart disease, and Down syndrome is associated with endocardial cushion defects.
  3. The most common congenital heart defects are listed in Table 18-4.
B. Atrial septal defect (ASD)
  1. Normal cardiac septation occurs between the third and sixth weeks of development.
  2. Prior to birth, a patent ostium secundum allows shunting of blood from the inferior vena cava to the left atrium. The increase in left atrial pressure at birth closes this pathway.
  3. This defect is the third most common congenital heart defect, occurring in 1 of 1,000 live births, and it accounts for 10% of congenital defects.
  4. Patent foramen ovale results from failure of fusion of the septum secundum and septum primum. This is present in 27% of the population at autopsy, and does not cause significant shunting. It may allow for paradoxical embolization.

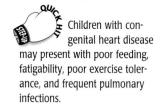

QUICK HIT Children with congenital heart disease may present with poor feeding, fatigability, poor exercise tolerance, and frequent pulmonary infections.

QUICK HIT Cyanotic heart disease is caused by the five Ts: tetralogy of Fallot, truncus arteriosus, total anomalous pulmonary venous return, tricuspid atresia, and transposition of the great vessels.

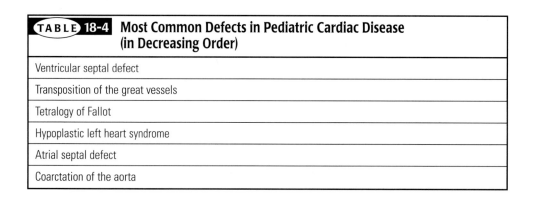

TABLE 18-4	**Most Common Defects in Pediatric Cardiac Disease (in Decreasing Order)**
Ventricular septal defect	
Transposition of the great vessels	
Tetralogy of Fallot	
Hypoplastic left heart syndrome	
Atrial septal defect	
Coarctation of the aorta	

5. Diagnosis
    a. Fixed splitting of S2, and a systolic ejection murmur at the left sternal border due to increased flow across a normal pulmonary valve.
    b. CXR cardiomegaly.
    c. EKG right axis deviation with incomplete right bundle branch block.
    d. ECHO confirms diagnosis and defines anatomy.
6. Treatment
    a. Intervention is recommended for all patients with symptomatic ASDs, and all asymptomatic patients with significant ASDs due to long-term complications.
    b. Repair usually occurs prior to school age.
    c. Transcatheter repair is possible for small to moderate secundum ASDs, and for patent foramen ovale.
    d. Surgical repair may be primary closure of the defect, or with Dacron, Gore-Tex, or pericardial patch.
C. Ventricular septal defect (VSD)
    1. VSDs are the most common congenital heart anomaly, with 4 per 1,000 live births.
    2. VSDs represent 40% of congenital anomalies.
    3. Some VSDs (30%) close spontaneously.
    4. VSDs are classified based on location into perimembranous (80%) versus inlet, outlet, and trabecular.
    5. Physiologic compensation.
        a. Increases pulmonary blood flow due to left-to-right shunting during systole, increasing volume load on the left heart. The right side of the heart is pressure loaded.
        b. After birth, the shunt volume is low, because pulmonary vascular resistance is high. As pulmonary vascular resistance falls, the volume will increase.
        c. Patients may be asymptomatic at birth, but develop cyanosis at several weeks of age.
        d. Most VSDs are restrictive, and tend to close spontaneously by 1 year.
        e. Large VSDs are not restrictive, and CHF symptoms develop by 2 months.
        f. Pulmonary vascular disease usually develops by 2 years of life.
        g. There is a small risk of endocarditis.
    6. Clinical features. Table 18-5 presents the signs and symptoms of VSDs.
    7. Treatment.
        a. Severe, symptomatic VSDs should be repaired early.
        b. If symptoms may be moderated with medical therapy, then surgical intervention can be delayed until school age to allow for possible spontaneous closure.
        c. Repair with patch: care is taken not to interrupt the conduction system.
D. Congenital aortic stenosis
    1. Left ventricular outflow obstruction.
    2. Aortic stenosis represents 4% of congenital heart disease.

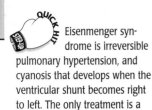

Eisenmenger syndrome is irreversible pulmonary hypertension, and cyanosis that develops when the ventricular shunt becomes right to left. The only treatment is a heart–lung transplant.

TABLE 18-5 Signs and Symptoms of Ventricular Septal Defect		
Tachypnea	**Hepatomegaly**	**Poor Feeding**
Failure to thrive	Holosystolic murmur (louder with small defects)	Increased vascular markings on chest x-ray
Electrocardiographic right ventricular hypertrophy	Echocardiography confirms diagnosis	Cardiac catheterization used in older children and adults in who elevated pulmonary vascular resistance is suspected.

3. 20% occur in conjunction with other cardiac defects, most commonly coarctation of the aorta, but also with patent ductus arteriosus, VSD, and mitral stenosis.
4. The male-to-female ratio is 4 to 1.
5. At birth, critical aortic stenosis is an emergency managed with intubation, inotropic support, and prostaglandins to maintain patent ductus arteriosus patency.
6. Physiologic compensation. Severe aortic stenosis is well compensated during development by increasing right ventricular output via a patent ductus.
7. Treatment
   a. Urgent intervention may be required.
   b. Treatment includes percutaneous balloon valvuloplasty, surgical valvotomy, or aortic valve replacement.
E. Tetralogy of Fallot
1. Tetralogy of Fallot is the most common congenital, cyanotic heart condition.
2. It consists of:
   a. Obstruction to right ventricular outflow.
   b. VSD.
   c. Hypertrophy of the right ventricle.
   d. Overriding aorta.
3. Resistance to right ventricular outflow exceeds systemic resistance, resulting in a right-to-left shunt with cyanosis and desaturation.
4. Clinical features
   a. Cyanosis in 30% of children at birth, and in 30% at 1 year.
   b. Presenting signs include cyanosis and dyspnea on exertion.
   c. Squatting temporarily alleviates symptoms by increasing systemic vascular resistance and increasing pulmonary flow.
   d. Cerebrovascular accidents and brain sepsis may be life-threatening events.
   e. Cardiac failure is rare.
5. Diagnosis
   a. Evaluation reveals cyanosis, clubbing, polycythemia, systolic murmur.
   b. A boot-shaped heart is revealed on CXR, due to right ventricular enlargement.
   c. CATH can determine the level of obstruction, and anatomy of pulmonary and coronary arteries.
6. Treatment
   a. Correction is performed at or after 2 years.
   b. Treatment is palliative, and systemic to pulmonary shunt may be performed prior to correction.
   c. Risk depends on age and degree of cyanosis.
   d. Dramatic improvement occurs after correction.
F. Transposition of the great arteries
1. Two separate and parallel circuits result from the aorta arising from the right ventricle, and the pulmonary artery arising from the left ventricle.
2. An anomalous communication is required for survival, such as an atrial septal defect, patent ductus arteriosus, or ventricular septal defect.
3. Diagnosis is based on ABG, CXR, and ECHO. An enlarged egg-shaped heart is seen on CXR.
4. Treatment involves septostomy to improve mixing followed by definitive correction.
G. Patent ductus arteriosus
1. In utero, prostaglandins E1 and E2, and hypoxia, keep the ductus open.
2. In normal-term infants, the pulmonary circulation causes increased oxygen levels with breakdown prostaglandins, resulting in duct closure in the first days of life.

3. Failure of closure may be asymptomatic, although a small number develop heart failure and pulmonary vascular disease.
4. Clinical features diagnosis
   a. Patients may present with signs and symptoms of congestive heart failure.
   b. Continuous machinery murmur is detected.
   c. Widened pulse pressure and bounding peripheral pulses are observed.
   d. Cyanosis is present, if associated with pulmonary vascular disease or other congenital anomalies.
5. Treatment
   a. Indomethacin is a prostaglandin inhibitor used to close the duct in preterm infants, with simple symptomatic patent ductus.
   b. Coil closure in the catheterization laboratory using a percutaneous approach.
   c. Surgical treatment is ligation of the ductus, and is indicated if patency persists after 2 to 3 years or if it causes symptoms of heart failure earlier.

H. Coarctation of the aorta
1. Severe narrowing of the aorta usually adjacent to the ductus arteriosus.
2. Occurs in males twice as often as in females.
3. A majority (60%) are associated with intracardiac defects.
4. Clinical features.
   a. May be asymptomatic for a variable length of time.
   b. Presenting symptoms and signs: CHF, headaches, dizziness, and lower extremity weakness.
5. Diagnosis
   a. Upper extremity hypertension with absent or diminished lower extremity pulses, and asystolic murmur are found.
   b. CXR in older individuals may show rib notching due to indentation by collateral circulation via intercostal arteries.
   c. ECHO and CATH further define anatomy, and evaluate for associated cardiac defects.
6. Treatment
   a. Surgical correction is indicated, although it may be delayed in asymptomatic patients.
   b. Correction may involve resection with end-to-end anastomosis, placement of a prosthetic graft, or use of subclavian artery used to enlarge the area of coarctation.
   c. Hypertension may persist postoperatively.
   d. Spinal cord ischemia is a rare complication of surgery.
   e. Mesenteric ischemia is a rare postoperative complication.

PULMONARY DISEASE

I. Spontaneous Pneumothorax

A. General principles
1. This occurs with rupture of a subpleural bleb, allowing lung collapse.
2. Incidence: usually occurs in young adults 18 to 24.
B. Clinical features. Presenting symptoms include chest pain and shortness of breath.
C. Diagnosis. The physical examination and CXR are the basis of diagnosis.
D. Treatment
1. Initial treatment is chest tube drainage.
2. Surgical videothoracoscopy with chemical and or mechanical pleurodesis is indicated for recurrent or persistent pneumothorax. Any bullae present are resected at the same time.
3. Tension pneumothorax is a clinical diagnosis based on tracheal deviation and absence of breath sounds, and is a life-threatening emergency.

QUICK HIT Prostaglandins act to maintain patency of the ductus. Indomethacin inhibits prostaglandins to promote closure of the ductus.

QUICK HIT Ebstein anomaly is a congenital anomaly associated with lithium during pregnancy. The tricuspid valve is placed low in the right ventricle, decreasing the size of the ventricle. The result is tricuspid regurgitation and decreased right-sided output.

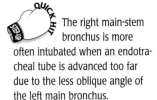

QUICK HIT The right main-stem bronchus is more often intubated when an endotracheal tube is advanced too far due to the less oblique angle of the left main bronchus.

CARDIOTHORACIC SURGERY

II. Disorders of the Pleura and Pleural Space

A. Empyema/abscess
1. Pus in the pleural space usually is secondary to pulmonary infection.
2. Forms in three stages:
   a. Acute phase: approximately 7 days, serous pleural fluid collection.
   b. Transitional phase: from day 7 to 21, characterized by fibropurulent fluid collecting in dependent areas.
   c. Chronic phase: after 21 days, organization of fluid collection with abscess formation.
3. Treatment
   a. Early-course treatment may involve aspiration, antibiotics, and sometimes fibrinolytic therapy.
   b. Late-course treatment requires continuous drainage or surgical debridement and decortication.

B. Mesothelioma
1. Mesothelioma is a pleural tumor, usually related to asbestos exposure.
2. Malignant mesothelioma usually presents with malignant pleural effusion.
3. The condition is usually fatal. Surgery has a limited role and is usually palliative.

III. Lung Lesion: Solitary Pulmonary Nodule

A. General principles
1. A small minority (5–10%) are malignant.
2. Risk factors for malignancy include size greater than 1 cm, indistinct margins, documented growth, and increasing age.
3. Half of lesions are malignant in smokers older than 50 years of age.

B. Diagnosis
1. If found incidentally, old films are reviewed. If the lesion is stable over 2 years, no further evaluation is needed.
2. Additional testing may include tuberculin skin testing, sputum cultures, chest CT, PET scan, CT-guided biopsy, and excisional biopsy.
3. Differential diagnosis includes infection, granulomatous disease, benign neoplasm, and malignancy.

C. Treatment
1. Lesions can be followed without a tissue diagnosis if they are stable over 2 years, or if popcorn calcifications (indicative of hamartoma) are present.
2. If a pulmonary nodule is present in the setting of hypertrophic osteoarthropathy, there is a 75% chance of carcinoma.

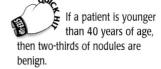 If a patient is younger than 40 years of age, then two-thirds of nodules are benign.

IV. Cancer

A. General principles (Table 18-6)
1. Lung cancer is the leading cause of cancer-related deaths, and the second cause of overall mortality.
2. The majority of patients present with distant disease.
3. Resection is the mainstay of treatment; however, only about 20% of cancers are resectable at presentation (stage I–IIIa).
4. Risk decreases to that of never smokers after 10 years.

B. Clinical features and diagnosis
1. Presenting signs and symptoms may include cough, hemoptysis, hoarseness, weight loss, fatigue, and recurrent infections.
2. CXR is not an effective screening tool, because lesions are not visible on the x-ray until they reach 1 cm. At that size, most neoplasms have metastasized.

C. Treatment. Lung cancer treatment can be divided into small-cell and non-small cell tumors.

D. Non-small cell lung cancer
1. Staging

Pancoast tumor is a tumor at the apex of the lung that may involve the brachial plexus, sympathetic ganglia, and vertebral body, leading to pain, upper extremity weakness, and Horner syndrome.

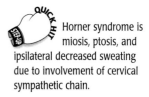 Horner syndrome is miosis, ptosis, and ipsilateral decreased sweating due to involvement of cervical sympathetic chain.

TABLE 18-6	Key Features of Pulmonary Cancers		
Squamous Cell	**Adenocarcinoma**	**Small (Oat) Cell**	**Large Cell**
Usually centrally located	Usually peripheral	Centrally located	Usually peripheral
Slow growing, late metastasis	Rapid growth with hematogenous and nodal metastasis	Highly malignant	Highly malignant
Associated with smoking	Associated with lung scarring	Strong association with smoking	
May be associated with Pancoast tumor			
		Neuroendocrine tumor	
		Usually unresectable	
		Treatment: chemotherapy and radiation	

   a. Stage I: any tumor size without extension to chest wall, mediastinum, pericardium, or diaphragm, with no nodes or metastasis, and at least 2 cm from the carina.

     (1) Treatment is surgical resection.

     (2) The 5-year survival is 65%

   b. Stage II: a stage I tumor with positive ipsilateral hilar or peribronchial nodes, and no distant metastasis.

     (1) Treatment is surgical resection.

     (2) The 5-year survival is 45%.

   c. Stage IIIa: any tumor size with local spread, not involving the heart, aorta, pulmonary artery, trachea, or esophagus, or with positive subcarinal or mediastinal nodes, and no distant metastasis.

     (1) Treatment is surgical resection, chemotherapy with or without radiation.

     (2) The 5-year survival is 30%.

   d. Stage IIIb: nodal involvement beyond that listed above, with mediastinal extension, and no distant metastasis.

     (1) Treatment is chemotherapy and radiation.

     (2) The 5-year survival is less than 10%.

   e. Stage IV: any tumor with distant metastasis.

     (1) Treatment is chemotherapy.

     (2) The 5-year survival is 0%.

2. Contraindications to surgical resection of lung cancer:

   a. Superior vena cava (SVC) syndrome.

   b. Supraclavicular or scalene node metastasis.

   c. Carinal involvement.

   d. Small-cell tumor.

   e. Poor pulmonary function (forced expiratory volume in 1 second [FEV_1] less than 1).

   f. Metastatic disease.

3. Risk assessment prior to resection includes cardiac evaluation, PFT, and room air ABG.

   a. An individual with a preoperative FEV_1 greater than 2 can tolerate pneumonectomy.

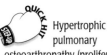

Hypertrophic pulmonary osteoarthropathy (proliferation of long bones and in the bones of the hand) is seen in 10% of patients with lung cancer.

    b. An individual who can climb five flights of stairs is likely tolerate pneumonectomy, but one who cannot climb one flight is unlikely to tolerate a pulmonary resection.

E. Surgical resection of pulmonary metastases
1. Pulmonary metastasis is a common presentation, and may be the only site of metastasis.
2. Resection of metastatic lesions may be part of a treatment protocol.

F. Benign tumors of the lung
1. Hamartoma is the most common benign lung tumor.
2. This presents as a solitary lung nodule.

G. Carcinoid syndrome
1. An amine-precursor uptake and decarboxylation tumor of the bronchus is slow growing, but may be malignant.
2. It may present with bronchial obstruction or stenosis.
3. Biopsy has to be undertaken with care, because significant hemorrhage is possible.
4. Carcinoid syndrome is rare with pulmonary carcinoid. This syndrome consists of episodic flushing, abdominal cramps, diarrhea, and right-sided heart valve damage.
5. Most bronchial adenomas have malignant potential. Other bronchial adenomas include mucoepidermoid carcinoma, mucous gland adenoma, adenoid cystic carcinoma.

V. Paraneoplastic and Other Cancer-Related Syndromes
A. These syndromes are associated with cancers with symptoms in distant parts of the body from the tumor. The cause may be endocrine activity of tumor cells, or may be unknown.
B. Manifestations of paraneoplastic syndromes include Cushing syndrome of inappropriate secretion of antidiuretic hormone (SIADH), hypercalcemia, Eaton–Lambert syndrome, cerebellar ataxia, hypertrophic osteoarthropathy, acanthosis nigricans, and thrombophlebitis.
C. Small-cell carcinoma can cause Lambert–Eaton syndrome, Cushing syndrome, or SIADH.
D. Hypercalcemia can result from parathyroid hormone production by a squamous cell tumor.
E. SVC syndrome results from compression of the SVC with impaired drainage. Patients present with edema and plethora of the head and neck, as well as central nervous system symptoms.

VI. Pulmonary Sequestration
A. Abnormal lung tissue with separate blood supply, and no communication with tracheobronchial airway.
B. Benign, may be asymptomatic, with possible recurrent infections.
C. Classified as interlobar (contained within visceral pleura) or extralobar (outside normal lung with separate pleural covering).
D. Treatment is resection if indicated.

VII. Mediastinum
A. Anterior mediastinal anatomy includes the thymus, extrapericardial aorta and its branches, great veins, and lymphatic tissue.
B. Anterior mediastinal masses
1. Thymoma
2. Teratoma
    a. Usually occurs in adolescents.
    b. The vast majority (80%) are benign.
    c. Derived from branchial cleft pouch.

The differential diagnosis of a mediastinal mass is based on anatomic location. The most common primary anterior mass in adults is a thymoma. The most common primary anterior mass in children is a teratoma.

CARDIOTHORACIC SURGERY

      d. Contain all tissue types.
      e. Treatment is surgical excision.
    3. Lymphoma
      a. Half of patients with lymphoma have mediastinal involvement, only 5% have isolated mediastinal disease.
      b. Present with cough, chest pain, fever, and weight loss.
      c. Diagnosis with imaging and lymph node biopsy.
      d. Treatment is nonsurgical.
    4. Germ cell
      a. Very rare mediastinal tumors present with vagus involvement.
      b. Treatment is resection.
  C. Middle mediastinal anatomy includes the heart, intrapericardial great vessels, pericardium, and trachea.
  D. Middle mediastinal masses
    1. Pericardial cysts
    2. Bronchogenic cysts
    3. Lymphoma
    4. Ascending aortic aneurysms
  E. Posterior mediastinal anatomy includes esophagus, vagus nerves, thoracic duct, sympathetic chain, and the azygous vein system.
  F. Posterior mediastinal masses: neurogenic tumors.
  G. Treatment for mediastinal masses
    1. Needle aspiration of suspected cysts.
    2. Resection either via minimally invasive techniques, or sternotomy/thoracotomy.

VIII. Chest Wall
  A. Thoracic outlet syndrome
    1. This compromised subclavian vessel flow is caused by a cervical rib or muscular hypertrophy.
    2. Presentation is unilateral upper extremity claudication.
    3. Treatment is surgical removal of obstruction (rib resection).
  B. Chest wall tumors
    1. Benign tumors
      a. Fibrous dysplasia of the rib may occur as part of McCune–Albright syndrome.
      b. Tumors are slow growing.
      c. Chondroma is the most common benign tumor.
      d. Osteochondroma is also a common benign tumor.
    2. Malignant tumors: fibrosarcoma, chondrosarcoma, osteogenic sarcoma, myeloma, and Ewing sarcoma.
    3. Treatment is wide excision with reconstruction of the chest wall.

 Differentiate thoracic outlet syndrome from subclavian steal syndrome by history. Subclavian steal presents with central nervous system symptoms, although both have unilateral upper extremity claudication.

 Fibrous dysplasia occurs posteriorly and laterally, chondromas occur anteriorly, and osteochondromas can occur anywhere.

 The majority (60–90%) of primary chest wall tumors are malignant. Chondrosarcoma is the most common, usually occurring in individuals 10 to 40 years of age.

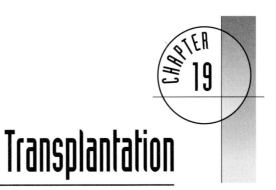

Transplantation

Christopher McCullough, MD
Giridhar Vedula, MD

IMMUNOBIOLOGY

I. Terminology
A. Types of grafts
  1. **Autograft (isograft):** transplantation of tissue from an individual to itself, usually a different site (e.g., split-thickness skin graft, parathyroid tissue, bone from iliac crest, autotransfusion of blood). An autograft requires no immunosuppression (Fig. 19-1A).
  2. **Allograft:** transplantation of tissue between genetically nonidentical individuals of the same species (e.g., solid organ transplants, allogeneic bone marrow transplants, cornea, blood transfusions). Allografts require immunosuppression to prevent rejection of the transplanted donor tissue by the recipient's intact immune system (Fig. 19-1B).
  3. **Xenograft:** transplantation of tissue between members of different species (Fig. 19-1C).
B. **B-cells**
  1. These lymphocytes arise and partially mature in bone marrow.
  2. They respond by directly binding antigen (Ag) to immunoglobulin (Ig) on the surface of the cell. Thus, activated B-cells proliferate (**clonal selection**) to terminally differentiate into antibody (**Ab**)-producing **plasma cells.**
    a. Antibodies are glycoproteins secreted by plasma cells.
    b. Antibodies are constructed from two **light** polypeptide chains, and two **heavy** polypeptide chains.
      (1) There are two **isotypes** of light chains: κ (kappa) and λ (lambda).
      (2) There are five isotypes of heavy chains: μ (mu), γ (gamma), ε (epsilon), α (alpha), and δ (delta) responsible for the five isotypes of circulating antibody: **IgM, IgG, IgE, IgA,** and **IgD.**
C. T-cells
  1. These lymphocytes arise in the bone marrow, and mature in the thymus.
  2. They are responsible for **cell-mediated immunity,** as well as facilitating B-cell response.
  3. They are broadly classified as **CD4+** or **CD8+.** CD is the abbreviation for **cluster determinant.**
    a. CD4+ T-cells have been termed **helper cells,** or **helper T-cells** (T_H), in that their function is crucial in promoting both B-, as well as T-effector function.
    b. Helper (CD4+) T-lymphocytes are further classified as **Th1** and **Th2,** depending upon the profile of cytokines they produce in response to antigen stimulation.
      (1) Th_1 cells produce interleukin-2 (IL-2) and interferon-gamma (IFN-γ) to stimulate macrophages, and cytotoxic T-cells.
      (2) Th_2 cells produce IL-4, IL-5, and IL-10 to increase production of immunoglobulin.
    c. CD8+ T-cells effect the T-cell response. This frequently involves direct cytotoxicity, and effector T-cells have also been termed **cytotoxic T-cells** (T_C).

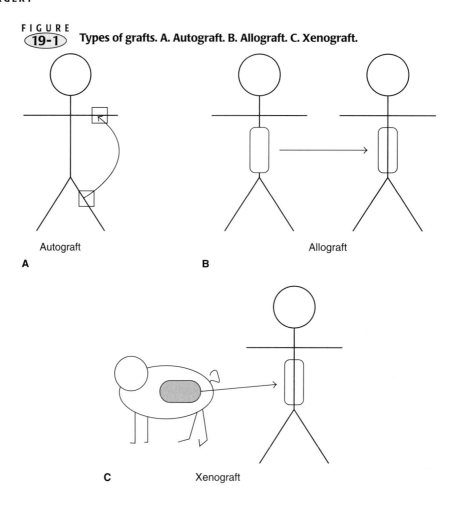

Autograft

A

Allograft

B

C   Xenograft

The human MHC is termed the human leukocyte antigen (HLA) complex. It is coded on the short arm of chromosome 6.

D. **Major histocompatibility complex**
  1. T-cells normally recognize (nonself) antigen only in the context of self major histocompatibility complex (**MHC**). Antigen is bound to the MHC molecule on antigen-presenting cells (**APCs**). This limitation on antigen recognition is referred to as **MHC restriction**.
  2. **MHC** is a cluster of genes found in all mammalian species, that allows an individual to differentiate **self** from **nonself**.
  3. This restriction of the T-cell recognition occurs during development and maturation in the thymus. At this stage, T-cells that would react to self antigens and T-cells that do not recognize self MHC as such are eliminated or inactivated (T-cell selection).
  4. Three genetic loci of the human MHC (HLA) are described—**class I, class II**, and **class III**. These loci code for class I, class II, and class III antigens.
    a. Class I and II region genes code for several highly polymorphic cell surface proteins (HLA antigens).
      (1) Class I is additionally subdivided into **HLA-A**, **HLA-B**, and **HLA-C**. Class I antigens are present on all nucleated cells.
      (2) Class II region genes code for **HLA-DR**, **HLA-DQ**, and **HLA-DP**. Class II antigens are present on B cells, dendritic cells (**DCs**), macrophages, and activated T-cells.
    b. Class III region genes code for some proteins of the complement system.
    c. Some other cell types (e.g., endothelial cells) may be induced to express class II antigen by cytokines (e.g., IFN-γ).
  5. HLA-A, HLA-B, and HLA-DR have been termed **major histocompatibility antigens**. These have been most closely associated with the host's immune response (rejection) to transplanted allogeneic tissue.

FIGURE
19-2

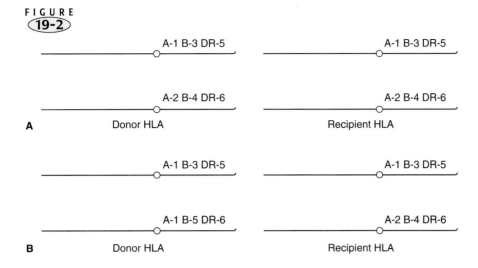

A   Donor HLA   Recipient HLA

B   Donor HLA   Recipient HLA

a. Because each individual has two # 6 chromosomes (one maternal and one paternal), there are potentially six distinct major HLA antigens expressed on cells.

b. If donor tissue and the recipient have the same HLA-A, HLA-B, and HLA-DR, this is referred to as a "six-antigen match" (Fig. 19-2A). An individual may be homozygous for any of these antigens (e.g., A-1) (see Fig. 19-2B).

6. Although in the above example, donor and recipient HLA are not identical, the donor is a "**zero antigen mismatch**" with the recipient, because the donor has no HLA antigens that mismatch with the recipient.

7. **APCs** process and present nonself antigen to T-cells in the context of MHC. APCs include macrophages (**Mϕ**), **DCs**, activated TH, and B-cells.

II. Rejection

A. Transplant rejection is the host response (antibody-mediated, cell-mediated or both) directed against nonself alloantigens (transplanted tissue).

B. **Hyperacute rejection**

1. This type of rejection is mediated by preformed (already present at the time of transplant) antibodies against donor antigen (HLA antigen). These antibodies may be IgG against HLA antigen, and/or IgM against an ABO mismatch. Hyperacute rejection is also controlled by activation of the complement system, which causes acute vascular injury, and activation of the coagulation cascade. Rapid and irreversible graft loss is due to ischemia from thrombosis.

2. Hyperacute rejection occurs within minutes to hours after organ reperfusion.

3. There are no effective treatments for hyperacute rejection. The clinical strategy is to avoid hyperacute rejection.

   a. **Pretransplant** cross-matches **are performed to detect preformed anti-HLA antibodies.** The rules regarding compatibility are generally the same as those for blood transfusion (Table 19-1).

   b. Hyperacute rejection is prevented by careful matching of ABO blood groups, and by screening for preformed anti-HLA antibodies with the pretransplant crossmatch.

   c. Blood group A may clinically present as A1 or A2. A2 individuals are clinically blood group A, but express significantly less A antigen. A2 organs have been successfully transplanted into blood group O and B recipients with low titers of anti-A antibody.

4. In the absence of meticulous preparation and manipulation of the immune response, transplantation across blood group compatibilities will fail with hyperacute rejection due to preformed antibodies.

TABLE 19-1 Renal Recipient versus Renal Donor Blood Type	
Donor	**Recipient**
O	O, A, B, AB
A	A, AB
B	B, AB
AB	AB

5. Experimental protocols to remove circulating antibody (plasmapheresis) and antibody producing cells (splenectomy and/or treatment with rituximab (anti-CD20) have had some success in permitting transplantation across blood groups.

C. **Accelerated acute rejection**
   1. This type of rejection is also antibody-mediated, but does not present clinically until 2 to 5 days after transplantation. This type of rejection is due to an **anamnestic** response from prior exposure (sensitization). Sensitization may result from previous blood transfusions, transplants, or pregnancy.
   2. Accelerated acute rejection has been successfully treated with plasmapheresis to remove antibody and intravenous IgG, anti-lymphocyte antibodies, or rituximab to manipulate further antibody production.

D. **Acute rejection**
   1. Most acute rejections are cell-mediated. Cell-mediated acute rejections are generally easier to reverse than antibody-mediated acute rejections.
   2. This type of rejection occurs days to months following transplantation.
   3. Acute rejection may present with fever, chills, arthralgias, and systemic toxicity (consistent with tumor necrosis factor-α and/or IL-1).
   4. With current immunosuppression protocols, acute rejection often lacks these clinical features, and presents as allograft dysfunction.
   5. The diagnosis of rejection is most definitively established by allograft biopsy. The **Banff classification** scheme is frequently used to describe and grade the severity of acute rejection on renal allograft biopsy specimens.

E. **Chronic rejection**
   1. This insidious process is the leading cause of late allograft loss.
   2. Chronic rejection likely encompasses both immunologic as well as non-immunologic (drug toxicity, infection, metabolic and biochemical alterations) factors.
   3. Chronic rejection may present differently in different transplanted organs.
   4. A Banff classification scheme can be used to grade the histopathology of chronic rejection in renal allografts.

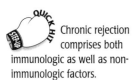

Chronic rejection comprises both immunologic as well as non-immunologic factors.

III. Immunosuppression

A. Current clinically applicable immunosuppression is nonspecific. Ideal immunosuppression would specifically suppress only those cellular subsets of the immune system that are genetically programmed to respond to donor antigen.

B. Except in the case of transplantation between monozygotic twins, allografts between individuals will elicit an immune response. Immunosuppressive drugs are administered to suppress the immune response.
   1. Although high-dose immunosuppressive therapy might eliminate rejection, it would be associated with an intolerable and unacceptable degree of morbidity and mortality.
   2. Giving no immunosuppressive therapy would be associated with no drug-related toxicity, but would lead to allograft loss from rejection.

C. Current immunosuppression protocols are designed to achieve acceptable allograft survival rates with minimal toxicities and side effects. The therapeutic window between lack of efficacy and toxicity/side effects is very narrow for most immunosuppressive medications.

   1. The calcineurin inhibitors (cyclosporine, tacrolimus) are metabolized by cytochrome P450 3A (CYP3A). Drugs that alter CYP3A activity can have significant effect on drug levels (efficacy/toxicity) of either calcineurin inhibitor.

   2. Increased CYP3A activity increases calcineurin metabolism, and decreases drug levels. Barbiturates, phenytoin, rifampin, and St. John wort may reduce calcineurin levels (decreased efficacy) by induction of CYP3A.

   3. Decreased CYP3A activity decreases calcineurin metabolism and increases drug levels. Ketoconazole, fluconazole, itraconazole, erythromycin, verapamil, and diltiazem increase calcineurin levels (increased toxicity) by decreasing CYP3A activity.

D. Complications of immunosuppression include an increased risk of infection and malignancy.

IV. Infection

A. General principles

   1. Immunosuppressed patients are susceptible to familiar bacterial infections (e.g., pneumonia, wound infection, line infection, urine infection), as well as unusual infections (e.g., viral, fungal, protozoal, atypical bacteria and mycobacteria). The time after transplant is an important factor in determining the etiology of an infection.

   2. Immunosuppressed patients frequently present with subdued clinical (and laboratory) signs and symptoms of infection. As a consequence, immunosuppressed patients may present later in the course of an infection.

   3. The key to successful management of infections in immunosuppressed patients is a high level of clinical suspicion, and an aggressive approach to diagnosis and treatment.

   4. Reduction of immunosuppression may be a necessary part of successful management of infection.

      a. The overall degree (intensity) of immunosuppression correlates with the risk and severity of infection.

      b. As the risk of certain ("unusual") infections is well known, drug prophylaxis protocols are used to reduce the risk of these infections.

B. Types of infections

   1. Cytomegalovirus (CMV)

      a. This member of the herpes family of viruses is a ubiquitous virus with many different serotypes. It can infect any cell type.

      b. In a nonimmunosuppressed individual, CMV usually occurs as a mild and self-limiting infection. An elevated anti-CMV IgG indicates previous CMV infection. The viral genome can persist without symptoms, for life.

      c. The CMV virus can be transferred with any solid organ transplant. CMV infection in transplant recipients has been associated with increased risk of rejection, increased risk of additional infections, and increased risk of malignancy (post-transplant lymphoproliferative disorder [PTLD]).

      d. In an immunosuppressed individual, CMV may occur as a primary or secondary infection.

         (1) A primary CMV infection occurs in a naïve, seronegative individual upon exposure to the CMV virus.

         (2) A secondary infection occurs in a seropositive individual. A secondary infection may represent **reactivation** from a latent virus or exposure to a new serotype.

      e. **CMV disease** denotes a more symptomatic infection (fever, "viral syndrome," leukopenia). **Invasive CMV** disease may cause serious pneumonitis, hepatitis, encephalitis, gastrointestinal invasion with bleeding and/or perforation.

f. CMV disease and invasive CMV is treated with ganciclovir or valganciclovir. CMV strains resistant to ganciclovir may be treated with foscarnet. Foscarnet has a significant renal toxicity.

g. Effective prophylaxis can reduce incidence and severity of CMV disease. Prophylaxis is provided by ganciclovir, valganciclovir, acyclovir, or CMV immune globulin.

2. Epstein–Barr virus (**EBV**)

a. This member of the herpes family of viruses most frequently infects B lymphocytes. It is the most common causative agent of mononucleosis. Elevated IgG against EBV viral capsid antigen, and/or EBV nuclear antigen indicate previous infection. The EBV genome may persist in lymphocytes.

b. Because all transplantable solid organs contain some donor lymphocytes, EBV may be transmitted by transplantation. EBV has been clearly associated with the development of PTLD (see below), especially in EBV-naive recipients.

c. Primary and secondary EBV infections may occur (as with CMV), but the severity is generally less.

d. Prophylaxis used for CMV (e.g., acyclovir, ganciclovir) may have some ameliorating effect on EBV.

3. Varicella zoster virus (**VZV**)

a. This a member of the herpes family of viruses. It is the etiologic agent of chickenpox. The virus persists for life in the dorsal root ganglia.

b. Reactivation of the VZV virus is responsible for clinical **shingles** (herpes zoster). Varicella zoster disease in immunosuppressed patients is due to reactivation. Disseminated disease is rare, and usually occurs in previously serologically naïve patients who are infected by the usual respiratory route.

c. Prophylaxis (like that for CMV) appears to be effective in that the incidence of clinical VZV disease is low during such prophylaxis.

4. Other

a. **Parvovirus B19** is the etiologic agent of fifth disease. In immunosuppressed individuals, parvovirus B19 can cause a profound and refractory anemia. The anemia may respond to intravenous IgG.

b. **BK virus** is a polyomavirus. In renal transplant patients, BK virus infection may present as progressive allograft dysfunction, mimicking acute rejection. It can be differentiated on biopsy and polymerase chain reaction. There are no specific, good therapies, and treatment usually is reduction of immunosuppression.

c. *Pneumocystis carinii* is the etiologic agent of pneumocystis pneumonia. Previously classified as a protozoan, *P. carinii* is now classified as a fungus.

(1) Treatment of pneumocystis pneumonia is with intravenous trimethoprim-sulfamethoxazole or intravenous pentamidine. The pentamidine is associated with a high incidence of side effects, including potentially severe pancreatitis.

(2) Effective prophylaxis is achieved with trimethoprim-sulfamethoxazole, dapsone, or inhaled pentamidine.

d. **Fungal infections** have increased incidence, and severity in immunosuppressed patients.

(1) Risk factors include indwelling catheters, diabetes, use of high dose steroids, intensity of immunosuppression, and use of broad-spectrum antibiotics.

(2) Invasive fungal infections may be treated with fluconazole, itraconazole, or amphotericin B.

(3) *Candida* infection, especially in the early post-transplant period, is most common. Effective prophylaxis against oral or esophageal candidiasis is provided by nystatin or clotrimazole.

V. Malignancy

A. There is an increased incidence and aggressiveness/virulence of certain tumors in immunosuppressed individuals.

1. This now appears to be more due to suppression of natural defenses than to direct oncogenic properties of individual immunosuppressive medications.

2. The incidence of these tumors is related to the intensity and duration of immunosuppression.

B. Malignant tumors, that may metastasize to the transplanted organ in a donor harboring a malignancy, may be transferred to the recipient of that organ.

1. Such tumors may exhibit aggressive behavior in the immunosuppressed host.

2. Potential organ donors with cancer are excluded (consideration may be given to prospective donors with nonmelanoma skin cancer and primary central nervous system [CNS] tumors).

C. Because immunosuppression may alter the innate defense against malignant cells, it is usually recommended that an individual not be transplanted/immunosuppressed until 2 to 5 years after curative therapy for cancer in a prospective transplant recipient.

D. Squamous cell carcinoma of the skin demonstrates the greatest increased incidence of these cancers. Prophylaxis against ultraviolet exposure (sunscreen, clothing), and appropriate dosing of immunosuppression are helpful preventive options.

E. Lymphoma has an increased incidence in immunosuppressed individuals. These are usually (greater than 90%) non-Hodgkin B-cell lymphomas.

F. PTLD has been ascribed to EBV infection of B-cells.

1. In immunocompetent patients, an EBV infection causes a polyclonal proliferation of B-cells. This proliferation may not be controlled in immunosuppressed individuals leading, through mutation, to an independent monoclonal expansion (lymphoma). Extranodal involvement (CNS, liver, kidney, intestines) is much more common than with lymphomas in immunocompetent individuals.

2. These lymphomas are much less responsive to standard chemotherapy and radiation treatments, which may increase the level of immunosuppression and worsen the prognosis.

3. These lymphomas may respond to aggressive reduction or cessation of immunosuppression. In some cases, antiviral (oligoclonal) therapy has been reported to be beneficial.

G. There is a moderate increased incidence of **Kaposi sarcoma** (herpes virus 8), and **cervical cancer** (human papilloma virus).

H. There is no increased incidence of common solid tumors such as colon, breast, and lung cancer.

ORGAN SUPPLY AND DEMAND

I. Organ Allocation

A. There is a large discrepancy between the demand (number of patients awaiting transplantation), and the supply (number of actual organ donors and transplantable organs). For deceased donor organs, there is also a discrepancy between the location of the donor and the potential recipient who, according to current algorithms, might best utilize these transplantable organs.

B. The **National Organ Procurement and Transplant Network (OPTN)** was established in 1984, through the National Organ Transplant Act, passed by the Congress of the United States. The intent of the act is to ensure that scarce transplantable organs are distributed equitable, safely, and efficiently.

C. The federal contract to administer the OPTN has been awarded to the **United Network for Organ Sharing (UNOS)**, which has its headquarters in Richmond, Virginia.

1. All organ transplant centers, organ procurement organizations, and tissue typing laboratories must meet and maintain standards set by UNOS to maintain membership in the network, and access to deceased donor organs.
2. UNOS maintains the national "**waiting list**" of patients awaiting a transplant.
   a. Each time a deceased donor organ becomes available for transplantation anywhere in the nation, this computerized database is searched, and transplant candidates are ranked according to predetermined parameters.
   b. It is important to note that the "list" is not merely a static ordinal rank of waiting time. The results of a **match run** is determined by multiple factors, of which waiting time is only one factor, not the most important factor for any organ.

D. The **Scientific Registry of Transplant Recipients (SRTR)** is responsible for maintaining a very extensive data base on all listed patients awaiting transplantation, and follow-up on all transplanted patients. SRTR data are easily accessible at **http://www.ustransplant.org**, and this website is a useful source of information for patients and health care providers.

E. Another useful resource is the **United States Renal Data System (USRDS)** (http://usrds.org), which maintains an extensive database on all patients who have enrolled in the End-Stage Renal Disease Program.

F. There is a different allocation algorithm for different deceased donor organs. These algorithms take in consideration multiple factors related to the **recipient, donor**, and **logistics**.
   1. Recipient factors include severity of illness for liver transplantation, loss of access for dialysis for renal transplantation, age (pediatric recipients receive a slight increased preference), and the likelihood of receiving a transplant (e.g., panel reactive antibody [PRA] for patients awaiting renal transplants).
   2. Donor factors include donor age, past medical history, social history, donor stability, and biopsy results of donor organs.
   3. Logistics primarily considers the distance (time of transport) between donor and recipient hospitals.

G. Organ procurement organizations (OPOs) identify potential deceased organ donors. The 57 nonprofit OPOs provide service to all 50 states and Puerto Rico.
   1. OPOs facilitate and coordinate organ recovery, preservation, and transport. Law requires that all deaths are reported to the OPO.
   2. OPOs are also charged with education of health care providers, and the lay public regarding organ donation.

II. Donor Organs from Diseased Individuals

A. Organ donation. Organs for transplantation may be recovered from individuals who meet the criteria for **brain death**, or from individuals who have massive and irreversible brain damage, and for whom an independent decision to withdraw life support has been made (**non-heart beating donor (NHBD)**, or **donation after cardiac death**).
   1. The basic legal framework for defining brain death is described in the **Uniform Determination of Death Act** (1980), which has been adopted by all states. In this act, brain death is defined as the "irreversible cessation of all functions of the entire brain, including the brainstem."
   2. Detailed specifics for clinical brain death (e.g., length of time for apnea), and requirements for confirmatory testing (e.g., electroencephalogram, cerebral blood flow studies) are the prerogative of individual hospitals.
   3. The standards to determine brain death are rigorous to exclude any conceivable potentially reversible factors (e.g., hypothermia, alcohol, drugs, severe metabolic abnormalities).
   4. The criteria for brain death include:
      a. A known and irreversible brain injury.
      b. Coma on a ventilator.

    c. Absent brain stem reflexes (e.g., pupillary, corneal, gag, vestibuloocular, oculocephalic).

    d. Apnea off a ventilator.

    e. Absence of exclusionary criteria.

5. Some hospitals require confirmatory tests (brain blood flow tests, electroencephalogram), although these have not been listed as mandatory in formal criteria.

6. NHBDs are comatose individuals with severe, irreversible damage, who do not meet all the formal criteria (usually, some remnant of brain stem activity) for brain death, and for whom an independent decision has been made to withdraw life support. Organ recovery is performed after there is cessation of cardiac function in the donor.

7. Recoverable solid organs for transplantation include the heart, lung, liver, pancreas (whole organ, or islets of Langerhans), kidney, and intestine. Donors may also donate tissue, including bone, tendons, heart valves, and corneas.

8. The criteria for what is considered an acceptable organ for transplant have expanded as the number of people awaiting transplant has increased. The clinical need of an individual patient is taken into account when deciding on the suitability of a given organ offer.

9. Contraindications to organ donation include malignancy, HIV, systemic infection, hepatitis B surface antigen positivity, hepatitis C antibody (many centers use organs from hepatitis C+ donors for hepatitis C+ recipients).

B. Organ preservation. Because the tolerance of transplantable organs to normothermic ischemia is measured in minutes, effective steps must be taken to protect against cell damage and cell death.

1. Normothermic cellular metabolism in the absence of oxygen, and the metabolic substrates supplied by an intact circulation leads to cell damage and death. The products of anaerobic cellular metabolism play a major role in **reperfusion injury** (e.g., oxygen free radicals) upon the reestablishment of normothermic circulation to the transplanted organ.

2. The strategy of organ preservation is to minimize cellular metabolism.

3. Hypothermia (less than 5°C) is a cornerstone of all organ preservation. Oxygen consumption is reduced by 95% at 5°C. Freezing, with intracellular ice crystal formation, must be avoided.

    a. Hypothermia does not totally stop metabolic processes, and the end products of metabolism accumulate over time. This is a major factor in the tolerable length of time between organ recovery and transplantation.

    b. Energy-independent cell functions are less affected by hypothermia (e.g., passive diffusion of extracellular sodium across thecal membrane). Organ preservation solutions approximate the intracellular environment with a high potassium and low sodium concentrations.

    c. Cellular swelling is a natural consequence of hypothermic storage, due to passive diffusion of water into the higher oncotic pressure of the cell. Impermeable oncotic agents (e.g., hetastarch, mannitol, raffinose) are included to prevent cell swelling.

4. Accumulation of lactic acid from low-level anaerobic metabolism leads to a progressively lower pH within the stored organ. Phosphates are the usual buffer for organ preservation solutions.

5. Several commercial organ preservation solutions with different components and concentrations have been approved for clinical use; including Collins, ViaSpan (University of Wisconsin Solution), and Custodiol (HTK).

6. Optimal organ preservation begins with careful clinical management of the deceased donor, with special attention to hemodynamic and metabolic parameters. Hypotension is common, and many donors have diabetes insipidus and marked hypernatremia. Severe hypernatremia in the donor has been associated with allograft dysfunction (especially liver allografts).

C. Organ recovery
   1. The operative approach is directed toward minimizing warm ischemia time, as well as surgical injury to the recovered organs.
   2. Proximal and distal control of the aorta for cold perfusion is carried out early in the operation. Access to the vena cava is required to vent blood and flush solution.
   3. In a stable donor, time may be expended to do a preliminary dissection: mobilizing individual organs and looking for anatomic variants (e.g., replaced right and/or left hepatic arteries). However, many transplant programs prefer to use a rapid technique of **en bloc excision** after cold perfusion with dissection and separation on the back table.

TRANSPLANTATION OF SPECIFIC ORGANS

I. Kidney
   A. Indications
      1. End-stage renal disease with a glomerular filtration rate (GFR) less than 20 mL/min$^{-1,}$ or maintenance hemodialysis are prerequisites for a deceased donor transplant.
      2. Pre-emptive renal transplant (GFR greater than 20 mL/min, or patient not yet on dialysis) may be performed using living donors.
      3. Conditions that are some of the more common causes of renal failure leading to renal transplantation, such as diabetic nephropathy, hypertensive nephropathy, glomerulonephritides, polycystic kidney disease, chronic pyelonephritis, obstructive uropathy, or congenital abnormalities.
   B. Contraindications
      1. Chronic, untreated infection. HIV, hepatitis B, and hepatitis C are no longer absolute contraindications to transplantation, but must be approached with a meticulous plan for long-term management.
      2. A recent malignancy (except small nonmelanoma skin cancer, and at some centers, carcinoma *in situ*) or metastatic cancer. A 2- to 5-year disease-free interval following curative treatment of a malignant tumor is required at most centers.
      3. Severe comorbid conditions that make the risk of surgery and/or chronic immunosuppression prohibitive.
      4. A history of recurrent noncompliance is a warning sign for inability to comply with the complicated postoperative management requirements.
   C. Preoperative evaluation
      1. A complete history and physical examination may identify many significant, but correctable, potential problems for transplantation. Evaluation of the lower urinary tract is often indicated based on history (e.g., recurrent infections, diabetes mellitus [neurogenic bladder]). Anuric patients have no voiding symptoms.
      2. Bilateral native nephrectomy is indicated for chronic infection, severe proteinuria, suspicion of cancer in the native kidneys, massively enlarged kidneys from polycystic kidney disease, with pain, infection, or bleeding. Bilateral native nephrectomy for refractory hypertension has been reported to be helpful in some cases.
      3. The patient has HLA typing and screening for preformed anti-HLA antibodies (PRAs) prior to being placed on the UNOS waiting list.
   D. Operation
      1. The kidney is transplanted into the heterotopic location of the iliac fossa. The renal artery and vein are anastomosed to the respective iliac artery and vein.
      2. Following reperfusion, the ureter is anastomosed to the urinary bladder. An antireflux maneuver (Litch technique [currently favored] or Politano–Lead [better] technique) is performed. The ipsilateral native ureter may be used.

E. Immediate postoperative care
1. Most aspects of management are the same as they would be for any general surgical patient. Attention to fluid and electrolyte management is particularly important. Hypovolemia (which can occur rapidly with a brisk diuresis) must be avoided.
2. Special attention must be paid to frequent monitoring of urine output. Approximately 20% of deceased donor renal transplants have delayed graft function with anuria or oliguria.
   a. Because serious and graft threatening technical complications (e.g., thrombosis, urine leak) may present with low urine output, this must be a diagnosis of exclusion, and causes of low urine output must be diligently sought and treated.
   b. Causes of low urine output include hypovolemia and hypotension, an occluded Foley catheter, arterial or venous thrombosis, hydronephrosis or urine leak, and antibody-mediated rejection.
F. Surgical complications
1. Urine leak may occur in as many as 10% of cases, and is most frequently caused by the poor blood supply to the distal transplant ureter. Urine leak may be diagnosed by biochemical analysis of fluid from the wound or nuclear scan.
   a. Urine leaks in the very early post-transplant period should be treated by surgical revision of the anastomosis.
   b. Urine leaks in the later post-transplant period should be evaluated with cystoscopy/retrograde or percutaneous nephrostogram, because such leaks are frequently associated with ureteral stenosis.
2. Lymphoceles are collections of lymph from divided lymphatic vessels along the iliac vessels. Lymphoceles have been reported to occur in as many as 20% of patients.
   a. Many of these collections are small, and have no clinical impact. These require no intervention.
   b. Large lymphoceles may cause allograft dysfunction (by compression or hydronephrosis), pain, or deep venous thrombosis (compression of iliac vein). Percutaneous drainage, sometimes combined with sclerotherapy of the cavity, may be adequate treatment. Lymphoceles may recur, and are treated with internal drainage between lymphocele cavity and the peritoneal cavity (fenestration). Fenestration may be accomplished by either open or laparoscopic approach.
G. Recurrent disease. Many of the diseases that cause end-stage renal disease in the native kidneys may recur in the transplanted kidney (Table 19-2). Recurrent disease does not always lead to allograft loss from recurrent disease.

TABLE 19-2 Renal Diseases and Their Risk of Recurrence

Renal Disease	Risk of Recurrence (%)
Oxalosis	75–100
Membranoproliferative glomerulonephritis (MPGN) type 2	80–100
Hemolytic uremic syndrome (HUS)	40–50
IgA nephritis	40–60
Focal segmental glomerulosclerosis (FSGS)	40–50
Membranoproliferative glomerulonephritis (MPGN) type 1	30–50
Diabetic nephropathy	75–100

TABLE 19-3 Kidney Donor Status and Survival		
Status of Donor	**1-Year Survival**	**5-Year Survival**
Living donor kidney transplant	95%	80%
Deceased donor kidney transplant	90%	65%

H. Long-term outcomes
   1. Current graft survival (dialysis independence) is shown in Table 19-3.
   2. There are no randomized prospective trials comparing chronic dialysis to transplantation.
   3. There are several "intent to treat" studies comparing outcomes of patients on dialysis awaiting transplant, and those actually transplanted. After the increased mortality associated with the operation itself, and early higher dose immunosuppression, the survival of transplanted patients is superior to dialysis after 8 months.

II. **Pancreas**
   A. Indications
      1. The majority of pancreas transplants are performed in patients with type I diabetes mellitus. Diabetes mellitus affects nearly 14 million Americans, and is the sixth leading cause of death (National Center for Health Statistics). It is a leading cause of blindness and renal failure.
      2. Pancreas transplantation is most frequently performed in combination with a kidney transplant ("simultaneous pancreas-kidney transplant" [**SPK**]). Pancreas may also be transplanted into non-renal failure diabetics ("pancreas transplant alone" [**PTA**]), or into diabetics with a previous renal transplant ("pancreas after kidney transplant" [**PAK**]).
   B. Contraindications
      1. Contraindications for pancreas transplantation are essentially the same as those for kidney transplantation.
      2. Because the incidence of atherosclerotic disease is so high in patients with diabetes, especially in patients with renal failure, an aggressive investigation of coronary and peripheral vascular disease should be performed.
   C. Operation
      1. The pancreas is transplanted with the adjacent duodenum, with which it shares a blood supply. The spleen is separated from the tail of the pancreas prior to transplantation.
      2. There have been multiple techniques of implantation of the pancreas graft. The two main considerations are the location of the vascular anastomoses, and the technique of managing exocrine drainage.
      3. The venous (portal) drainage is still most frequently into the systemic circulation (iliac vein or inferior vena cava). Several centers advocate drainage directly into the portal venous system (superior mesenteric vein or splenic vein). There is good clinical evidence that portal drainage is associated with a lower incidence of rejection.
      4. Enteric drainage may be either into small bowel (Roux-en-Y or side-to-side anastomosis), or into the urinary bladder. Enteric drainage is now the favored technique for enteric drainage.
      5. Bladder drainage is associated with metabolic acidosis, due to obligatory loss of the high pH pancreatic secretions, dehydration, "reflux pancreatitis," cystitis, and bleeding. Monitoring of urinary amylase excretion may aid in the diagnosis of rejection, and the pancreas graft can be biopsied cystoscopically.
      6. A functioning pancreas allograft rapidly establishes euglycemia, and "rebound hypoglycemia" is rare.

D. Long-term outcomes
1. The potential of normalized glucose control (as reflected by a normal **hemoglobin A1C**) to prevent the severity and progression of the complications of diabetes, has been well demonstrated by the Diabetes Control and Complications Trial (DCCT) (see *New England Journal of Medicine* 1993; 329[14]).
2. Successful pancreas transplantation can establish euglycemia, and a normalized Hgb A1C. Current data suggest that successful pancreas transplantation can improve peripheral neuropathy, and stabilize or even reduce diabetic retinopathy. There is no evidence that successful pancreas transplantation reverses macrovascular disease.
E. Islet transplantation
1. The whole pancreas transplanted to correct diabetes mellitus contains less than 2% of its mass, the insulin producing islets of Langerhans. Experimental studies demonstrating that isolated islet transplantation can correct diabetes were published by Lacy and Ballinger more than 30 years ago. Clinical attempts to use islet transplantation had low success rates of marginal durability. The **Edmonton Protocol** (*New England Journal of Medicine* 2000; 343[4]) is a new immunosuppression protocol that uses daclizumab, tacrolimus, sirolimus and is **steroid-free.** Seven consecutive patients were insulin independent, with median follow-up of 1 year.
2. Islets of Langerhans can be isolated from the pancreas using a combination of mechanical and enzymatic techniques. The isolated islets are injected into a branch of the portal vein in the liver. Islets from two to three donor pancreases are usually needed to achieve sufficient islet mass to correct diabetes.

III. Liver
A. General principles
1. Indications for liver transplantation include acute hepatic failure and chronic liver failure.
2. Before the advent of surgery, the 1-year mortality for patients with decompensated liver failure reached more than 50%. Since transplantation has been available, the survival reaches 85% at 1 year, and 70% at 5 years.
B. Transplantation for acute liver failure
1. Acute liver failure is defined as acute decompensation of hepatic function, with the time from onset of jaundice to encephalopathy in less than 8 weeks.
2. The most common reasons for fulminant liver failure in the United States are acetaminophen (Tylenol) overdose (20%), followed by non-A or non-E hepatitis (also called cryptogenic liver failure) (15%), and drugs (12%).
3. Presentation and accurate diagnosis begins with a thorough history and physical examination.
   a. Most patients are encephalopathic on presentation, and history can be obtained from the family.
   b. Identify findings of depression and medication overdose.
   c. Additionally, patients may have anorexia and malaise.
   d. Symptoms are suggestive of a viral syndrome.
4. Prompt treatment includes admission to the intensive care unit with appropriate resuscitation.
   a. Follow liver function tests and chemistries closely.
   b. Initiate lactulose therapy early when patient is encephalopathic.
   c. Treat acetaminophen overdose with N-acetyl cysteine.
   d. Early referral to transplant center is critical for successful outcomes.
5. Kings College and Clichy criteria identify the degree of disease, and the appropriate candidates that would benefit from transplantation in a patient with acute hepatic failure.
6. Research interest: some centers use artificial liver support systems to bridge a patient to liver transplantation. These are temporary measures.

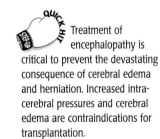
Treatment of encephalopathy is critical to prevent the devastating consequence of cerebral edema and herniation. Increased intracerebral pressures and cerebral edema are contraindications for transplantation.

QUICK HIT

Identify the main portosystemic shunts via the esophageal veins (causing esophageal varices), short gastric veins (causing gastric varices), umbilical vein (causing caput medusae), and rectal veins (causing hemorrhoids).

QUICK HIT

The degree of liver dysfunction is determined by the Child–Turcotte–Pugh classification. This scoring system takes into account the degree of ascites, hepatic encephalopathy, serum bilirubin, prothrombin time, and albumin.

QUICK HIT

Priority on the waiting list is determined by the model for end-stage liver disease score (MELD score). This involves a complex mathematical equation that places patients with greatest metabolic disturbance higher on the list.

QUICK HIT

With liver transplantation, the donor organ is placed in the same area as the previous diseased liver, and therefore, such a placement is termed orthotopic transplantation. With kidney and pancreas transplantation, the donor organ is placed in the pelvis, and therefore, it is termed heterotopic transplantation.

C. Transplantation for chronic liver failure
  1. In the United States, common reasons for transplantation in a patient with chronic liver failure include alcohol-induced cirrhosis, and the myriad of viral hepitides. Other causes of liver failure include primary sclerosing cholangitis, primary biliary cirrhosis, hepatocellular carcinoma, biliary atresia, metabolic disorders such as hemochromatosis, Wilson disease, and enzymatic deficiencies in the urea cycle.
  2. The pathophysiology of chronic liver failure involves two basic concepts: portal hypertension and hepatocyte damage. The increased portal venous blood flow through the liver, results in blood flow via the physiological portosystemic shunts, as a compensatory mechanism to increased portal blood flow. Hepatocyte damage results from insult at a cellular level by the virus or other toxins.
  3. Selection for liver transplantation involves identification of contraindications (HIV, advanced age, disseminated cancer), degree of liver disease, availability of psychosocial support group (to assist in postoperative care), and financial ability (postoperative care requires strict adherence to immunosuppressive regimens that may be expensive).
D. Surgical techniques
  1. Surgery can be especially difficult in a patient who is coagulopathic, and has evidence of portal hypertension.
  2. The native liver is mobilized by releasing the attachments from the diaphragm. The portal triad, which includes the bile duct, portal vein and the hepatic artery, are skeletonized in preparation of the donor organ. The suprahepatic inferior vena cava (IVC) is mobilized. Following this, these structures are clamped and transected, releasing the liver from the bed.
  3. The donor organ is prepared in a similar way, followed by end-to-end anastomosis of the suprahepatic and infrahepatic IVC. The portal vein, hepatic artery, and finally the bile duct anastomosis are completed in that order.
  4. Occasionally, a split liver transplant may be performed in a child, wherein an adult liver cannot be accommodated into the abdomen.
E. Postoperative complications
  1. Bleeding: usually occurs when coagulopathy is not adequately addressed.
  2. Primary nonfunction of the liver: this disastrous situation occurs when the liver is unable to function after transplantation. This condition warrants urgent retransplantation.
  3. Reperfusion injury: this scenario is common when the ischemic time on the organ is prolonged. The treatment is primarily supportive.
  4. Vascular complications: following the hepatic arterial anastomosis, the artery may thrombose, leading to elevations of the transaminases, abscess formation, and biliary tract strictures. This usually results from a technical error.
     a. Acute portal hypertension after transplant should alert the physician to this complication.
     b. Treatment may be angiography with lytic therapy and stenting. Rarely portal vein thrombosis may occur.
  5. Biliary tract stricture: strictures in the tract occur primarily due to ischemia of the tract. These can be treated with endoscopic retrograde cholangiopancreatography and stent placement.
  6. Rejection: early rejection can occur if immunosuppressive therapy is not initiated early. The patient may be asymptomatic, or may have a rise in the transaminases and bilirubin.
     a. The presence of inflammatory cells and lymphocyte-mediated bile duct injury as seen in the biopsy can be diagnostic. The diagnosis is confirmed by biopsy.
     b. This condition warrants the administration of immunoglobulin or high-dose steroids.

7. Infection: most commonly, CMV infection may result. One must always maintain a very low threshold for infection in a post-transplant patient. Work up includes blood, urine, and stool cultures for bacteria, fungi, and viruses.

8. Recurrence of native disease: patients that are transplanted for hepatitis B and hepatitis C are prone to infecting the donor organ. Primary sclerosing cholangitis, biliary cirrhosis, hemochromatosis, and autoimmune hepatitis may occur in the donor organ.

9. PTLD: as mentioned earlier in the chapter, post-transplant patients may be susceptible to this malignancy.

F. Outcome. Since the advent of transplantation, approximately 10,000 liver transplants have been performed. This population has a 1-year patient survival rate of 90%, and a 5-year patient survival rate of 75%. More importantly, these patients have a dramatic improvement in their quality of life.

IV. Small Bowel

A. The importance of bowel transplantation has been recognized for decades, and yet the first successful transplant was not performed until 1988, in Germany. Very few centers in the United States currently undertake the daunting task of intestinal transplant.

B. Indications for this operation involve cases of short gut (less than 50 cm), intestinal disorders, or malabsorption syndromes. These include Crohn disease, trauma with multiple bowel resections, necrotizing enterocolitis, gastroschisis, intestinal atresia. It is important to understand that there is no specific disease entity that warrants intestinal transplant.

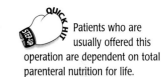 Patients who are usually offered this operation are dependent on total parenteral nutrition for life.

C. The procedure involves the removal of the donor bowel, maintaining the superior mesenteric artery (SMA) and celiac axis. The transplant is conducted by anastomosis of the SMA to the aorta, with venous drainage into the IVC or the portal vein. The maximal ischemia time for bowel is about 6 hours.

D. Complications are failure of graft, infection, and rejection.

TRANSPLANTATION

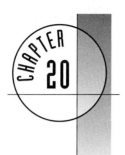

Acute Abdomen

Syed Hashmi, MD
Muhammad Nazim, MD

SEVERE ABDOMINAL PAIN

I. Definition

A. Acute abdomen is defined as severe, persistent abdominal pain usually of sudden onset that is likely to require surgical intervention to treat its cause. Although the severity of the pain is a guide to its seriousness, it is critical to decide what patients need surgery, because not all of them require an operation to treat their pain.

B. It is one of the most common reasons for presentation to emergency departments and physician offices.

II. Embryology of the Gastrointestinal Tract

A. The organs of the gastrointestinal tract are externally lined by a layer of mesodermally derived cells called the visceral peritoneum.

B. This is continuous with the inner layer of the abdominal wall called the parietal peritoneum.

C. The gastrointestinal tract is divided by blood supply into three areas:

1. Foregut: consists of the oropharynx down to the proximal duodenum, and includes the pancreas, liver, biliary tract, and spleen. Its blood supply is the celiac axis.

2. Midgut: consists of the distal duodenum down to the proximal two-thirds of the transverse colon. Its blood supply is the superior mesenteric artery.

3. Hindgut: consists of the colon and rectum. It is supplied by the inferior mesenteric artery.

III. Physiology of Abdominal Pain

A. Visceral pain: due to stimuli affecting the visceral peritoneum (overlying the organs of the gastrointestinal tract).

1. It is mediated by the autonomic nervous system and appreciated at the level of the thalamus.

2. It is stimulated by pulling, stretching, distention, or spasm. It is not stimulated by touch or heat.

3. Chemical stimuli including substance P, serotonin, prostaglandins, and hydrogen ions can also cause pain by stimulating the visceral chemoreceptors.

4. Pain is often a dull ache and is poorly localized. It is frequently described in the midline, because of the bilateral innervation of the viscera. Because it is not affected by movement, patients are often restless.

B. Parietal pain: pain appreciated in the parietal peritoneum covering the abdominal cavity, which is innervated by peripheral nervous system.

1. These stimuli are transmitted by the central nervous system, and are interpreted at a specific cortical level.

2. It is induced by touch, pressure, heat, and inflammation.

3. Localized by great accuracy, it is often described as sharp or cutting. Pain is affected by movement, so patients tend to lie still.

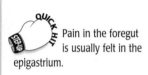
Pain in the foregut is usually felt in the epigastrium.

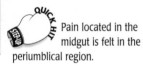
Pain located in the midgut is felt in the periumblical region.

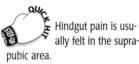
Hindgut pain is usually felt in the suprapubic area.

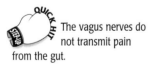
The vagus nerves do not transmit pain from the gut.

C. Referred pain: pain felt at a site distant from the diseased organ, but sharing a common development.

1. Splenic disease is felt at the tip of the left shoulder, because splenic pathology irritates the diaphgram, which is supplied by the phrenic nerve. The phrenic nerve itself comes from the trunks of the fourth cervical nerve, and pain in its distribution is felt in the skin distribution of the fourth cervical nerve.

2. Right subscapular pain is the referred site of pain, due to biliary colic or perforated ulcer.

3. Back pain often occurs with patients with pancreatitis or ruptured aortic aneurysms.

D. Combined pain: visceral and parietal pain can often be combined when there is an alteration of the relationship, and proximity of the two types of peritoneum.

1. Contact between an organ with inflamed visceral peritoneum and its pain-sensitive parietal peritoneum, results in the perception of pain over the site of the parietal peritoneum.

2. Rebound tenderness is appreciated when an examiner presses down on the patient, and then lets go to see if this movement elicits pain. By doing this, the examiner alters the relationship between the two peritoneal surfaces, and attempts to elicit contact between the parietal peritoneum and the visceral peritoneum.

IV. Etiology and Pathology of Abdominal Pain

A. Etiology. Sources of abdominal pain are listed in Table 20-1. The most common causes of acute abdominal pain requiring hospital admission include:

1. Acute appendicitis.
2. Nonspecific abdominal pain.
3. Pain from genitourinary organs.
4. Intestinal obstruction.
5. Biliary tract disease.

B. Pathology

1. Peritonitis is intra-abdominal inflammation.

   a. Inflammation of the peritoneal cavity causes increased secretion of fluid containing protein and leukocytes into the peritoneal cavity.

   b. Ongoing inflammation leads to increased secretion, and resultant hypotension.

   c. If peritoneal defenses are adequate, an exudate is formed that causes adherence between bowel loops or omentum to wall off the area of inflammation, causing an intra-abdominal abscess, which causes localized findings on examination. If these defenses are overwhelmed, there is diffuse peritonitis, which usually requires surgery.

   d. Intra-abdominal pain can have extra-abdominal pathology.

> **QUICK HIT**
> The subdiaphragmatic, subhepatic, paracolic, and pelvic areas are the most common sites of abscess formation.

TABLE 20-1 **Sources of Abdominal Pain**

Abdominal
- Abdominal wall
- Intraperitoneal organs
- Retroperitoneal organs and tissues
- Pelvic organs

Extra-Abdominal
- Intrathoracic organs
- Systemic dysfunction
- Functional abdominal pain

(Reprinted, with permission, from Sterns EE. *Clinical Thinking in Surgery*. Norwalk, CT: Appleton & Lange; 1988.)

TABLE 20-2 Key Historical Features in Acute Abdominal Pain
Age
Time and mode of onset of pain
Duration of symptoms
Character of pain
Location of pain and site(s) of radiation
Associated symptoms and their relation to pain
Nausea or anorexia
Vomiting
Diarrhea or constipation
Menstrual history

(Reprinted, with permission, from *Greenfield's Surgery: Scientific Principles and Practice*, 4th ed. Baltimore:Lippincott Williams & Wilkins; 2006:1210.)

2. Types of peritonitis
   a. Primary or spontaneous peritonitis is inflammation of the peritoneum from a source outside the abdomen. For instance, cirrhotic patients can develop spontaneous bacterial peritonitis.
   b. Secondary peritonitis is inflammation of the peritoneum from an intra-abdominal pathology, such as perforation of the appendix causing appendicitis.
   c. Tertiary peritonitis is the persistent and ongoing infection that results after inadequate treatment for secondary peritonitis.

V. Diagnosis of Abdominal Pain
A. A systemic approach is critical in diagnosing abdominal pain, starting with a thorough history, physical examination, laboratory testing, and then radiological testing as needed.
B. History (Table 20-2)
   1. With regard to the pain, it is critical to document:
      a. Location: assists in defining the anatomic area that may be involved in the disease (Table 20-3).
      b. Nature of the pain: dull pain more likely to be visceral, whereas sharp pain more likely to be parietal pain.
      c. Mode of onset and duration: sudden sharp, severe pain with hypotension suggests a surgical emergency such as perforated ulcer or a rupture of an abdominal aortic aneurysm. Progessive pain over a few hours to days is more consistent with a process, such as appendicitis or bowel obstruction.
      d. Quality and intensity.

> **QUICK HIT**
> Abdominal pain of more than 6 hours duration is likely to require surgical intervention.

TABLE 20-3 Most Common Causes of Pain by Quadrants	
Right Upper Quadrant Pain	**Left Upper Quadrant Pain**
Biliary tract disease	Splenic disease
Liver disease	Perforated gastric ulcer
Pulmonary disease	Pulmonary disease
Renal disease	Myocardial infarction
Right Lower Quadrant Pain	**Left Lower Quadrant Pain**
Appendicitis	Colonic disease
Renal disease	Renal disease
Pelvic inflammatory disease	Pelvic inflammatory disease
Ovarian torsion	Ovarian torsion

e. Exacerbating or relieving factors, such as relation to meals (e.g., exacerbation of right upper quadrant pain by fatty foods is suggestive of cholelithiasis).

f. Radiation: flank pain going to the groin is suggestive of renal calculus disease, whereas right lower quadrant pain going to the back is more suggestive of appendicitis.

g. Associated factors: anorexia, nausea, vomiting, or change in bowel habits in relation to the pain.

   (1) Most patients with abdominal pain of surgical causes lose their appetite.

   (2) In surgical patients, vomiting usually follows the development of abdominal pain, unlike patients with medical conditions such as gastroenteritis. It is important to characterize the vomitus.

      (a) Bilious vomiting suggests an obstruction distal to ampulla of Vater.

      (b) Feculent or foul-smelling vomiting suggests a long-standing small bowel obstruction.

   (3) Change in bowel habits can also give clues to the etiology of abdominal pain. Progressive constipation suggests an obstruction, whereas bloody diarrhea suggests inflammatory bowel disease.

2. Other important historical factors are:

a. In women: thorough menstrual history.

b. Timing of the last meal: this affects anesthetic management.

c. Past medical history and surgical history.

d. Review of current medications is also essential.

   (1) If patients are taking steroids, the immunosuppressive effects can modify the inflammatory reaction such that these patients may have minimal findings on examination. They require steroid supplementation if an operation is planned to prevent adrenal insufficiency.

   (2) Anticoagulants may cause bleeding.

e. Family history (e.g., patients with familial Mediterranean fever or acute porphyria may have recurrent attacks of abdominal pain).

f. Social history, including substance abuse. Cocaine can cause visceral ischemia.

C. Physical examination

1. Vital signs

a. Elevated temperatures are rare in most surgical patients. They are more common in patients with urinary tract infection or gynecological pathology.

b. Tachycardia or hypotension suggest significant volume deficits, and an aggressive disease process.

2. Observe and inspect the patient

a. Start by observing their position in bed: patients with renal colic are restless, whereas patients with perforation and peritonitis tend to lie still, because movement irritates the parietal peritoneum.

b. Inspect the abdomen for distention, scars, hernias, or masses.

c. Auscultate the abdomen, which allows for the detection of bowel sounds, but also to listen for abdominal bruits.

   (1) Hypoactive bowel sounds suggest ileus.

   (2) Hyperactive bowel sounds suggest obstruction.

d. Palpate the abdomen.

   (1) Should be gentle, and start away from the area of pain.

   (2) Should include all four quadrants, and search for hernias (see Table 20-3).

   (3) Assess for presence of guarding (when patient resists movement by tensing abdominal muscles) and rebound tenderness. Percussion of the abdomen is also a useful adjunct because it is a more gentle way to elicit rebound tenderness.

e. Perform a rectal examination to assess for blood, masses, and tenderness.

f. Perform a gynecologic examination to assess for tenderness in the adnexa, cervical discharge, and ovarian enlargement.

    g. Elderly, alcoholic, or immunosuppressed patients may have minimal findings on physical examination despite having serious illness.

    h. Special signs:

       (1) **Murphy sign:** right subcostal pain upon palpation with an inspiratory arrest, is elicited by having patient take a deep breath, and is suggestive of acute cholecystitis.

       (2) **Rovsing sign:** palpation of the left lower quadrant causes pain in the right lower quadrant, and is suggestive of acute appendicitis.

       (3) **Iliopsoas sign:** pain of passively extending the hip, and is suggestive of acute appendicitis.

       (4) **Obturator sign:** pain on internal or external rotation of the flexed hip, and is suggestive of acute appendicitis.

D. Laboratory tests

  1. Assist in diagnosis, but rarely provide it.

  2. Include the following:

    a. Complete blood count, which allows assessment of inflammation and anemia.

    b. Serum electrolytes, where patients have alteration if they have been vomiting or are dehyrated.

    c. Serum amylase/lipase levels in patients suspected of having pancreatitis, where the serum lipase is more sensitive. These can also be elevated in conditions other than pancreatitis, such as small bowel infarction.

    d. Liver function tests, which include bilirubin, alkaline phosphatase, serum transaminases, in patients with right upper quadrant pain.

    e. Human chorionic gonadotropin in all women of child-bearing age.

    f. Urinanalysis in all patients to check for blood or urinary tract infection.

    g. Electrocardiogram (EKG) in patients with heart disease, because myocardial infarction can be confused with abdominal pain.

E. Radiologic studies

  1. Is an important adjunct to clinical diagnosis.

  2. X-rays are useful as a screening tool, and three x-rays are usually taken.

FIGURE 20-1 **Free air.**

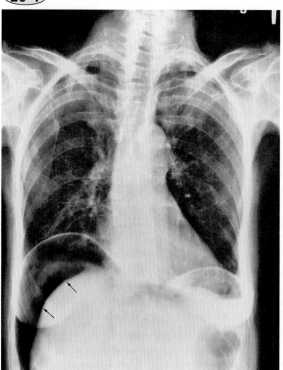

(Reprinted, with permission, from Blackbourne LH. *Surgical Recall,* 4th ed. Baltimore: Lippincott Williams & Wilkins; 2006:185.)

TABLE 20-4	Conditions Characterized by Diffuse Abdominal Pain
Peritonitis	
Mesenteric ischemia	
Diabetic ketoacidosis	
Uremia	

      a. Chest x-ray to look for free air suggestive of visceral perforation or pneumonia causing abominal pain.

      b. Abdominal x-ray (erect and supine views) to look for:

          (1) **Free air**, which suggests perforation of a viscus (Fig. 20-1).

          (2) **Air–fluid levels** suggestive of bowel obstruction.

          (3) Abnormal calcification: 90% or renal calculi, and 10% of gallstone calculi have enough calcium to be detected by x-rays. If it is not possible to take upright films, lateral decubitus films can be done to look for free air.

3. Ultrasound

      a. Allows low-cost evaluation of patient with abdominal pain.

      b. Best used to detect liver, gallbladder, or gynecologic pathology.

      c. Is both operator and patient dependent (difficult to obtain good windows in the obese).

4. Computed tomography (CT) scans

      a. Allows anatomical evaluation of the patient with abdominal pain.

      b. Usually done with oral and intravenous contrast. (CT scans for renal calculi are done without contrast).

      c. CT improves diagnostic accuracy, but may not need to be performed in all patients.

      d. Best used in the elderly, immunosuppressed, or obese patients with suspected disease and minimal signs.

      e. IV contrast may be contraindicated, if there is history of anaphylaxis or renal disease.

5. Other tests such as hydroxy-iminodiacetic acid (HIDA) scans are performed more selectively depending on clinical circumstances. (Tables 20-4 to 20-6).

TABLE 20-5	Most Common Causes of Midline Abdominal Pain
Epigastric	
Peptic ulcer Pancreatitis Myocardial ischemia Cholecystitis	
Periumblical	
Early appendicitis Intestinal obstruction Pancreatitis Ruptured abdominal aortic aneurysm	
Infraumblical	
Appendicitis Diverticulitis Ovarian torsion Cystits	

(TABLE 20-6) Warning Signs in Patients with Abdominal Pain
History
Severe, sudden, sharp continous pain Elderly Immunosuppressed
Physical Examination
Changes in vital signs espically tachycardia, or hypotension Hypoxia Altered mentation Peritoneal signs, especially a rigid abdomen Abdominal pain out of proportion to physical findings
Laboratory Testing
Anemia Leukocytosis Renal failure Acidosis Elevated liver enzymes
Radiology
Free air Bowel obstruction with air fluid levels Air in the portal venous system

(Adapted, with permission, from Flasar MH, Goldberg E. Acute abdominal pain. *Med Clin North Am.* 2006;90:481–503.)

VI. Management

A. It is critical to decide whether a patient needs an operation, and when he or she needs it.

B. Patients who will probably need an operation include:

1. Patients with peritoneal signs such as tenderness, guarding, or rebound.
2. Patients with sepsis or worsening abdominal pain.
3. Patients with free air.

C. If signs are equivocal, patients can be admitted and observed for progression of pain.

D. Preparation for an operation involves:

1. Fluid hydration.
2. Making sure that the patient is nil per os (NPO), or nothing by mouth.
3. Analgesia.
4. Antibiotics, depending on circumstances.
5. Consent.

E. Choice of an operation is up to the operating surgeon.

1. Laparotomy involves open exploration of the abdominal contents.
2. Laparoscopy involves using a laparoscope to evaluate intra-abdominal contents in a less invasive fashion.

VII. Special Patient Populations

A. Pregnant women

1. Acute abdominal pain can also occur during pregnancy.
2. Timing of surgery:
   a. First trimester: operations should be avoided secondary to risk to the fetus.
   b. Second trimester: this is the safest time for operation.
   c. Third trimester: operations carry the risk of premature labor.
3. Cholecystitis also can complicate pregnancy.

      a. Generally an operation is not indicated, unless the patient has severe, constant pain.

      b. If an operation is needed, it should be done in the second trimester.

    4. Appendicitis complicates 1 in 1,500 pregnancies.

      a. This condition is difficult to diagnose, because the enlarging uterus may push the appendix laterally into the flank or right upper quadrant.

      b. Ultrasound can aid in diagnosis, and it also prevents radiation exposure.

B. Geriatic patients

    1. One-third of all geriatric patients with acute abdominal pain require surgical intervention.

    2. These patients have more medical conditions.

    3. There is a higher rate of misdiagnosis, due to subtle or confusing presentations.

    4. Objective findings may or may not be present.

    5. Medication can alter response to pain or alter the examination, such as beta-blockers blunt the tachycardia of the stress response.

    6. It is essential to perform a thorough examination, and obtain an EKG to evaluate for myocardial ischemia.

    7. The threshold for intervention should be low.

C. Immunosuppressed individuals

    1. Patient populations, who may have varying degrees of immunosuppression include:

      a. Elderly.

      b. Those who are malnourished.

      c. Those with diabetes.

      d. Those with renal failure.

      e. Those with a current malignancy, especially if they are on chemotherapy.

      f. Those who are on immunosuppressive medications such as steroids, chemotherapy agents, and antirejection medicines for transplants.

      g. Those with HIV and CD4 counts less than 200/mL.

    2. Symptoms are vague, and the threshold for intervention needs to be high.

    3. Causes are likely to be either unusual fungal infections or unusual tumors.

    4. Common diseases are gastrointestinal non-Hodgkin lymphoma, acute appendicitis, cytomegalovirus colitis, and mycobacterium intracellular colitis.

D. Patients with medical conditions

    1. Some conditions may complicate evaluation of abdominal pain, and should be considered in the differential diagnosis.

    2. Urinary tract infection may mimic appendicitis, which is why it is critical to do a urinalysis on all patients.

    3. Patients with pneumonia may complain of right or left upper quadrant pain.

    4. History and physical examination assist in diagnosing these conditions.

ACUTE APPENDICITIS

I. Epidemiology

A. One of the most common abdominal emergencies: at least 250,000 cases per year.

B. Incidence: 10 in 100,000 population.

C. Overall lifetime risk: 7%.

II. Embryology and Anatomy

A. The appendix is a vestigial organ, which develops as an outpouching of the cecum. The base of the appendix is located at the union of the taenaie of the colon.

B. It contains large amounts of lymphoid tissue.

C. Histologically, cells are similar cells to those of the colon.

D. It is located in a retrocecal position in two-thirds of patients, although it can also be in pelvic brim or in the pelvis, which can cause delay in diagnosis because of the lack of peritoneal irritation.

E. Arterial blood comes from the appendicular artery, a branch of the ileocolic artery.

F. Venous drainage is via ileocolic veins to the portal vein.

G. Lymph drainage is to the ileocolic nodes, which are often inflamed during an acute attack.

III. Pathology

A. Initial process: luminal obstruction occurs by lymphoid hyperplasia or by fecaliths.

B. Early appendicitis: obstruction leads to mucosal edema with rising intraluminal pressure. This is appreciated by the visceral nerve fibers. Due to bilateral innervation, patients feel pain at the periumblical region.

C. Suppurative appendicitis: intraluminal pressure exceeds perfusion pressure, causing ischemia of the appendiceal wall. This leads to bacterial penetration of the appendiceal wall. When the inflamed appendix touches the abdominal wall, there is a migration of pain to the right lower quadrant.

D. Gangrenous appendicitis: the rising pressure in the appendix impedes venous outflow and then arterial inflow, which can then lead to perforation.

E. Appendiceal abscess: an appendiceal perforation can by walled off the surrounding bowel or by the greater omentum, leading to abscess formation.

IV. Diagnosis

A. The typical presentation (80% of cases) starts with:
   1. Periumbilical pain
   2. Anorexia
   3. Right lower quadrant pain
   4. Fever
   5. Leukocytosis
   6. Can also complain of urinary symptoms due to irriation of the urethra or bladder

B. An algorithm showing the workup of acute appendicitis is shown in Figure 20-2.

C. Examination
   1. Almost all patients have some degree of tenderness in right lower quadrant, especially at **at McBurney point** (one-third of the distance from the anterior superior iliac spine to the umbilicus), corresponding roughly to the position of the appendix.
   2. A pelvic appendix may elicit minimal peritoneal signs, but can be appreciated on rectal examination.
   3. Other signs that can help in detecting appendicitis include the iliopsoas, obturator, and Rovsing's signs.

D. Laboratory tests
   1. Leukocytosis is common, but very high white blood cell count is rare.
   2. Important to get a urinanalysis, and a human chorionic gonadotropin level.

FIGURE 20-2 **Workup of acute appendicitis.**

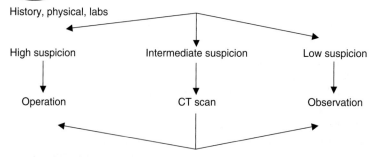

(Adapted, with permission, from *Greenfield's Surgery: Scientific Principles and Practice*, 4th ed. Baltimore: Lippincott Williams & Wilkins; 2006.)

ACUTE ABDOMEN ● 321

E. Radiology
 1. Plain x-rays are rarely helpful, but may help rule out other pathology, such as renal calculi.
 2. Ultrasound has been shown to have variable benefit in diagnosis of acute appendicitis. It is affected by operator experience and patient's body habitus.
 3 Clinical picture is a typical lesion or a noncompressible structure in right lower quadrant.
 4. It is helpful, if it is thought that pelvic pathology is causing the pain.
 5. A CT scan of the abdomen and pelvis is performed with oral and intravenous contrast, and the area of the appendix is scanned with thin cuts of the appendix.
  a. CT appears to be the most sensitive test to diagnose appendicitis.
  b. However, in classic presentation it should rarely be needed. It is associated with a significant exposure to radiation.
  c. CT scan findings of appendicitis (Fig. 20-3):
   (1) Include lack of contrast in appendix.
   (2) Appendiceal enlargement.
   (3) Inflammation around the appendix (i.e., inflammtory stranding).

V. Management

A. In the typical presentation, an operation is required after giving broad-spectrum antibiotics.
B. The operation can be performed in two ways, and the choice is usually made by surgeon preference.
 1. Open appendectomy.
  a. An incison is made at the McBurney point.
  b. Even if no appendicitis is found, the appendix is removed, and a search is made for other causes of pain:
   (1) Ileocecal inflammatory disease such as Crohn disease.
   (2) Meckel's diverticulitis, which is an outpouching of the ileum, located 2 feet from the ileocecal valve.
   (3) Gynecological causes in women.
 2. Laparoscopic appendectomy.
  a. Uses a minimally invasive approach to remove the appendix.
  b. Allows more complete examination of the peritoneal cavity.

FIGURE

Acute appendicitis in a 53-year-old woman with fever and right lower quadrant pain and tenderness. Note the thick-walled, fluid-filled appendix with surrounding inflammation. A gangrenous appendix was found at operation.

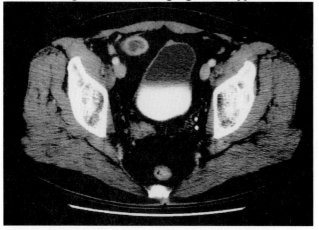

(Reprinted, with permission, from *Greenfield's Surgery: Scientific Principles and Practice*, 4th ed. Baltimore: Lippincott Williams & Wilkins; 2006:1217.)

C. Appendiceal mass
1. When appendiceal inflammation is contained by surrounding tissue, patients develop inflammatory mass or abscess.
2. This leads to delayed presentation, because these patient have minimal signs.
3. This usually occurs 5 days or so after acute attack.
4. Treatment is nonoperative, with antibiotics and drainage of abscess as needed.
5. Affected patients should go undergo appendectomy 6 to 8 weeks after an acute attack to allow for resolution of the inflammatory changes.

ABDOMINAL PAIN IN WOMEN

I. **Epidemiology.** More than two-thirds of the patients who present with abdominal pain to emergency departments in the United States are women.

II. **Diagnosis**
A. A thorough history is essential, including details of menstrual cycle, prior pregnancies, and surgeries.
B. Examination should focus on the abdomen, rectum, and pelvis.
C. Investigations should include checking for pregnancy, and checking vaginal cultures.

III. **Differential Diagnosis.** It is necessary to keep a broad differential diagnosis in mind.
A. Ectopic pregnancy
B. Pelvic inflammatory disease (PID)
C. Tubo-ovarian abscess (TOA)
D. Ovarian torsion

IV. **Specific Disease States**
A. Ectopic pregnancy
1. Ectopic pregnancy is the third leading cause of death of pregnancy-related deaths.
2. The risk is 1 in 200 but increases to 20 to 100 times, if the patient has a history of PID, history of tubal pregnancy, or an intrauterine contraceptive device.
3. The most common site is the oviduct, especially in the distal ampulla, abdomen, and ovary.
4. Classical symptom triad is amenorrhoea, vaginal bleeding and pain, but this is not always present.
5. If rupture occurs, the patient may present with hypotension and acute abdomen.
6. In stable patients, consider transvaginal ultrasound.
B. PID
1. Annually, there are about 1 million cases in United States, and about 150,000 require surgical intervention.
2. The spectrum of disease ranges from salpingitis to pelvic peritonitis, and tubo-ovarian abscess (TOA).
3. Presentation can be subtle or asymptomatic.
4. Organisms include *Neisseria gonorrhoeae, Chlamydia trachomatis, Mycoplasma pneumoniae, Ureaplasma urealyticum,* and uncommonly anaerobes.
5. Management.
a. Currently, the Centers for Disease Control and Prevention recommend empirical treatment for sexually active women with cervical motion tenderness, when no other cause for pain can be found.
b. The mild form can be treated on an outpatient basis with 250 mg ceftriaxone intramuscularly (single shot), followed by 100 mg of doxycycline twice daily for 14 days.

  c. Additional criteria for starting treatment include:
   (1) Temperature greater than 101°C.
   (2) Abnormal vaginal discharge.
   (3) Presence of white blood cells on saline "prep."
   (4) Laboratory documentation of *N. gonorrhoeae* or *C. trachomatis*.
   (5) Most specific: endometrial biopsy and/or laparoscopy.
  d. Indication for admission: pregnancy, nulliparity, failure of treatment, TOA, noncompliance.
C. TOA
 1. Incidence is 1% to 4%, and ruptured TOA has about 8% mortality.
 2. Half of patients have a recent history of PID.
 3. Presenting factors include lower abdominal pain and an adnexal mass, and patients tend to have more pain than those with PID. Patients may also present with peritonitis and shock.
 4. Bacteria include mixed aerobes and anaerobes, mostly bacteroides. *N. gonorrhoeae* and *C. trachomatis* are common, but in 33% of patients no organisms are cultured.
 5. Diagnosis is by ultrasound and laparoscopy.
 6. TOA usually requires admission and treatment with broad-spectrum antibiotics, such as ampicillin/sulbactam and intravenous doxycycline. Patients may also require an operation.
D. Ovarian pathology. This can also cause abdominal pain, usually from torsion or cyst rupture.
 1. Torsion, which is most likely due to enlargement of the ovary beyond 6 cm.
  a. Presentation is usually abrupt, with a sharp, localized, knife-like pain.
  b. The pain is often precipitated by exercise.
  c. Physical examination shows tender adnexal mass.
  d. However, there also may be minimal findings.
  e. Prompt surgical intervention is necessary to protect fertility.
 2. Rupture of ovarian cysts.
  a. This condition can present like torsion.
  b. Adnexal or abdominal tenderness may be present.
  c. If it is associated with bleeding, there may be distention and hypotension.
  d. Ultrasound may help with diagnosis.
  e. If the patient is unstable, operative exploration is needed.

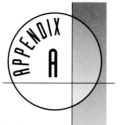

Next Step Questions

Clinical Scenario 1. A 30-year-old man sustains blunt head trauma and is unconscious. His urine output exceeds 1,500 mL per hour despite only receiving maintenance intravenous fluids. He becomes profoundly hypernatremic. Which of the following is the next step in the initial management of this patient?

Answer. This patient has blunt head trauma and diabetes insipidus, characterized by high volume, low osmolality urine. This, untreated, may result in profound dehydration and hypernatremia. Treatment is conservative, with replacement of free water intravenously.

Clinical Scenario 2. An 18-year-old man with hemophilia A presents to the emergency room with a large hemarthrosis of his left knee. His vital signs are stable and he complains only of pain and swelling in the left knee. What is the next step in management?

Answer. This patient has classic hemophilia, or hemophilia A, manifested by a deficiency in factor VIII. It can be treated with either factor VIII or cryoprecipitate intravenously.

Clinical Scenario 3. A 66-year-old woman with metastatic breast cancer presents to the emergency room sleepy with a serum calcium of 12.9 mg/dL. What is the next step in management?

Answer. This patient has symptomatic hypercalcemia. Initial management is adequate hydration and diuresis with a loop agent, such as furosamide.

Clinical Scenario 4. A 25-year-old man presents after a motor vehicle accident (MVA). He has severe facial fractures and deformities, is bleeding, and moans only in response to stimulus. What is the first action to take?

Answer. Assess and secure the airway via endotracheal intubation but be prepared for a surgical airway.

Clinical Scenario 5. A 20-year-old woman presents after a skiing accident. She is alert and talking but not moving. Her blood pressure is 80/55 mm Hg, and her pulse is 80 beats/minute. What is the etiology of her shock, and what should the workup include to aid in the diagnosis?

Answer. Neurogenic shock from a probable cervical spine fracture. Workup should include a complete spine evaluation.

Clinical Scenario 6. An elderly man presents to the emergency department after a fall. On examination he opens his eyes to pain, is confused, and withdraws to painful stimulus. What is his Glasgow Coma Score (GCS)?

Answer. His GCS is 10: (eye) opening to pain, 2; (verbal) confused, 4; (motor) withdraw to painful stimulus, 4.

Clinical Scenario 7. A patient presents after a motor vehicle accident. He is intubated. Initial systolic blood pressure is 80 mm Hg, but he responded to fluid administration. However, his blood pressure just dropped again to 80 mm Hg. His chest x-ray (CXR) is normal, and his pelvis has bilateral inferior rami fractures. A diagnostic peritoneal lavage (DPL) is performed and produces 15 mL gross blood initially. What is the diagnosis and treatment?

Answer. The patient has shock from bleeding in the abdomen. The DPL is grossly positive. He needs urgent laparotomy.

Clinical Scenario 8. A man is brought to the emergency department after an explosion in a confined area. The skin is dark and leathery around his entire torso and his entire left arm. What should be initially done and what is the extent of the burn?

> **Answer.** The patient should be intubated for airway protection; there is a high risk of airway compromise in explosions in a confined area. The burn as described is a 45% total body surface area burn. The next step would be initiate fluid resuscitation and transfer to a burn center.

Clinical Scenario 9. A 79-year-old man presents with a painful incarcerated inguinal hernia. After intravenous fluids and antibiotics are administered, what is the next step in his management?

> **Answer.** The patient has a painful irreducible hernia. After initial resuscitation, surgical reduction and repair is required. A laparotomy may be required if necrotic viscera are found within the hernia sac.

Clinical Scenario 10. A 45-year-old woman presents with a reassurance diastasis recti. What is the initial management?

> **Answer.** Reassurance diastasis recti are a benign widening of the linea alba and do not require surgical intervention.

Clinical Scenario 11. A 60-year-old man develops a complete small bowel obstruction. Physical examination reveals a small and freely reducible nontender left inguinal hernia. What are the next steps in the management of this patient?

> **Answer.** The patient has a complete bowel obstruction and an unrelated hernia. The next step is laparotomy to address the life-threatening condition of small bowel obstruction.

Clinical Scenario 12. A 55-year-old man comes to clinic with complaints of progressive dysphagia and a 20-pound weight loss over the past 3 to 6 months. On further questioning, he describes daily regurgitative symptoms and a long history of heartburn symptoms that he has treated with over-the-counter medications. On physical examination, halitosis is noted but no other significant findings are present. What are the likely diagnoses, and what should the initial management be?

> **Answer.** This patient is describing symptoms of esophageal obstruction. Esophageal cancer, achalasia, and gastroesophageal reflux disease with peptic stricture should be high on the list of potential diagnoses. Initial diagnostic measures should include a barium esophagram along with flexible esophagoscopy with biopsy.

Clinical Scenario 13. A 75-year-old woman is admitted with anemia. On history, she reports dysphagia, positional regurgitative symptoms, and chest pain with meals. She has been admitted three times over the past year with pneumonia and bronchitis. What is the best test to arrive at a diagnosis for this patient? Why is the patient anemic? What surgical option would you offer this patient?

> **Answer.** This patient has symptoms of a paraesophageal hernia. Diagnosis can be made with a barium esophagram. Flexible esophagoscopy is also useful in evaluation of paraesophageal hernias, and in this case would likely show linear ulcerations in the hernia portion of stomach known as Cameron ulcers. Because this patient is symptomatic with anemia, dysphagia, and recurrent pulmonary complications (aspiration pneumonia and bronchitis), relocation of the stomach to the abdomen, repair of the hernia, and an esophagogastric fundoplication make up the components of a reasonable surgical approach to her problem.

Clinical Scenario 14. A 46-year-old man presents with burning epigastric pain of 8 months duration. The pain is somewhat relieved by eating. He has found mild relief with an over-the-counter H_2-receptor antagonist. He smokes one pack of cigarettes per day and drinks alcohol socially. Endoscopy reveals a shallow-based ulcer just proximal to the pylorus. What type of ulcer is this? Is this ulcer associated with acid hypersecretion?

> **Answer.** This is a type III ulcer, called a "prepyloric" or "channel ulcer." It is associated with acid hypersecretion, as are type II ulcers (gastric ulcers in conjunction, synchronous or metachronous with duodenal ulcers).

Clinical Scenario 15. A 54-year-old man presents with anemia and mild epigastric pain. Endoscopic evaluation of stomach with biopsy reveals mucosa-associated lymphoma tissue. What will be the initial treatment?

> **Answer.** *Helicobacter pylori* eradication utilizing antibiotics and protein pump inhibitors.

Clinical Scenario 16. A 25-year-old man presents to the emergency department with a history of 6 months of variable right lower quadrant abdominal pain, which acutely worsened over the past 12 hours so that he now rates it as 8 on a scale of 10, with 10 being the most painful. He also reports that he has been having diarrhea and low back pain for about 3 months. Computed tomography scan shows stranding of the mesentery in the right lower quadrant. On insertion of a laparoscope, you note that the terminal ileum and cecum are markedly inflamed, with some fat wrapping of the terminal ileum, although the appendix appears normal. What is your next step in this operation?

> **Answer.** Close the camera incision and treat the patient for Crohn disease. Even if the base of the cecum is uninvolved, appendectomy is contraindicated in the presence of Crohn disease due to an unacceptably high rate of enterocutaneous fistulization.

Clinical Scenario 17. You are consulted by internal medicine regarding a 51-year-old woman with abdominal distension and moderate diffuse abdominal pain. Her history is significant for almost 2 years of hospital admissions for partial small bowel obstructions, all of which have resolved without the need for exploration. She is thought to have an adhesive small bowel obstruction secondary to her hysterectomy. On examination, the patient is extremely distended and tender to palpation. A three-way abdominal series shows no free air but a high-grade distal small bowel obstruction. You take the patient for laparotomy and find, on entering the abdomen, that there is a 10-cm diameter area of inflammatory fibrosis that is obstructing the distal jejunum. What should you do next?

> **Answer.** This is a classic presentation of small bowel carcinoid, which causes a profound desmoplastic response in the soft tissues adjacent to what is often a small primary tumor. You should resect the mass, the involved bowel, and any enlarged adjacent lymph nodes, and perform primary anastomosis. The liver should be examined for metastatic disease. The entire gastrointestinal tract should be examined, because there is a high incidence of synchronous carcinoids **and** adenocarcinoma, the latter especially in the colon.

Clinical Scenario 18. A 90-year-old man who lives in a nursing home is brought to the emergency department for feculent vomiting. The man is in the skilled nursing facility for dementia and can give no history. The patient is afebrile but moderately hypotensive and tachycardic, although he does respond to fluid resuscitation. His abdomen is massively distended, with the skin glassy and taut, although he does not exhibit much tenderness on examination. There are multiple incisions on his abdomen, but there is no one to inform you as to what operations this man has undergone. The abdominal series shows pneumobilia and a distal small bowel obstruction. After establishing an adequate urine output, you take the patient to the operating room. You encounter massively dilated small bowel with a transition point about 20 cm proximal to the ileocecal valve. At the transition point, there is a smooth intraluminal mass without any abnormalities of the serosal surface of the bowel. What is the appropriate course of action?

> **Answer.** This is the stereotypical presentation of gallstone ileus. The distended bowel should be opened proximal to the impacted gallstone (do not cut down on the ischemic bowel in which the gallstone is lodged) and the gallstone milked back into the proximal bowel and extracted. The bowel should be examined for any other gallstones that may be proximal to the obstruction. Given the tenuous health of this patient, it is best to leave the cholecystoduodenal fistula takedown for a second operation.

Clinical Scenario 19. A 45-year-old man had a 6-cm gastrointestinal stromal tumor (GIST), high grade and *c-kit* oncogene positive, of the proximal ileum resected 3 years prior. He is being followed with serial computed tomography (CT) scans of the abdomen and chest x-rays (CXRs) every 6 months. His most recent CT scan demonstrates a 5-cm lesion in segment VI of the liver, which when biopsied is consistent with metastatic GIST. The remainder of the CT and the CXR show no other sites of disease. What treatment should this man be offered?

> **Answer.** Although he could be treated with the tryosine kinase inhibitor Gleevec due to his expressing the *c-kit* oncogene, metastectomy of this solitary lesion would be more appropriate. The fact that the patient avoids systemic therapy for a resectable isolated metastasis and the fact that his long disease-free interval would predict for a more favorable prognosis following [extirpation] of the liver metastases also favor metastectomy.

Clinical Scenario 20. A 73-year-old woman undergoes a computed tomography (CT) scan for abdominal pain and is found to have thickening of the terminal ileum. She is also noted to have multiple mesenteric lymph nodes that are enlarged to more than 2 cm. A colonoscopy is performed that shows no abnormalities of the colon, but when the terminal ileum is entered, a friable intraluminal mass is encountered. The biopsies of this mass are read as diffuse large cell non-Hodgkin lymphoma. Positron emission tomography and CT confirm involvement of the terminal ileum but are also read as showing multiple mediastinal nodes involved with the disease. Bone marrow aspiration is negative for lymphoma. Should this patient undergo a wide resection of the diseased terminal ileum prior to starting chemotherapy?

Answer. No. The patient has stage III non-Hodgkin lymphoma and should be treated with chemotherapy and possibly radiotherapy to the mediastinum. The only indication for surgical exploration in this patient would be if she should start bleeding from the terminal ileum or if the involved area should perforate.

Clinical Scenario 21. A 28-year-old man complains of anorectal pain with bowel movements. He believes that he has a lump in his anorectal area. He notes blood on the toilet tissue after bowel movements. He has no prior medical or surgical history. What is the next step in the examination of this patient?

Answer. This patient may have hemorrhoids. The next step in the evaluation is inspection for skin abnormalities, masses, protrusions, and sites of drainage. Once completed, palpation of the perineum, anal canal, and lower rectum should be undertaken with a gloved, well-lubricated finger.

Clinical Scenario 22. A 79-year-old nursing home resident presents to the emergency department complaining of abdominal distension and pain. He has passed no gas per rectum and has not had a bowel movement in 1 week. Physical examination of the abdomen reveals tympany in all four quadrants as well as distension. What is the next step in the evaluation of this patient?

Answer. This patient may have sigmoid volvulus. The condition is common in nursing home residents. Patients may present with abdominal pain, distension, and obstipation. The next step for this patient should be abdominal radiograph which may reveal a massively distended loop of bowel. This procedure should be performed immediately.

Clinical Scenario 23. A 39-year-old woman complains of right upper quadrant pain. She also has nausea and fatigue. She has a history of ulcerative colitis. Physical examination reveals icteric sclera. Laboratory studies reveal elevated transaminases. What is the next step in the management of this patient?

Answer. This patient likely has primary sclerosing cholangitis. This condition results in stenosis or obstruction of the ductal system. ERCP may reveal thickening and stenosis of the biliary ductal system.

Clinical Scenario 24. A 4-year-old boy with progressive jaundice is found to have cystic involvement of the intrahepatic biliary ducts. Physical examination reveals icteric sclera and jaundice. What is the next step in the evaluation and management of this patient?

Answer. This patient needs liver transplantation. There is evidence of type IV choledochal cystic disease in this patient. This condition is a congenital malformation of the paocreaticobiliary tree.

Clinical Scenario 25. A Caucasian man aged 68 was admitted to the hospital with severe epigastric pain radiating to the back and vomiting. He denies alcohol consumption. Serum amylase is 3,000 IU/L. CT scan showed gallstones and peripancreatic inflammatory stranding. A diagnosis of acute pancreatitis is made, and the patient is managed with NG decompression, IV fluids, and analgesia. He improves initially, but 48 hours later develops high fever and labored breathing. What is the next step?

Answer. The patient needs to be cared for in the intensive care unit (if not already there). A chest radiograph and blood gases should be obtained to rule out ARDS. An urgent abdominal CT should also be performed to assess pancreatic viability. If extensive pancreatic necrosis is seen, the patient may need pancreatic debridement and wide drainage.

Clinical Scenario 26. A 75-year-old man is transferred to your tertiary care facility from a peripheral hospital 10 days after a bout of acute pancreatitis. He was managed conservatively but did not show significant improvement. Over the last 24 hours he deteriorated with fever to 103°F, WBC count of 24,000/UL, and worsening abdominal pain. CT scan shows a 4 × 6 cm fluid collection in the pancreatic bed with air. What is the next step?

> **Answer.** This man has a pancreatic abscess until proven otherwise. An urgent image-guided FNA should be done and the aspirate sent for Gram stain. Presence of microorganisms mandates surgical exploration with debridement and wide drainage. Pancreatic abscesses are generally not treated adequately with percutaneous drainage.

Clinical Scenario 27. A 50-year-old patient returns to clinic 1 month after an attack of pancreatitis complaining of abdominal fullness and early satiety. An ultrasound obtained by the primary physician shows a 4-cm fluid collection at the head of the pancreas. You obtain a CT, which shows a pancreatic pseudocyst compressing the duodenum. What is the next step?

> **Answer.** Most pseudocysts resolve with time. Once they reach approx 6 cm in diameter or become symptomatic (as in this case), intervention is required. The patient should be admitted and fed enterally with a naso-jejunal tube. If the pseudocyst does not shows signs of resolution, an ERCP should be performed to look for communication with the pancreatic duct. Cysts are allowed to mature for at least 6 weeks before attempting some form of internal drainage, mostly into the stomach.

Clinical Scenario 28. A 45-year-old woman presents to the ER with acute on chronic epigastric pain and steatorrhea . She has a history of excessive alcohol consumption and has had similar episodes in the past. On examination she looks emaciated and has loss of sensation in the feet with absent ankle jerk reflexes. Serum amylase is normal. Abdominal CT shows atrophic pancreas with "calcifications" in the pancreatic duct. What are the next steps in management?

> **Answer.** Supportive care with analgesia, discontinuation of alcohol, and pancreatic enzyme supplements. Assess for diabetes mellitus. She will need an ERCP to evaluate the pancreatic duct and determine if she is a candidate for a drainage procedure.

Clinical Scenario 29. An African-American man aged 70 was admitted complaining of 30-pound weight loss over 6 weeks. He also reports a loss of appetite, "indigestion," dark-colored urine, and pale stools. On clinical examination he appears jaundiced. Serum bilirubin is 15 mg/dL. CT shows a pancreatic head mass with intra- and extrahepatic biliary duct dilatation. An attempt at ERCP for cytology and stenting the CBD is unsuccessful. A percutaneous transhepatic cholangiogram (PTC) is requested. What is the next step?

> **Answer.** Ensure that patient's prothrombin time is normal. It may be prolonged because of failure to absorb fat soluble vitamin K. The factors influencing resectabilty of the mass should also be evaluated. These include mass size (ideally <2 cm), invasion of surrounding vascular structures, and presence of distant metastases.

Clinical Scenario 30. A 19-year-old woman had thyroid lobectomy for a 1.5-cm papillary thyroid cancer at a local hospital and presents requesting a second opinion as to whether she should have completion thyroidectomy. What do you recommend as the next step?

> **Answer.** Based on the AMES risk stratification (age, metastases, extent, size), a young woman with a well-differentiated cancer of small size, the risk of recurrent disease with careful thyroid suppression (maintaining low thyroid-stimulating hormone level but not inducing osteoporosis or heart disease) is very low, and the patient does not need complete thyroidectomy.

Clinical Scenario 31. A 40-year-old woman who underwent subtotal thyroidectomy is now in the recovery room having difficulty in breathing. Oxygen saturation is 92% on a 40% facemask. Physical examination of the neck reveals enlargement of the tissues underlying the incision line. Some active bleeding is noted through the dressing. What is the next step in the management of this patient?

> **Answer.** This patient has postoperative hemorrhage after thyroidectomy. This may be due to hypervascularity of the overactive thyroid gland. This can lead to airway obstruction and laryngeal edema. Treatment is surgical exploration, clot evacuation, and coagulation of bleeding vessels.

Clinical Scenario 32. A 7-year-old boy is evaluated for progressive speech difficulties. He is otherwise healthy and approximates the 50th percentile for height and weight. Physical examination reveals a mass in the posterior aspect of the tongue. What is the next step in the management of this patient?

Answer. This patient has a glottic thyroid gland. Patients often present with speech difficulties. Diagnosis is by inspection or indirect laryngoscopy. Radioactive thyroid scan will identify this mass as containing thyroid tissue.

Clinical Scenario 33. A 38-year-old woman presents to her primary care physician with unilateral bloody discharge from her right breast. She explains that for the last several months, her right breast became tender, especially in the region of the nipple which itself became swollen. Biopsy reveals a diagnosis of invasive ductal carcinoma with marked nuclear atypia within the nipple. Which of the following lymph nodes would the metastatic cells next spread to?

Answer. 75% of the breast, including the entire nipple and most of the lateral segment, drains lymph to the pectoral node, with minor amounts going to the remaining axillary nodes. Lymph from the pectoral node then drains into the central axillary node, along with contributions from the posterior and lateral axillary nodes. Lymph from the central axillary node then drains into the apical axillary node, which lies along the subclavian artery. The remaining 25% of the breast drains into the parasternal nodes, which lie along the internal thoracic artery.

Clinical Scenario 34. A 44-year-old woman with a right breast mass has an elevated alkaline phosphatase level. Physical examination reveals a mass in the right upper quadrant. What is the next step in the evaluation and management of this patient?

Answer. This patient may have distant metastasis from breast cancer. When alkaline phosphatase is elevated, this will raise the suspicion of hepatic metastasis. A liver imaging study should be obtained. The best study would be a CT scan. Liver ultrasound could also be considered.

Clinical Scenario 35. A 25-year-old man is transferred to the hospital with second-degree burns to the left forearm. There are numerous blisters associated with the injury. After resuscitation, how would you treat the blisters?

Answer. The blisters associated with second-degree burns should be unroofed. The dermal appendages are normally colonized with bacteria, and the serous fluid within a blister provides as excellent medium for the bacteria to grow.

Clinical Scenario 36. In the course of managing a wound that has been allowed to heal by secondary intention, it appears that the granulation tissue, although clean, is beginning to mound higher than the surrounding normal skin. What is this, and how do you approach this situation?

Answer. This phenomenon is known as "proud flesh" and is the result of overactivation of the fibroblasts forming the granulation tissue. This "proud flesh" is concerning because it inhibits wound healing by delaying contracture and epithelialization. The granulation tissue can be painted with silver nitrate to halt the overgrowth.

Clinical Scenario 37. A man presents with a chronic wound on the plantar surface of the right foot. He states that this wound has been present for several months. He has been followed for this by his primary care physician for diabetic control and wound care. What are some of the factors that would impair the healing of this wound? How should this wound be managed?

Answer. Wounds in areas with decreased sensation delay healing, because the patient is unable to sense overt pressure or irritation. If this patient has poorly controlled diabetes and a history of neuropathy, this can be an especially profound problem. Furthermore, wounds in areas subjected to pressure or shear forces can contribute to delayed wound healing.

Management entails alleviating the pressure points, culturing the wound, debriding the wound if necessary, accurate diabetic control, determining the nutritional status of the patient, and evaluating the vascular supply to the extremity.

Clinical Scenario 38. During workup of dyspepsia and gallstones in a 66-year-old man, the sonographer notices that the infrarenal abdominal aortic diameter is 3.6 cm × 2.5 cm. The patient does not report abdominal pain and is otherwise healthy. How would you manage this patient?

Answer. The patient should receive a follow-up sonogram in 6 months to a year.

Clinical Scenario 39. A 72-year-old woman is being evaluated for lower back pain, and she has a 6 cm × 5.5 cm infrarenal abdominal aortic aneurysm. She has chronic obstructive pulmonary disease, and her blood pressure is 172/96 mm Hg. What would you tell this patient?

Answer. She is at high risk for complications of abdominal aortic aneurysm, especially rupture, and should be offered elective surgical repair.

Clinical Scenario 40. What is the preferred operative approach for a 72-year-old man with a 6-cm infrarenal abdominal aortic aneurysm? His past history includes multiple abdominal operations, including colostomy and radiation therapy for cancer.

Answer. Endovascular aneurysm repair is the most appropriate operative technique.

Clinical Scenario 41. The diagnosis of esophageal atresia is made soon after birth in a male infant. Respiratory distress was noted immediately after birth. Physical examination reveals excessive drooling and tachypnea. Chest x-ray reveals a blind upper pouch. Which of the following is the next step in the preoperative management of this patient?

Answer. This patient has evidence of esophageal atresia as evidenced by the physical examination findings of drooling, tachypnea, and the x-ray revealing a blind upper pouch. This newborn requires decompression of the proximal pouch with a sump tube using constant suction.

Clinical Scenario 42. A 30-year-old Caucasian man is transported to the emergency department from the scene of a trauma that occurred approximately 30 minutes ago. He was the restrained driver in a single-vehicle crash into a tree. He did not lose consciousness and presents to the emergency department with a GCS of 15. He is adequately transported on a backboard by EMTs and presents wearing a cervical collar. His right lower extremity is in a splint and is covered with gauze. The EMTs inform the trauma staff that he sustained an open fracture of the right distal tibia. After transfer of the patient to the hospital bed, what is the next most appropriate step?

Answer. Begin ATLS protocol. In most trauma situations, many different actions are taking place simultaneously. It is important to remember that ATLS protocol must be followed in all trauma situations. The term "life before limb" must be remembered, even in situations that are considered orthopaedic emergencies. Protocols ensure that certain key vital steps are performed. Once ATLS protocol has been followed, the patient's history can be obtained quickly, followed by a complete physical examination, focusing on the musculoskeletal system. At that time the dressings can be removed, and the fracture can be documented. This ensures that the patient receives appropriate care for his known injuries, and that other injuries the patient sustained can be addressed. Once the fracture is known and the proper imaging is obtained, a consent form can be signed for surgery.

Clinical Scenario 43. A 28-year-old woman is referred to the emergency department by an outside facility, who diagnosed a closed bimalleolar ankle fracture. AP and mortise view x-rays accompany the patient; they reveal a fracture of the medial malleolus and a Weber B fracture of the lateral malleolus. The woman reportedly twisted her left ankle and fell 2 hours ago. ATLS protocol has been followed, and this appears to be an isolated injury. She presents in a well-padded splint. Her toes are warm and pink, and her dorsalis pedis pulses are equal and asymmetric in her bilateral lower extremities. After obtaining a complete history from the patient and performing a thorough physical examination, and finding no other injuries, what is the next most appropriate step?

Answer. A lateral x-ray of the ankle is necessary. It is important when imaging fractures that two orthogonal (90-degree angles to each other) views are obtained. In this case, the patient actually had a trimalleolar ankle fracture that was missed at the outside facility because a lateral ankle x-ray was not taken. Once the patient has been adequately imaged and the diagnosis is secure, a consent form can be signed. CT and MRI studies are typically not needed in ankle fractures. A vascular injury would be relatively rare in this scenario and would manifest itself with decreased pulses in the affected extremity.

Clinical Scenario 44. A 50-year-old Caucasian man is transported to the emergency department from the scene of a trauma. He was the unrestrained driver in a motor vehicle crash. He did not lose consciousness, and presents to the emergency department with a GCS of 15. He is adequately transported on a backboard by EMTs and presents wearing a cervical collar. ATLS protocol is followed. A thorough history is taken, and a physical examination is performed. The patient is found to have a bimalleolar ankle fracture that is repaired by open reduction and internal fixation in the evening of his injury. The next day, during morning rounds, the patient states that his left wrist has been hurting since the accident. The wrist is minimally tender to palpation and only minimally swollen compared to the unaffected side. What is the next most appropriate step?

> **Answer.** Obtain x-rays of the left wrist. Part of the tertiary examination requires repeat examinations to ensure that injuries are not missed. When a patient has a significant injury, other injuries may be missed by the patient during questioning due to the patient concentrating on their major injury. The major injuries are called "distracting injuries." In this case the patient also had a minimally displaced fracture of the radial styloid.
>
> The patient should not have lost enough blood during ankle surgery to cause anemia unless he was anemic at baseline. Deep venous thrombosis of the upper extremity usually presents with pain and swelling. If the patient was examined, x-rayed, and found to be free of injury, then a presumptive diagnosis of wrist sprain can be made and a removable splint can be applied. The patient had a credible mechanism for injury to the wrist that should not be mistaken for malingering.

Clinical Scenario 45. A 27-year-old man unrestrained driver is involved in a motor vehicle accident. He is ejected from the vehicle. You are evaluating him on the scene of the accident. He is conscious but not alert to time, place, or person. He is breathing. He complains of neck pain. Blood pressure is 100/60 mm Hg, pulse is 80 beats/minute, and respirations are 22/minute. Which of the following is the next step in the initial management of this patient?

> **Answer.** Immobilization of the cervical spine in a hard collar. This patient received blunt trauma as a result of ejection from the vehicle. He may have a neck injury. Immobilization of the spine in the field is required before transport to the hospital. Up to 25% of patients suffer from improper manipulation of the spine between the time of the accident and arrival at the hospital. The patient should be placed on a spine board. Administration of methyprednisolone may be effective in treatment of spinal cord injury but should be considered after immobilization of the spine. Arm and leg restraints should not be placed. The administration of mannitol is not indicated in this patient at this time.

Clinical Scenario 46. A 41-year-old man complains of progressive tinnutis, vertigo, and hearing loss. Physical examination of the head and neck are normal. The patient has an absent left sided corneal reflex. Audiometry reveals a left-sided high-frequency sensorineural hearing loss. What is the next step in the management of this patient?

> **Answer.** This patient likely has an acoustic neuroma on the basis of symptoms of tinnitus, vertigo, and hearing loss. The physical examination finding of absent corneal reflex is also suggestive. Audiometry in these patients will reveal high-frequency sensorineural hearing loss. The next step in the management is imaging of the cerebellopontine angle with MRI. Ultrasound is unlikely to be of benefit in this patient. CT scan could also be considered, but it must include the head. Brain stem evoked response will not add additional information necessary for this diagnosis. There is no reason to repeat audiometry in this patient.

Clinical Scenario 47. A 32-year-old man with a history of asthma and aspirin allergy presents with recurrent episodes of nasal congestion and drainage, fever, fatigue, and headache. On physical exam, he has a temperature of 101°F and purulent drainage from his left nasal passageway. What pathologic process is occurring and what is the next step is treatment?

> **Answer.** The patient is displaying signs and symptoms of the Samter triad, which consists of asthma, aspirin sensitivity, and nasal polyposis. These patients often have sinus symptoms exacerbated by the use of aspirin, while the nasal polpys disrupt the normal drainage of the sinuses. He should be treated medically for the episode of sinusitis and also be referred to a otolaryngologist for surgical treatment of his nasal polyps if present.

Clinical Scenario 48. A 5-year-old boy presents to the pediatrician with a 2-day history of fever (102°F), fatigue, and a severe sore throat. He denies a cough. Physical exam reveals anterior cervical lymphadenopathy, palatal petechiae, and a gray exudate on his tonsils. What is the diagnosis and what should you do for this child's illness?

Answer. This child has pharyngitis. To confirm the diagnosis, a rapid antigen test should be performed. Treatment should be with antibiotics.

Clinical Scenario 49. A 9-year-old girl presents with swelling and pain on the left side of her neck while recovering from a common cold, which was managed symptomatically. On physical exam, she has significant swelling in her left lateral neck at the level of the hyoid bone and is audibly stridorous. What is most likely diagnosis and what should the next step in treatment be?

Answer. The patient probably has a branchial cleft cyst. To confirm the diagnosis, imaging of the neck should be performed. Ultrasound is a very good modality for this, but because of the patient's symptoms (stridor), a CT or MRI should be ordered to evaluate the proximity to her airway. She should be treated with antibiotics and taken to the OR for excision of the cyst.

Clinical Scenario 50. A 4-year-old girl presents to the ER with a 2-day history of fever, drooling, and severe odynophagia. When you go to see the patient, she is sitting up in bed with her neck extended and supported with both her arms. A lateral neck x-ray is read as a possible "thumb sign." What is your working diagnosis and next step in treatment?

Answer. This patient is showing signs of epiglottitis. You should avoid doing anything with the patient that may cause her to become upset, which can trigger respiratory compromise. The patient should be taken immediately to the OR by the otolaryngologist and anesthesiologist. Once epiglottitis is confirmed by physical examination, the patient can be treated with antibiotics alone or may need intubation depending on the severity of the illness.

Clinical Scenario 51. A 10-month-old girl is brought to the clinic with a 4-cm bright red lesion with sharp borders that involves most of her right cheek and auricle. You note no other lesions anywhere on the child. It feels rubbery on palpation, and is nontender. Further physical examination reveals clear lung fields and no heart murmur that is readily appreciated. The mother is very worried that this might be cancer because it has grown so quickly over the past few months. What should be done about this child's problem?

Answer. Watchful waiting. This lesion is most likely an infantile hemangioma. After 1 year of life, this lesion should slowly regress. The mother should be instructed, however, to take note of any stridorous breathing that may suggest subglottic involvement.

Clinical Scenario 52. A 5-year-old girl presents to her pediatrician with a 1-day history of fever and midline neck swelling which has become red and tender. She is otherwise asymptomatic. On exam, it is noted that the mass is fluctuant and elevates when she is asked to swallow. There is no thyromegaly noted. What is the appropriate treatment for this child?

Answer. She has a thyroglossal duct cyst, which has become infected. This infection should be treated with appropriate antibiotics. She should then be taken for surgery to remove the cyst and center of the hyoid bone, which is involved in the migration of the thyroid gland from the tongue to the anterior neck.

Clinical Scenario 53. In the newborn nursery, a 2-week-old girl presents with a very large mass on the right side of her neck. The mass transilluminates when backlit with a penlight. The mass has caused some torticollis in the patient's neck. What is the mass, and how should her care be managed?

Answer. This is most likely a type of lymphatic malformation know as cystic hygroma. A CT or MRI should be performed to evaluate for its affects on the airway. Cystic hygroma can be seen in certain syndromes (e.g., Turner), and further workup to evaluate for comorbidities can be useful.

Clinical Scenario 54. An 85-year-old diabetic nursing home resident is in your clinic complaining that his hearing aid in his right ear doesn't work well. On examination, his temperature is 102°F and there is granulation tissue filling the external ear canal. There is also significant swelling around the auricle, which is tender to any traction placed on it. What is your concern in this clinical setting, and what should be done for this patient?

Answer. In an elderly patient with diabetes who is suspected to have otitis externa, one must be highly suspicious for osteomyelitis of the temporal bone, also known as malignant otitis externa. A CT scan should be performed to see if there is any involvement of the temporal bone around the EAC. A patient with malignant otitis should be taken to the OR for debridement of the temporal bone and admitted for IV antibiotics.

Clinical Scenario 55. An 18-month-old child who was found to be pulling at his right ear over the past 2 days has a fever of 102°F. The tympanic membrane was retracted and fluid was seen behind it as well. He was diagnosed with otitis media and given a prescription for amoxicillin. Four days later, the patient has no change in symptoms. Why has this child had no improvement in his symptoms?

Answer. This child most likely has drug resistant *Streptoccus pneumoniae*. Drug resistance has been steadily increasing with these bacteria. The child should be switched to a different antibiotic, such as amoxicillin clavulonate or a cephalosporin.

Clinical scenario 56. A 23-year-old student presents with abdominal pain that started about 2 days ago around her umblicus and now has moved to the right lower quadrant. It is associated with anorexia and a low-grade fever. On examination, she has tenderness in the right lower quadrant with rebound. What is the diagnosis?

Answer. Acute appendicitis. The appendix is supplied by the automomic nervous system (which has bilateral innervation); thus pain is first localized to the periumbilical region. Only when the appendix touchs the parietal peritoneum does the pain localize to the right lower quadrant.

Clinical Scenario 57. A 60-year-old woman with a history of arthritis for which she has been taking over-the-counter nonsteroidal anti-inflammatory drugs (NSAIDS) presents with severe abdominal pain. When you examine her, she has diffuse tenderness and rebound. Her chest x-ray shows free air. What is the next step in management?

Answer. With her use of NSAIDs, this patient is at a very high likelihood for having peptic ulcer disease. Her examination and chest x-ray findings now suggest a perforation of a peptic ulcer. She needs hydration and an urgent operation.

Clinical Scenario 58. A 75-year-old nursing home patient with a history of atrial fibrilliation presents with worsing abdominal pain and bloody diarrhea. Examination shows diffuse abdominal tenderness and rebound. What is the most likely diagnosis?

Answer. Mesenteric ischemia. Her atrial fibrillation most likely led to formation of a clot in the left atrium, which became dislodged and entered the mesentric circulation causing ischemia. She needs prompt surgical evaluation and possibly an operation.

Clinical Scenario 59. A 45-year-old man who smokes presents with progressively increasing cough, sputum production, and fever for the past 4 days. In the past day he has also noticed the development of right upper quadrant abdominal pain. On examination, he has diminished breath sounds at the right base, with dullness to percussion. Abdominal examination shows minimal tenderness in the right upper quadrant, with no Murphy sign. What is the diagnosis?

Answer. He most likely has a right lower lobe pneumonia irritating his diaphragm, which is leading to his right upper quadrant pain.

Clinical Scenario 60. A 57-year-old African-American man comes to clinic for an annual physical examination. He reports no problems, but upon digital rectal examination, a 1.5-cm rock-hard discrete nodule is palpated. What is the next appropriate step in the management of this patient?

Answer. This patient may have prostate cancer and needs a prostate needle biopsy. Prostatic cancer incidence increases with age and has been found to be most common in African-American men. Adenocarcinoma of the prostate typically arises at the periphery of the gland, and therefore digital rectal examination is one of the best screening tests for prostate cancer. Upon palpation of a mass, transrectal needle biopsy should be used to comfirm the diagnosis. Spread of prostate cancer is by local extension, with the most common location of metastasis being the axial skeleton. Widespread bone metastases may respond to several therapies including androgen ablation, orchiectomy, LHRH agonists, or anti-androgens such as flutamide.

Clinical Scenario 61. A 91-year-old man who is wheelchair bound and in a nursing home has a urinary catheter placed because of a prolonged history of enuresis and daytime urinary incontinence. His current medical problems include diabetes mellitus, hypertension, and congestive heart failure, and he has a history of myocardial infarction 2 years ago. His current medications include glyburide, atenolol, and lasix. On a recent urine culture in the nursing home the patient is noted to have 75,000 colony-forming units of *Escherichia coli*. What is the next opportunity for this patient to receive antibiotic therapy?

> **Answer.** All patients with an indwelling catheter will eventually develop bacteriuria. After the catheter has been in place for approximately 10 days, nearly all patients will have asymptomatic bacteriuria. This patient should not receive antibiotic therapy unless he becomes symptomatic and develops fever or chills. Treatment of patients with bacteriuria without symptoms will lead to development of resistant organisms, which will ultimately become a problem when the patient develops a true urinary tract infection.

Clinical Scenario 62. A 31-year-old woman complains of a 3-day history of left otalgia. She has no prior medical or surgical history. Physical examination of the left ear reveals grouped vesicles in various stages of development on the pinnae. Motor function of the facial nerve is intact. What is the next step in the treatment for this individual?

> **Answer.** This patient has evidence of herpes zoster. This condition is characterized by intense ear pain and the appearance of grouped vesicles. Treatment involves systemic corticosteroids such as methylprednisolone and oral acyclovir. Pain control is important, as these lesions are typically quite painful.

Clinical Scenario 63. A 23-year-old man is seen in the emergency department after a motor vehicle accident. He was an unrestrained passenger. He is able to breathe on his own but tells you that each breath is extremely painful. You note that a segment of his chest wall appears to sink inwards with each respiration, and that when he exhales this same segment does not move with the rest of the chest wall. Vital signs are stable. The patient has no other obvious traumatic injuries. The arterial blood gas reads as follows: 7.3/55/85/25. What is the most appropriate next step in management?

> **Answer.** This is a classic vignette describing flail chest. This occurs when four or more ribs are fractured in at least two locations, leading to paradoxical movement of the chest wall during respiration. This commonly occurs after trauma such as a motor vehicle accident. The true danger in patients with flail chest is the frequent underlying pulmonary contusion. In this patient we see a blood gas indicative of a decreased respiratory effort, suggesting that he is not properly respiring. The ABCDEs of trauma must be adhered to in any trauma situation, particularly flail chest. We would need to inubate this patient and provide mechanical ventilation in light of the marked respiratory distress.

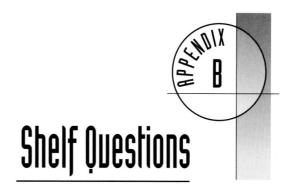

Shelf Questions

Directions: *Each of the numbered items or incomplete statements in this section is followed by answers or by completions of the statement. Select the **one** lettered answer or completion that is **best** in each case.*

1. A postoperative patient with protracted vomiting is like to have:
  A. Metabolic acidosis.
  B. Respiratory acidosis.
  C. Metabolic alkalosis.
  D. Lactic acidosis.
  E. Microcytic anemia.

2. Indications for total parenteral nutrition (TPN) include:
  A. Standard postoperative recovery after inguinal hernia repair.
  B. Massive enterectomy (resection of small bowel).
  C. Pneumothorax.
  D. Inadequate peripheral venous access.
  E. Age >65.

3. The commonly used anticoagulant heparin:
  A. Has a half-life of 6 hours.
  B. Is administered orally.
  C. Activity is measured by PTT.
  D. Works by inhibiting platelet aggregation.
  E. Inhibits factors V and VII.

4. An adult patient with both legs severely burned and his anterior trunk also burned has what percentage total body burn?
  A. 45%.
  B. 54%.
  C. 60%.
  D. 90%.
  E. 74%.

5. Chance fractures are associated with:
   A. Skiing injuries.
   B. Hanging injuries.
   C. Lap belts.
   D. Ankle dislocation.
   E. Blunt urethral injuries.

6. A 23-year-old welder sustains an airway thermal injury after a fire in the warehouse:
   A. An upper airway injury occurs more often than a lower airway injury.
   B. Diagnosis is best confirmed by direct esophagoscopy.
   C. Symptoms usually do not manifest until 24 hours after injury.
   D. The most sensitive sign is tongue swelling.
   E. Endotracheal intubation is indicated if posterior pharyngeal swelling, mucosal sloughing, or carbonaceous sputum is present.

7. Risk factors for inguinal hernias in adults include:
   A. Sedentary lifestyle.
   B. Chronic obstructive pulmonary disease.
   C. Anorexia nervosa.
   D. Hypertension.
   E. Irritable bowel syndrome.

8. Incarceration of the antimesenteric portion of the bowel wall is referred to as which of the following?
   A. Umbilical hernia.
   B. Richter hernia.
   C. Femoral hernia.
   D. Indirect inguinal hernia.
   E. Hiatal hernia.

9. The most lateral femoral structure in the anatomic position of the groin is:
   A. Artery.
   B. Lymphatics.
   C. Empty space.
   D. Nerve.
   E. Vein.

10. A hernia that arises lateral to the inferior epigastric vessels is which of the following?
   A. Indirect inguinal hernia.
   B. Direct inguinal hernia.
   C. Femoral hernia.
   D. Obturator hernia.
   E. Sliding hernia.

11. Repair of an inguinal hernia that approximates the conjoined tendon and transversalis fascia to the inguinal ligament is known as which of the following?

 A. McVay repair.

 B. Shouldice repair.

 C. Laparoscopic preperitoneal repair.

 D. Lichtenstein repair.

 E. Bassini repair.

12. The borders of the Hesselbach triangle do not include:

 A. The lateral border of the rectus muscle.

 B. The inguinal ligament inferiorly.

 C. The semilunar line superiorly.

 D. The inferior epigastric vessels.

13. Treatment for trichobezoars involves:

 A. Gastrectomy.

 B. Splenectomy.

 C. Endoscopic therapy.

 D. Vagotomy and pyloroplasty.

 E. Proton pump inhibitors and two antibiotic therapies for 3 weeks.

14. An example of a pulsion diverticulum is:

 A. Zenker diverticulum.

 B. Traction mid-esophageal diverticulum.

 C. True diverticulum.

 D. Meckel diverticulum.

 E. Esophageal leiomyoma.

15. Mallory–Weiss syndrome:

 A. Is usually fatal.

 B. Is best treated with surgery.

 C. Requires CT scanning for diagnosis.

 D. Can usually be treated endoscopically.

 E. Mandates *Helicobacter pylori* testing.

16. Persons diagnosed as having Peutz–Jeghers syndrome:

 A. Have a double recessive gene disorder.

 B. Should undergo GI surveillance starting at age 10.

 C. Rarely manifest hamartomas of the small bowel.

 D. Have an increased cancer risk due to malignant transformation of the hamartomas of the bowel.

17. Intussusception of the small bowel in the adult:

 A. Is associated with a discernible lead point in <25% of cases.

 B. Presents with symptoms similar to that seen in the toddler with intussusception.

 C. Can generally be successfully reduced by barium enema.

 D. Is most often caused by benign neoplasms of the small bowel.

18. Regarding the Meckel diverticulum:
   A. Most of the symptomatic Meckel diverticula are lined with colonic mucosa, which results in a high incidence of diverticulitis.
   B. It is a remnant of the urachus.
   C. The ratio of males:females with symptomatic Meckel diverticulum is 1:5.
   D. Internal herniation associated with a mesenterodiverticular band should be treated with resection of the band and the Meckel diverticulum.

19. Conditions such as Crohn disease that interfere with function of the terminal ileum may result in all of the following except:
   A. Bile acid diarrhea.
   B. Decreased incidence of rectal carcinoid tumors.
   C. Propensity for forming bilirubin gallstones.
   D. Microcytic anemia.

20. Celiac disease (gluten enteropathy) is NOT associated with an increased risk of:
   A. Small bowel adenocarcinoma.
   B. Esophageal adenocarcinoma.
   C. Melanoma.
   D. Squamous cell cancer of the skin.
   E. Small bowel lymphoma.

21. A 29-year-old woman complains of left lower quadrant pain, cramps, and bloody diarrhea. She has been symptomatic for 1 year. She has a 20-pound weight loss. Her primary care physician diagnosed her with irritable bowel syndrome. Physical examination reveals minimal left lower quadrant tenderness. Stool cultures are negative for ova and parasites. What is the most appropriate next step in the management of this patient?
   A. Abdominal x-rays.
   B. Repeat stool culture for ova and parasites.
   C. Proctoscopy.
   D. Small bowel contrast study.
   E. Reassurance.

22. A 71-year-old woman in good health complains of anal pain, mucus discharge, and anal incontinence. Physical examination reveals protrusion of the full thickness of the rectum. What is the most appropriate treatment for this patient?
   A. Antibiotics.
   B. Low anterior resection with rectopexy.
   C. Rectal fixation to sacrum with mesh.
   D. Left hemocolectomy with colostomy.
   E. Reassurance.

23. A 38-year-old man is brought to the emergency department complaining of anorectal pain and drainage of pus and blood. Physical examination reveals swelling and fluctuance in the left anorectal area approximately 2 cm from the anal verge. His white blood cell count is 14,000/mm³. What is the most appropriate treatment for this patient?

A. Lateral internal sphincterotomy.

B. Stool softeners and sitz baths.

C. Oral antibiotics.

D. Incision and drainage.

E. Rubber band ligation.

24. A 47-year-old man with multiple medical problems and recurrent cholecystitis is being considered for laparoscopic cholecystectomy. Physical examination reveals an obese man with right upper quadrant tenderness to palpation. Which of the following is the most significant potential contraindication to this procedure for this patient?

A. Generalized peritonitis.

B. Systemic hypertension.

C. History of smoking.

D. Hypercholesterolemia.

E. Prior history of wound infections.

25. A 47-year-old woman with recurrent bouts of acute cholecystitis is hospitalized on the medicine service. Physical examination reveals right upper quadrant pain to palpation. Ultrasound reveals evidence of pericholecystic fluid and gallstones. Which of the following laboratory studies is most likely to be abnormal in this patient?

A. AST.

B. Lipase.

C. Amylase.

D. Bilirubin.

E. Alkaline phosphatase.

26. A 40-year-old woman with a long history of oral contraceptive use complains of chronic abdominal pain. Ultrasound reveals a well circumscribed 3-cm lesion in the right lobe of the liver. Angiography of the mass reveals hypervascularity. Liver biopsy reveals normal hepatocytes without evidence of hemorrhage or necrosis. Which of the following laboratory findings would be expected in this patient?

A. Elevated AST.

B. Elevated ALT.

C. Elevated alkaline phosphatase.

D. Elevated lipase.

E. Normal amylase.

27. A 40-year-old man is admitted to the hospital with upper abdominal pain after binge drinking. Serum amylase is 1,900 IU/L. His laboratory values are as follows: WBC count 14,000/mm³, blood glucose 300 mg/dL, serum LDH 500 U/L, and AST 200 U/L. His fiancé has heard that pancreatitis can be lethal and asks you what his risk of mortality is. Based on the available information, you will quote a rate of:
   A. 2%.
   B. 20%.
   C. 50%.
   D. 100%.

28. The following is the primary stimulant for pancreatic bicarbonate secretion:
   A. Cholecystokinin.
   B. Enterokinase.
   C. Secretin.
   D. Somatostatin.

29. A 60-year-old woman with recent onset of diabetes mellitus undergoes an abdominal CT as part of a trauma evaluation and is found to have an incidental 5-cm mass in the tail of the pancreas. Which of the following would confirm the suspicion of a glucagonoma?
   A. C-peptide assay.
   B. Erythematous skin rash.
   C. Hypokalemia.
   D. Watery diarrhea.

30. An 8-year-old boy is recently diagnosed with ITP. Which of the following statements is true?
   A. Splenectomy is more often necessary in adults than children.
   B. Platelet transfusions are necessary prior to splenectomy in order to keep a count above 50,000.
   C. Adults are more susceptible to overwhelming post-splenectomy sepsis (OPSI).
   D. Early splenectomy can avert sickling crises in sickle cell anemia.

31. A 65-year-old man is seen in the clinic with a history of central abdominal pain, jaundice, and weight loss. A CT scan shows an irregular mass in the head of pancreas. Which of the following is NOT indicated?
   A. Serum CA 19-9 and CEA assay.
   B. Percutaneous image-guided biopsy of the mass for tissue diagnosis.
   C. Endoscopic ultrasound to assess respectability.
   D. ERCP with CBD stent placement for relief of obstructive jaundice.

32. A 43-year-old woman with a history of hypertension complains of polyuria and polydipsia. Physical examination reveals parched lips and dry oral mucous membranes. Cardiac, pulmonary, and abdominal examinations are within normal limits. Laboratory values reveal a plasma aldosterone/plasma renin activity ratio >30 and plasma aldosterone >20. CT scan shows multiple bilateral 1-cm adrenal nodules. CT-guided biopsy reveals adrenal hyperplasia. What is the most appropriate treatment for this patient?

A. Right adrenalectomy.

B. Left adrenalectomy.

C. Bilateral adrenalectomy.

D. Spironolactone.

E. Watchful waiting.

33. A 52-year-old woman with chronic diarrhea, weight loss, and lower abdominal pain undergoes exploratory laparotomy. Findings include an intense desmoplastic reaction causing fibrosis, intestinal kinking, and obstruction at the level of the cecum and appendix. The lesion measures 3 cm in size. Preoperatively, her laboratory values included elevated urinary levels of 5-hydroxyindoleacetic acid in 24-hour urine and serum chromogranin A. What is the most appropriate treatment for this patient?

A. Segmental intestinal resection.

B. Wide excision of bowel and mesentery.

C. Right hemicolectomy.

D. Local excision.

E. Pancreaticduodenectomy.

34. A 45-year-old white man complains of fatigue and weight gain during the past few months. He is worried because his first cousin was diagnosed as having thyroid carcinoma last year. Physical examination reveals a nodule in the upper lobe of the right thyroid gland. Serum electrolytes are as follows: sodium 135 mEq/L, potassium 5 mEq/L, chloride 104 mEq/L, and calcium-6.1 mg/dL. What is the most likely diagnosis?

A. Anaplastic carcinoma of the thyroid gland.

B. Follicular carcinoma of the thyroid gland.

C. Hashimoto thyroiditis.

D. Medullary carcinoma of the thyroid gland.

E. Papillary carcinoma of the thyroid gland.

35. A 26-year-old nulligravid woman complains of bilateral nipple discharge that she describes as milky and sticky. She has been having this problem for the past 4 weeks, and it seems to be getting worse. She states that her menses have been of normal timing, duration, and quality, with her last menstrual period occurring 6 days ago. Urine BHCG is negative, and lab studies reveal serum prolactin of 45 ng/mL and TSH is 7I U/mL. What is the most likely diagnosis?

A. Ductal carcinoma *in situ*.

B. Duct ectasia.

C. Metochlopramide being taken for gastric stasis.

D. Hypothyroidism.

E. Pituitary adenoma.

36. A 39-year-old woman undergoes bilateral mastectomy after the diagnosis of infiltrating ductal carcinoma is made. Her mother, aunt, and three other relatives have had similar procedures performed, also in attempts to treat infiltrating ductal carcinoma in one or both breasts. Which of the following is the most likely etiology of the cancer in this woman?

A. A decrease in the expression of the [c-erb] allele.

B. A mutant p53 allele.

C. A mutant Rb allele.

D. Expansion of a CCG trinucleotide repeat.

E. Loss of a specific enzyme in the excision repair system.

37. A 39-year-old woman presents to her family physician complaining of a rash that has recently developed on the areola of her left breast. She states that the lesion has recently become itchy and has been accompanied by a watery red discharge for the last couple of days. Physical examination reveals that the lesion appears eczematous and the left nipple feels more solid and warm than the right. What is the most likely diagnosis?

A. Intraductal papilloma.

B. Invasive ductal carcinoma.

C. Medullary carcinoma.

D. Nipple adenoma.

E. Phyllodes tumor.

38. A physician wishes to deliver a local anesthetic subcutaneously to a patient. Which of the following epidermal skin layers will the physician penetrate first?

A. Stratum basale.

B. Stratum corneum.

C. Stratum granulosum.

D. Stratum lucidum.

E. Stratum spinosum.

39. A 65-year-old man presents to his physician with a lesion present on his nose. Examination reveals a raised, shiny, papular lesion with small blood vessels. What is the most likely diagnosis?

A. Basal cell carcinoma.

B. Squamous cell carcinoma.

C. Malignant melanoma.

D. Merkel cell carcinoma.

E. Histiocytosis X.

40. A patient with dysplastic nevus syndrome presents to clinic with a brown papular lesion on his neck. What is the most likely diagnosis?

A. Basal cell carcinoma.

B. Squamous cell carcinoma.

C. Malignant melanoma.

D. Merkel cell carcinoma.

E. Histiocytosis X.

41. A 64-year-old man is discovered to have an asymptomatic left carotid bruit. He asks about the significance of this:

A. He should be told that it is highly associated with carotid stenosis.

B. It is found in over 30% of his age-matched cohorts.

C. Is treated with surgery in most cases.

D. Aspirin will lower the risk of TIA.

E. The use of long-term anticoagulants (warfarin or heparin) is indicated.

42. The most significant risk factor for abdominal aortic aneurysm rupture is:

A. Male sex.

B. Obesity.

C. History of smoking.

D. Aneurysm diameter.

E. Aneurysm length.

43. A 56-year-old mailman complains of two block left calf claudication. Which of the following is true about his condition?

A. He is most likely to have type III claudication.

B. His ankle–brachial index (ABI) will be 0.35.

C. Urgent femoral artery to popliteal artery bypass is indicated.

D. He is very unlikely to ever need an amputation of the affected limb.

E. An initial period of bed rest is warranted.

44. A patient with chronic splanchnic (mesenteric) ischemia is likely to:

A. Gain weight.

B. Have postprandial pain.

C. Have occlusion of one of the three major arteries—the superior mesenteric artery, the celiac artery, or the inferior mesenteric artery.

D. Present with Leriche syndrome.

E. Have a mycotic aneurysm.

45. An 18-year-old boy presents to his primary care physician after being involved in a motor vehicle accident. He was in the emergency department the previous evening, and was discharged in good condition. He reports that he hit his head on the dashboard and has a contusion on the right side of his temple. He was told that he suffered a contrecoup injury and is asking you to explain what that means. You proceed to tell him that it is a:

A. Nonpenetrating head wound on the right side of the brain.

B. Nonpenetrating head wound on the left side of the brain.

C. Penetrating head wound on the left side of the brain.

D. Penetrating head wound on the right side of the brain.

E. Penetrating head wound with minimal hemorrhage.

46. A 23-year-old woman driving her automobile is struck by another driver, the force of impact causing her to strike the temporal area of the skull against the window. She develops a mild headache but does not lose consciousness. Several hours later, she develops a severe headache with nausea and vomiting. Which is the most likely diagnosis?

A. Bacterial meningitis.

B. Berry aneurysm of the circle of Willis with rupture.

C. Epidural hematoma.

D. Subarachnoid hemorrhage.

E. Subdural hematoma.

47. A 32-year-old man presents to the ambulatory care clinic with new-onset seizures. He also complains of headaches, nausea, and emesis. Surgical resection is performed, and specimens are sent to pathology. The resected tumor demonstrates closely packed cells with large round nuclei surrounded by clear cytoplasm. What is the most likely diagnosis?

A. Acoustic neuroma.

B. Ependymoma.

C. Medulloblastoma multiforme.

D. Meningioma.

E. Oligodendroglioma.

48. An infant is found to have herniation of the intestine through a small defect to the right of the umbilical cord. This infant was the first born to a 29-year-old woman who did not present for prenatal care until week 24 of gestation. The small bowel of the newborn appears normal but is covered by a thickened peel. The most likely diagnosis is:

A. Gastroschisis.

B. Omphalocoele.

C. Patent omphalomesenteric duct.

D. Patent urachus.

E. Umbilical hernia.

49. A 7-year-old boy presents to the emergency department with a history of passing a large, bloody bowel movement. Vital signs are stable. Further workup using a technetium scan localizes ectopic gastric mucosa in the lower abdomen. Failure to obliterate which structure in the developing fetus gives rise to this anomaly?

A. Cardinal veins.

B. Ductus venosus.

C. Vitelline duct.

D. Omphalomesenteric duct.

E. Stenson duct.

50. A 4-year-old boy is brought to the emergency room where his mother explains that her son fell while playing in the house. The mother gives a history of prior fractures, and also notes that her son has bilateral hearing loss. On examination, the arm is erythematous, swollen, and extremely tender to palpation. A radiograph illustrates a fracture of the radius, as well as characteristics of old, healed fractures. What is the most likely explanation for the pattern of fractures?

A. Abnormal FGF receptor.

B. Abnormal synthesis of type I collagen.

C. Abuse by the caregivers.

D. Deficiency in vitamin D.

E. Underlying bone tumor.

51. A 5-year-old boy with progressive gait abnormality is referred for evaluation. Physical examination reveals decreased range of motion of the right femur with muscle strength reduction of 20% as compared with the left lower extremity. The child is in the 30th percentile for head circumference, height, and weight. Cardiac evaluation reveals a regular rate and rhythm. Pulmonary evaluation reveals no evidence of rales or ronchi; however, some decreased breath sounds were noted at both bases. Gastrointestinal examination revealed no evidence of guarding or rebound tenderness. MRI reveals a metaphyseal fluid-filled cavity in the right femur and evidence of a pathologic fracture. The most likely diagnosis is:

A. Adamantinoma.

B. Aneurysmal bone cyst.

C. Chordoma.

D. Metastatic tumor of bone.

E. Unicameral bone cyst.

52. A 74-year-old man with a history of diabetes mellitus and hypothyroidism presents for evaluation of intermittent gross hematuria with small clots noted upon urination. He complains of nocturia 3 times/night and decreased force of urinary stream with hesitancy. He is a nonsmoker but admits to 1 beer/week for the past 20 years. His medications include an oral hypoglycemic agent and a synthethic thyroid hormone preparation. Physical examination reveals no evidence of rubs, murmurs, or gallops. Pulmonary auscultation reveals decreased breath sounds at the lases bilaterally. Gastrointestinal examination reveals some tenderness along the sigmoid colon without evidence of guarding or rebound tenderness. Rectal examination is guaiac positive with stool in the vault. A small internal hemorrhoid is noted in the left lateral position. Urine analysis reveals +2 hematuria with no evidence of leukocytes or nitrates. Kidney and bladder sonography reveal no evidence of hydronephrosis. The bladder is smooth walled with few trabeculations. Which of the following is the most likely diagnosis?

A. Bacterial prostatitis.

B. Carcinoma of the urinary bladder.

C. Benign prostate hyperplasia.

D. Urinary tract calculi.

E. Urinary tract infection.

53. A 16-year-old boy presents to the emergency department with severe acute onset of right testicular pain that began 2 hours ago. There was no history of trauma to the testicle and the patient reports being in good health with no recent illness. Upon examination, the patient was afebrile, and the right testicle was swollen, painful, and high riding with a horizontal lie. Elevation of the testicle by the examiner provided some relief of pain. What is the most likely diagnosis?

A. Epididymitis.

B. Bacterial prostatitis.

C. Henoch–Schönlein purpura.

D. Testcular carcinoma.

E. Testicular torsion.

54. On the second postoperative day you notice that one of the patients you are caring for while on surgery rotation sounds hoarse. He recently underwent a thyroidectomy to remove a cancerous lesion. Throughout his hospital stay you observe that his voice remains hoarse and does not improve with time. Which of the following structures was most likely injured during the operation?

A. Superficial branch of the laryngeal nerve.

B. Cricothyroid nerve.

C. Superior thyroid nerve.

D. Recurrent laryngeal nerve.

E. Accessory laryngeal nerve.

55. A 4-year-old girl presents to the ER with a 2-day history of fever, drooling, and severe odynophagia. When you go to see the patient, she is sitting up in bed with her neck extended and supported with both her arms. A lateral neck x-ray is read as possible "thumb sign." What is the most likely diagnosis?

A. Epiglottitis.

B. Laryngeal carcinoma.

C. Thyroid carcinoma.

D. Recurrent laryngeal nerve palsy.

E. Lymphoma with cervical adenopathy.

56. A mother of an 8-month-old girl comes to the clinic complaining that her infant does not seem to be gaining weight, is irritable, and appears to be easily fatigable. Physical examination reveals that the child is pale, has spooning nails, is tachycardic with a systolic ejection murmur, and has glossitis. What is the next appropriate laboratory test/tests that would help to determine the cause of this patient's physical findings?

A. TSH cascade.

B. Lead level.

C. TIBC, serum iron, and serum ferritin.

D. Urinalysis.

E. Hematocrit.

57. A 46-year-old female with polycystic kidney disease is receiving a kidney transplant. Within minutes of the anastomoses of the graft vasculature, the kidney rapidly regains a pink coloration and normal tissue turgor and promptly begins excreting urine. However, 1 month after the transplant she has a serum creatinine of 3.9 mg/dL. Urine output is 20 mL/hour. Biopsy of the transplant shows extensive mononuclear cell infiltrate, edema, and mild interstitial hemorrhage. What is the most likely explanation for these findings?

A. Acute rejection.

B. Chronic rejection.

C. Graft versus host disease.

D. Hyperacute rejection.

E. Normal post-transplant process.

58. A 12-year-old boy with leukemia has received a bone marrow transplant. Within 1 week of the transplant the boy begins experiencing a rash, fever, jaundice, and hepatosplenomegaly. There is little infiltration of the affected tissues with lymphocytes. What is the most likely explanation for these findings?

A. Acute graft rejection.

B. Chronic graft rejection.

C. Graft versus host disease.

D. Hyperacute graft rejection.

E. Normal, expected, post-transplant process.

59. A 39-year-old man with advanced renal carcinoma undergoes a protocol of immunotherapy. He is to receive combination immunotherapy with external-beam radiotherapy over a 6-month time period. Immunotherapeutic agents given will include interleukin-1, interleukin-2, and interleukin-6. Which of the following describes the potential of interleukin-2 as the key agent in this therapeutic trial?

A. Ability to cause proteolysis.

B. Ability to serve as an endogenous pyrogen.

C. Ability to serve as an immunostimulant.

D. Ability to stimulate the hypothalamus.

E. Ability to synthesis hepatic acute phase proteins.

60. A cadaver kidney becomes available for transplantation into a 39-year-old man with end-stage renal disease. The next step is to determine which of the following is an absolute contraindication to use of this organ for transplantation. Which would prohibit transplantation of this cadaver kidney?

A. AB incompatibility.

B. Cold ischemia lasting more than 36 hours.

C. HLA tissue typing with a poor match.

D. Positive T-cell cross-match.

E. Prior positive T-cell match but currently negative.

61. A 52-year-old executive and heavy smoker tells you in the emergency room that he developed sudden overwhelming epigastric pain at 8:15 AM. His skin feels clammy and he is tachycardic, and his abdomen is rigid. The most likely diagnosis is:
   A. Appendicitis.
   B. Pelvic inflammatory disease.
   C. Perforated peptic ulcer.
   D. Acute cholecystitis.
   E. Right lower lobe pneumonia.

62. A sign useful in the diagnosis of acute cholecystitis is:
   A. Rosving sign.
   B. Murphy sign.
   C. Obturator sign.
   D. Iliopsoas sign.
   E. Chandelier sign.

63. Visceral pain:
   A. Is mediated by the central nervous system, coordinated at the hypothalamic level.
   B. Is stimulated by pulling, stretching, and distension.
   C. Does not involve visceral chemoreceptors.
   D. Is affected by movement, so patients lie still.
   E. Is a manifestation of sympathetic overdrive.

64. The safest time to operate on a pregnant patient for acute appendicitis is:
   A. First trimester.
   B. After an induced delivery, even if premature.
   C. Second trimester.
   D. Third trimester.
   E. Early morning.

1. **Answer: C.** Protracted vomiting leads to loss of hydrogen ions and a metabolic alkalosis.

2. **Answer: B.** Massive enterectomy leads to loss of most of the GI absorptive capacity for nutrients and fluids. TPN is indicated for such patients.

3. **Answer: C.** Heparin is an intravenous or subcutaneous administered anticoagulant, and works by accelerating the effects of antithrombin III.

4. **Answer: B.** 54%. Each leg is 18% and anterior trunk is 18% of body surface area.

5. **Answer: C.** Chance fractures are transverse lumbar spine fractures and are often associated with lap belt wearing and have a high association with retroperitoneal and bowel injuries.

6. **Answer: E.** Airway thermal injuries are usually upper airway, confirmed by direct laryngoscopy, manifest within 6 hours, and airway protection and maintenance is paramount if thought to be severe by the criteria in answer E.

7. **Answer: B.** Heavy straining and increased pressure are contributory factors to the development of inguinal hernias. Chronic obstructive pulmonary disease leads to chronic forceful coughing, which can lead to increased pressure. Hypertension is not known to be a predisposing factor for hernias.

8. **Answer: B.** Richter hernia is a hernia at any site that involves only a portion of the antimesenteric wall of the bowel. Because the lumen is only partially involved, obstruction rarely occurs. However, strangulation of the involved segment is common.

9. **Answer: D.** One can use the mnemonic NAVEL (nerve, artery, veil, empty space, lymphatic) to remember the position of groin structures from lateral to medial.

10. **Answer: A.** An indirect inguinal hernia arises lateral to the epigastric vessels, a direct hernia arises medial to the vessels, a femoral hernia is found through the femoral canal, an obturator hernia protrudes through the obturator canal, and a sliding hernia is any hernia where a portion of the sac is made up of the wall of an intra-abdominal organ.

11. **Answer: E.** A Bassini repair joins the conjoined tendon and transversalis fascia to the inguinal ligament. A McVay repair sews the transverses aponeurosis to the Cooper ligament, a Shouldice repair combines the McVay and Bassini repairs, the preperitoneal repair involves placing a piece of mesh over the defect in the preperitoneal space, and the Lichtenstein repair uses a piece of mesh in an open repair.

12. **Answer: C.** The structure not included in the borders of the triangle is the semilunar line. The semilunar line is related to Spigelian hernias.

13. **Answer: C.** Trichobezoars are accumulations of swallowed hair in the stomach and are usually treated with endoscopic therapy.

14. **Answer: A.** A Zenker diverticulum is a pulsion, or false diverticulum. All the other answers are true, that is, containing all layers of the visceral wall. An esophageal leiomyoma is a benign tumor, not a diverticulum.

15. Answer: D. Mallory–Weiss Syndrome, a condition of bleeding from a mucosal rent at the gastroesophageal junction, has a fairly benign course and can almost always be diagnosed and treated with endoscopic hemostatic maneuvers. It is not associated with *H. pylori* infection.

16. Answer: B. Peutz–Jeghers is an autosomal dominant genetic disorder characterized by muco-cutaneous pigmentation and multiple benign GI hamartomas. It is also associated with an increased incidence of adenomatous lesions of the GI tract; it is from these "bystander" polyps that the increased risk of GI malignancy arises. Intensive GI screening of the entire GI tract is started at age 10.

17. Answer: D. Lead points are present in over 90% of adult intussusception, while most pediatric cases are idiopathic in etiology. The classic presentation of acute onset abdominal pain, with the child drawing up the knees and severe paroxysms of abdominal colic, is rarely present in the adult. Even the "currant-jelly stool" seen in the child is a rarity among adults. Because of the presence of the lead point, barium enema reduction is not likely to be successful in the adult. Small bowel intussusception is most often caused by benign neoplasms (lipomas, hemangiomas) of the bowel, although among the malignant etiologies, GIST is the most frequently seen.

18. Answer: D. Most Meckel diverticula are symptomatic in the young male child due to GI bleeding, indicating the presence of ectopic gastric mucosa. It is an embryonic remnant of the omphalomesenteric duct. The M:F ratio in symptomatic Meckel diverticula is about 3:1. Because the blood supply to the diverticulum may travel in the mesenterodiverticular band, both the band and the diverticulum should be resected in preference to simply lysing the band, which might lead to ischemia and perforation of the Meckel diverticulum if it is left *in situ.*

19. Answer: B. Loss of terminal ileal function results in decreased recovery of bile salts from the intestinal lumen, increasing their entry into the colon and leading to the irritative bile acid diarrhea. Depletion of the bile salt pool (loss of the enterohepatic circulation) results in supersaturation of the bile with cholesterol and formation of gallstones. Inability to absorb vitamin B_{12} causes macrocytic (megaloblastic) anemia.

20. Answer: C. There is no association of celiac disease and melanoma.

21. Answer: C. This patient likely has ulcerative colitis on the basis of her chronic history of left lower quadrant abdominal pain, bloody diarrhea, and weight loss. On the basis of this information, her diagnosis of irritable bowel syndrome should be questioned. Proctoscopy is a valuable test for diagnosis of ulcerative colitis, which should be suspected in this patient. It may reveal mucosal inflammation above the level of the dentate line. Biopsies can be taken to confirm the diagnosis.

22. Answer: B. This patient has rectal prolapse. She is in good health. Her most appropriate treatment should be low anterior resection with rectopexy. An alternative choice may be rectal fixation to sacrum with mesh. However, this procedure can be associated with difficulty in stool elimination. Colostomy is not indicated in this patient.

23. Answer: D. This patient has an anorectal abscess. The treatment of choice is incision and drainage and should be performed immediately. Lateral sphincterotomy is a treatment for anal fissure. Stool softeners are indicated for patients with hemorrhoids.

24. Answer: A. Relative contraindications to laparoscopic cholecystectomy include coagulopathy, cirrhosis, portal hypertension, and generalized peritonitis. In addition, pregnancy, adhesions from prior surgery, and severe cardiopulmonary disease may complicate laparoscopic cholecystectomy.

25. Answer: D. Serum bilurubin is elevated in approximately 50% of patients with acute cholecystitis. Serum AST is elevated in nearly 40% of patients. Serum alkaline phosphatase is elevated in 25% of patients. Finally, amylase is elevated in nearly 15% of patients. Lipase is not elevated in patients with acute cholecystitis.

26. Answer: E. This patient likely has hepatocellular adenoma. This tumor is common in women who take oral contraceptives. Pathology reveals normal hepatocytes. Laboratory studies in these patients reveal normal liver function testing. Angiography is present from hypervascularity.

27. Answer: A. Mortality rates correlate with the number of Ranson criteria present. These range from 0 to 2 criteria = 2% mortality; 3 to 4 criteria = 15% mortality; 5 to 6 criteria = 40% mortality; 7 to 8 criteria = 100% mortality. This man has only 2 criteria present.

28. Answer: C. Pancreatic acini secrete enzymes in response to cholecystokinin. Bicarbonate rich solution is secreted by centroacinar cells in response to secretin. The concentration of bicarbonate in the pancreatic juice increases with the rate of secretion. Enterokinase activates trypsinogen in the duodenal lumen. Somatostatin is an inhibitor of gastrointestinal secretions.

29. Answer: B. C-peptides assays are elevated in insulinomas. Hypokalemia and watery diarrhea are features of VIPomas. Necrolytic migratory erythema is typical of glucagonomas, which in turn are mostly located n the tail of pancreas.

30. Answer: A. Only one-fourth of adult patients respond to medical treatment and most require splenectomy for cure. Platelet transfusions are not required because they are consumed and do not confer any benefit. Children are more likely to die from OPSI than adults. Sickle-cell patients undergo "auto-splenectomy" as a consequence of multiple splenic infarcts. Splenectomy therefore has no role in the management of sickle cell anemia.

31. Answer: B. CA 19-9 is a tumor marker sensitive for pancreatic cancer. Endocopic ultrasound can help in identifying locally advanced disease and is also useful for obtaining biopsies. Percutaneous biopsies of pancreatic masses can seed tumor in the biopsy.

32. Answer: D. This patient has evidence of bilateral adrenal nodules. These are likely due to bilateral adrenal hyperplasia. [Her reveal a plasma aldosterone/plasma renin activity ratio >30 and plasma aldosterone >20.] The most appropriate treatment for nodular adrenal hyperplasia or bilateral masses is non-surgical. However, if pathology reveals adenoma, the treatment is adrenalectomy.

33. Answer: B. This patient has pathologic evidence of a large small-bowel carcinoid tumor. Treatment for tumors larger than 1 cm, multiple tumors, or lymph node involvement is wide excision of bowel and mesentery. Tumors less than 1 cm without evidence of metastatic disease can be treated with segmental intestinal resection. Tumors in the terminal ileum are managed with right hemicolectomy, while large duodenal tumors are managed with pancreaticoduodenectomy

34. Answer: D. This patient most likely has medullary carcinoma of the thyroid because he has a relative with thyroid cancer and a decreased calcium level on laboratory analysis. The medulla of the thyroid produces calcitonin, which inhibits osteoclast destruction of bone and helps to keep blood calcium levels low. This patient's calcium level was 6.1, which is below the normal range of 8.4 to 10.2, and makes a calcitonin-producing tumor of the thyroid most likely. Anaplastic carcinoma presents more commonly in the elderly and has the poorest prognosis of the thyroid cancers. Follicular carcinoma also has a poor prognosis and can metastasize through the blood to the lungs and bones, among other locations. Hashimoto thyroiditis is a noncancerous hypothyroid condition, which is more common in females and can be detected by antithyroglobulin or antithyroid peroxidase antibodies. Papillary carcinoma is the most common thyroid cancer, has a good prognosis, spreads by lymph nodes metastases, and has a ground glass appearance histologically with Psammoma bodies.

35. Answer: C. The lab results in this case are the deciding factor as to the etiology of the discharge. Always when assessing suspected galactorrhea, the prolactin and TSH levels should be obtained. If prolactin levels are elevated, the next step should be to examine for medications that could be interfering with the normal dopaminergic suppression of prolactin secretion. In this case, that medication is metochlopramide. The TSH level is within normal range, ruling out secondary hypothyroidism and making a pituitary adenoma unlikely. The absence of irregular menses also suggests that the etiology is not an adenoma. Mammary duct ectasia, while often bilateral, most often presents with a serosangineuous nipple discharge and normal prolactin levels. *In situ* ductal carcinoma is most often unilateral, and also presents with serosanguineous nipple discharge and normal prolactin levels.

36. Answer: B. The presence of bilateral cancerous lesions, especially in such a young woman, is highly suggestive of a germ-line mutation. Of those listed, a derangement of the p53 allele is most highly correlated with the development of breast cancer. Genes implicated in the development of breast cancer include BRCA-1, BRCA-2, and p53. The c-erb allele is a growth factor receptor gene and is upregulated in some breast cancers. Increased trinucleotide repeats, Rb, and the excision repair system have yet to be implicated in the pathogenesis of breast cancers.

37. Answer: B. An eczematoid lesion of the nipple or areola is characteristic of Paget disease of the breast, which almost always signifies an underlying invasive ductal carcinoma of the breast. It is thought that the intraductal carcinoma undergoes retrograde extension into the overlying epidermis through mammary duct epithelium. The large cells of the eczematous lesion have a typical histologic feature of being surrounded by a clear, halo-like area. None of the other options are related to Paget disease of the breast. Intraductal papilloma is a benign lesion of the lactiferous ducts that also produces a serosanguinous discharge. Medullary carcinoma is a highly malignant breast cancer containing little stroma and a fleshy histologic appearance. Nipple adenoma is a benign tumor of the nipple that produces a serosanguinous discharge and is often mistaken for malignancy. Phyllodes tumor is a large tumor of variable malignancy, often causing an ulceration of the overlying skin.

38. Answer: B. Histologically, the epidermis has five layers, which are demarcated based upon microscopic morphology. The most superficial layer, the stratum corneum, is characterized by anucleate cells filled with keratin filaments. Beneath the stratum corneum is the stratum lucidum which is only seen well in thick skin and is considered to actually be a subdivision of the stratum corneum. The stratum granulosum is beneath the stratum lucidum and contains keratohyalin granule-containing cells. The stratum spinosum, beneath the stratum granulosum, is composed of spiny-looking cells. Finally, the stratum basale, the deepest layer of the epidermis, is composed of a single layer of stem cells from which keratinocytes arise.

39. Answer: A. Basal cell carcinomas are the most common skin tumors. They tend to involve skin-exposed areas most often in the head and neck. Grossly, they are characterized by a pearly papule with overlying telangiectatic vessels. The lower lip is actually the most common site for a tobacco user to develop squamous cell carcinoma. Malignant melanomas are the most likely primary skin tumors to metastasize systemically.

40. Answer: C. While normal individuals will develop nevi (moles) in sun-exposed areas, patients with dysplastic nevus syndrome have an increased risk of spontaneously developing malignant melanoma. Malignant melanomas are the most likely primary skin tumors to metastasize systemically. Patients who chew tobacco for a large period of time are at an increased risk of developing squamous cell carcinomas near or in the oral cavity.

41. Answer: D. Aspirin therapy decreases the risk of TIA and coronary events in patients with asymptomatic carotid bruit. Neither surgery nor anticoagulation is indicated, and there is a weak association between bruits and significant carotid stenosis.

42. Answer: D. The risk of abdominal aortic aneurysm rupture is most dependent upon its diameter, with diameter greater than 5.5 cm at higher risk.

43. Answer: D. Claudication is usually a manifestation of type II disease, ABIs range from 0.5 to 0.9, and surgery—bypass and especially amputation—is rarely indicated.

44. Answer: B. Postprandial pain, or intestinal angina, is seen in chronic splanchnic ischemia, wherein patients develop a fear of eating and lose weight. Two of the three major arteries must be occluded, and Leriche syndrome and mycotic aneurysm are not associated with this condition.

45. Answer: B. A contrecoup is a nonpenetrating injury to the brain, located on the opposite side of the skull impact. The location of the impact is on the right temple, and therefore it would be expected that the contrecoup injury would be located on the left side of the brain. (Coup injuries are located on the same side as the area of impact.)

46. Answer: C. Epidural hematoma results from hemorrhage into the potential space between the dura and skull. The hemorrhage most likely results from rupture to a meningeal artery, which travels within this plane; the middle meningeal artery is most common, which branches off the maxillary artery in the temporal area. Normally, the patient experiences a "lucid interval," an asymptomatic period of a few hours following the trauma.

47. Answer: E. Oligodendroglioma is a slow-growing neoplasm that usually presents in middle age. Patients typically present with new-onset seizures, headache, nausea, and vomiting. The tumors are morphologically characterized by a "fried egg" appearance of the cells and most likely arise in the cerebral hemispheres. Ependymoma is a common neoplasm in childhood that most frequently occurs in the fourth ventricle. Medulloblastoma multiforme is the most common primary intracranial neoplasm in adults, and morphologically demonstrates "pseudopalisading arrangement" of cells. Meningioma originates from arachnoid cells of the meninges and is characterized histologically by laminated calcified psammoma bodies.

48. Answer: A. Gastrochisis represents rupture of the umbilical cord at the site of the right resorbed umbilical vein. The intestine herniates through this small defect. In females, the fallopian tube may also herniate through this orifice. Intestinal atresia may also be noted. The intestine may appear normal but may be covered by a thickened peel. Treatment often involves primary closure under general anesthesia. Omphalocoele is herniation of the abdominal contents into the umbilical cord. Liver and colon herniations are often seen. Patent omphalomesenteric duct connects the ileum to the yolk sac via the umbilical cord and may persist as Meckel diverticulum. Patent urachus is a communication between the bladder and the umbilical cord. Urine may be seen eminating from the umbilicus. Umbilical hernia results from failure of closure of the umbilical ring. Repair is undertaken surgically.

49. Answer: C. Meckel diverticulum is a congenital sacculation of the distal ileum. It is usually located within 2 feet of the ileocecal valve and varies in length from 1 to 6 inches. Normal obliteration of the vitelline duct usually occurs around the seventh week of fetal development. If the ileal portion of this structure is not obliterated, a Meckel diverticulum forms. It is a true congenital diverticulum and therefore contains heterotopic tissue of the digestive tract. Bleeding is often profuse but not life threatening. The most severe complication is intestinal obstruction. Treatment involves surgical resection.

50. Answer: B. Osteogenesis imperfecta is a group of related genetic disorders that result from abnormal synthesis of type I collagen. Clinical characteristics include a history of multiple fractures, blue sclera of the eyes, conductive hearing loss, and short stature. Abnormal FGF receptor is the etiology of achondroplasia, which manifests as dwarfism. Child abuse must be considered in this case, but nothing in the history or physical examination indicates abuse. Deficiency in vitamin D causes rickets in children, and would manifest with characteristic bowing of the legs. There is no evidence that the patient has an underlying bone tumor.

51. Answer: E. Unicameral bone cyst is an expansile, benign, bone lesion of childhood. Usually affecting the femur or humerus, this fluid-filled cavity can be associated with pathologic fractures. The lesion often resolves spontaneously after bone maturity occurs. Adamantinoma is a tumor that arises in the diaphyses or metaphyses of long bones such as the tibia. Aneurysmal bone cyst is a vascular lesion in the metaphysis of young children and may respond to radiation therapy. Chordoma is a tumor of notochord remnants and affects the sacrum or coccyx in middle aged adults. Tumors that are metastatic to bone include breast, prostate, lung, thyroid, and kidney. Pathologic fractures are the usual presenting symptom.

52. Answer: C. In this patient of greater than 70 years of age, there is a 70% chance that he has benign prostatic hyperplasia. In addition to urinary obstructive symptoms such as nocturia, frequency, urgency, and decreased force of stream, intermittent gross hematuria is also possible. Bacterial prostatitis can be associated with intermittent gross hematuria but is more frequently associated with fever, low back pain, and a tender prostate upon digital rectal examination. Bladder carcinoma can be associated with either gross or microscopic hematuria as well as irritative or obstructive urinary symptoms. This patient has a normal kidney/bladder sonogram and is a nonsmoker, which places him at low risk for this disease. Urinary tract calculi are usually associated with hydronephrosis or hydroureter as well as the presence of a stone on sonography. Microhematuria is more commonly seen with this condition. Urinary tract infection is unlikely given the urinanalysis findings of negative nitrates and leukocytes.

53. Answer: E. Testicular torsion is the correct answer in this scenario, and is indeed a urologic emergency. A high-riding testicle in a horizontal lie in which elevation of the testicle provides relief is the classic presentation of testicular torsion. The critical time of ischemia for testicular torsion is 4 hours and if a gangrenous testicle is missed, the patient will be at a high risk of sterility due to his body mounting an autoimmune response to his own sperm. Appropriate management is immediate bilateral orchiopexy because the contralateral testicle is also at an increased risk of torsion. Epididymitis is unlikely in this scenario due to the lack of fever or systemic illness in this patient. Epididymitis is not a urologic emergency and can be treated with IV antibiotics. If this patient presented with epididymitis, some examiners would still use a sonogram of the testicle to rule out testicular torsion.

54. Answer: D. The recurrent laryngeal nerve has been injured. Thyroidectomy is the treatment of choice for patients diagnosed with thyroid cancer. Although this is a rare complicaion (occurring in only 1% of patients), it soon becomes apparent when the patient assumes a husky and hoarse voice. This injury may cause temporary voice pathology lasting 6 to 12 months or it may be a permanent issue. This type of injury is more common when surgeons are dealing with large invasive or recurrent tumors.

55. Answer: A. This patient is showing signs of epiglottitis. You should avoid doing anything with the patient that may cause her to become upset, which can trigger respiratory compromise. The patient should be taken immediately to the OR by the otolaryngologist and anesthesiologist. Once epiglottitis is confirmed by physical examination, the patient can be treated with antibiotics alone or may need intubation, depending on the severity of the illness.

56. Answer: C. This patient's most likely diagnosis by her physical findings is iron-deficiency anemia. It is the most common cause of anemia during childhood and is usually seen between 6 and 24 months of age. It may result from a nutritional iron deficiency usually with rapid growth or from blood loss (e.g., microscopic intestinal hemorrhage). Mild iron deficiency is relatively asymptomatic. With moderate to severe iron deficiency, infants may develop anorexia, irritability, apathy, and fatigability. On physical exam patient may appear pale and sallow, have glossitis, angular stomatitis, spoon nails, and tachycardia with a systolic ejection murmur at the left sternal border. Very severe anemia may result in signs of CHF. If this is high on the differential, a serum iron level, TIBC, and ferritin level are needed for analysis. Other helpful tests include a CBC with differential and red blood cell indices, reticulocyte count, and blood smear.

57. Answer: A. Acute rejection typically occurs days to months after transplantation and is characterized by lymphocytic and macrophage infiltration. Acute rejection is primarily T-cell mediated. These patients typically present with symptoms of acute renal failure. Hyperacute rejection occurs within minutes or hours of the transplantation and is primarily antibody mediated. In a hyperacute kidney rejection the graft would rapidly become cyanotic, mottled, and flaccid and does not produce urine. It is typically due to the presence of preexisting antibodies to donor antigens. A chronic rejection is primarily due to antibody-mediated vascular damage and occurs months to years after transplantation. Patients typically present clinically with a progressive rise in serum creatinine levels over a 4- to 6-month period.

58. Answer: C. Rash, fever, jaundice, and hepatosplenomegaly are typical clinical features of graft versus host disease. Graft versus host disease occurs most commonly following a bone marrow transplant. Symptoms arise within days to weeks of the transplant and occur due to donor T-cells reacting against the recipient's cells. Principal target organs are the liver, skin, and gastrointestinal mucosa leading to the common symptoms of jaundice, rash, mucosal ulceration, bloody diarrhea, hepatosplenomegaly, and fever.

59. Answer: C. Interleukin-2 is a true lymphokine because it has the ability to serve as a T-cell growth factor. Production of this immunoglobulin is impaired in patients with thermal injuries. Interleukin-1 has the ability to induce proteolysis. Interleukin-1 has the ability to serve as an endogenous pyrogen. Interleukin-1 stimulates the hypothalamic–pituitary axis. Interleukin-6 promotes the synthesis of hematic acute phase proteins.

60. Answer: D. A current positive T-cell cross-match indicates the presence of circulating antibodies against class I antigens, and the certainty of a hyperacute rejection reaction. This represents an absolute contraindication to transplantation.

61. Answer: C. Perforated peptic ulcer. Patients who perforate a hollow viscus can often remember the exact time it occurs, based on the suddenness of onset and intensity of pain. The other choices would have more gradual onset of pain and associated symptoms.

62. Answer: B. Murphy sign is seen in acute cholecystitis. It consists of a brief inspiratory arrest or cessation of a requested deep breath as the right upper quadrant is palpated.

63. Answer: B. Visceral pain is dull, achy, poorly localized, and can be stimulated by pulling, stretching, distension, or spasm.

64. Answer: C. The second trimester is the safest interval to operate on a pregnant woman.

Index

Page numbers followed by *f* and *t* indicate figures and tables, respectively.